OLDER PEOPLE

issues and innovations in care

4th edition

OLDER PEOPLE

issues and innovations in care

Rhonda Nay
Emeritus Professor, La Trobe University
Honorary Professorial Fellow, National Ageing Research Institute
(NARI), Melbourne, Victoria

Sally Garratt
Aged Care Consultant, Adjunct Associate Professor
Australian Centre for Evidence Based Aged Care
La Trobe University, Melbourne, Victoria

Deirdre Fetherstonhaugh
Director, Australian Centre for Evidence Based Aged Care
La Trobe University, Melbourne, Victoria

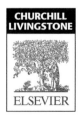

CHURCHILL LIVINGSTONE

ELSEVIER

Sydney Edinburgh London New York Philadelphia St Louis Toronto

Churchill Livingstone
is an imprint of Elsevier

Elsevier Australia. ACN 001 002 357
(a division of Reed International Books Australia Pty Ltd)
Tower 1, 475 Victoria Avenue, Chatswood, NSW 2067

ELSEVIER

This edition © 2014 Elsevier Australia

3rd edition 2009; 2nd edition 2004; 1st edition published by Maclennan and Petty 1999

eISBN: 978-0-7295-8163-9

National Library of Australia Cataloguing-in-Publication Data

Older people: issues and innovations in care / Rhonda Nay,
Sally Garratt, Deirdre Fetherstonhaugh.

4th edition.
9780729541633 (paperback)
Previous edition: Sydney: Churchill Livingston Elsevier, c2009.
Includes bibliographical references and index.

Geriatric nursing—Australia.
Older people—Care—Australia.

Nay, Rhonda.
Garratt, Sally.
Fetherstonhaugh, Deirdre.

610.73650994

Publishing Director: Luisa Cecotti
Senior Content Strategist: Libby Houston
Senior Content Development Specialist: Liz Coady
Project Managers: Martina Vascotto, Rochelle Deighton and Prasad Subramanian
Edited by Matt Davies
Proofread by Forsyth Publishing Services
Cover and internal design by Tania Gomes
Index by Robert Swanson
Typeset by Toppan Best-set Premedia Limited
Printed in China by China Translation and Printing Services

CONTENTS

ABOUT THE AUTHORS

Rhonda Nay
PhD, MLitt, BA, RN
Prior to retiring this year Rhonda Nay was director of the Australian Institute for Primary Care and Ageing and the Dementia Training Studies Centre Victoria & Tasmania. She was previously director of the Institute for Social Participation and the Australian Centre for Evidence Based Aged Care (ACEBAC). Rhonda has held various senior nursing positions, advised state and national governments and been actively involved in a number of professional and industry organisations. She was a director on the Aged Care Standards and Accreditation Agency Board and is a member of the Minister's Dementia Advisory Group.

Sally Garratt
DipAppSc (NsgEd), BEd, MScN, DNsg, DLF, CNA
Prior to her retirement Sally Garratt held a position between Caulfield General Medical Centre, Bayside Health and Gerontic Clinical Nursing School, La Trobe University as an Associate Professor of Gerontic Nursing. She has been involved in nurse education in aged care for many years, has practised as a director of nursing in aged care facilities and has develop quality programs for several facilities. Sally has served on the board of Alzheimer's Australia (Tasmania) for eight years and maintains an interest in the delivery of services for people with dementia.

Deirdre Fetherstonhaugh
PhD, MA (HlthSc), BA (SocSc), DipAppSc (Nsg),
Renal Certificate, RN
Deirdre is the director of the Australian Centre for Evidence Based Aged Care (ACEBAC) at La Trobe University in Victoria. Her research focuses on: the translation and implementation of research evidence into practice; the ethical implications of clinical practice; decision making in dementia; and the reality of person-centred care.

ACKNOWLEDGMENTS

We wish to thank all our wonderful contributors—all very busy people and experts in their fields—for their time spent on updating or completely re-writing the chapters in this book. There has been a generous commitment from all involved to provide the reader with relevant current information about the care of older people.

We thank Lisa Derndorfer for her administrative role and trying to keep Rhonda organised! Libby Houston and Elizabeth Coady from Elsevier were very patient and we thank Elsevier for supporting this fourth edition.

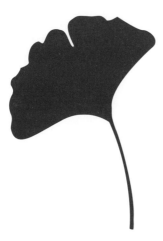

The ginkgo tree is classified as a living fossil, being one of the oldest living plants on the planet. The properties of the ginkgo are believed to improve memory and wellbeing. A very positive symbol for ageing!

FOREWORD

The fourth edition of a book is testament to its utility and popularity. It is clear to see why. *Older People: Issues and innovations in care (4th edition)* presents a rich tableau of topics relevant to the care of older people. The book is grounded in current Australian practice; it is scholarly yet practical and very readable, enlivened by quotes and vignettes sprinkled through each chapter. The reflective questions challenge readers to give deeper consideration to issues and to their own practices. The scope of the 25 chapters is comprehensive and the content is up to date with current developments in aged care such as the Australian aged care reform and Living Longer Living Better, as well as medical developments. The authors, who are leaders in aged care in Australia, are highly regarded. *Older People: Issues and innovations in care* differs from most geriatric books in that it focuses on applied and organisational issues relevant to everyday practice.

Now, more than ever, we need books like this to enhance knowledge and improve aged care practice. The media frequently highlights negative stories such as the epidemic of ageing, the tsunami of dementia, scandals in nursing homes, egregious examples of elder abuse, crises in aged care and bed blockers in hospitals. Admittedly there are current gaps in services and room for improvement and there is a need for more skilled professionals and better policies; however, Australians can rejoice and take pride in stories of positive ageing (e.g. see Chapter 3 on centenarians), the excellence and humanity in the provision of quality care and the advances in practice that are occurring.

Population ageing is a global phenomenon. In the next generation about one in four people in the developed world will be older than 65 years of age and there will be twice as many older people as there are children. The developing world is catching up quickly; China and India between them will have half the world's population with dementia by 2050. Aged care is core business in healthcare and the lessons from this book are relevant beyond Australia.

Professor Henry Brodaty AO
Scientia Professor of Ageing and Mental Health
Director, Dementia Collaborative Research Centre
Co-Director, Centre for Healthy Brain Ageing at University of New South Wales
August 2013

PREFACE

The previous editions of this book were well received by health professionals, students and others involved in providing care to older people and undertaking research into ageing and dementia. Subsequently there was a need for a fourth edition to update the knowledge from new research and acknowledge government policy changes that have occurred. We have endeavoured to do this through our contributors and by including new chapters and a greater emphasis on dementia.

We have maintained the use of vignettes, study questions and innovative approaches to care delivery that enable the reader to test their knowledge and to appreciate how others change their practices. Critical reflection on practice is acknowledged as a fundamental instrument for change and we hope this book will encourage this in daily work.

This is not a 'how-to' book, but rather a text that will encourage the reader to explore care issues and use evidence-based practice to improve the care of older people and their families.

Person-centred, evidence-based, interdisciplinary care is the foundation for successful care outcomes, whether it is delivered at home, in acute care, in residential aged care facilities, in palliative or in rehabilitative units. Older people often have multiple chronic healthcare problems that lead to complex care needs. Assessment and interdisciplinary discussion, ensuring that the person's goals and strengths are central to that discussion, is the best way to plan interventions and monitor outcomes.

Family members, with the consent of the older person, are collaborators in care. They are not difficult interruptions. Issues of advanced care planning and substitute decision making for people who have cognitive impairment should be discussed early in the care process. Regular involvement of family or significant others, together with the older person, can assist timely detection of changes, enable alterations in care planning and delivery and ensure collaborative decision making.

Issues such as lack of medical specialists, care staff with only basic skills, monitoring of funding and insufficient professional staffing levels are still evident. Quality care may be very different from quality of life but one impacts on the other and both should be monitored closely. This text does not propose any particular model of care or tools for assessments but rather encourages the reader to examine what is available and suitable for the purpose they want to achieve.

At the time of writing this text the National Disability Insurance Scheme had been through the political process and legislation is now completed. The actual implementation of the scheme is yet to unfold so the reader will need to examine what is happening in each state and territory as the work progresses. Our understanding is that older people will continue to receive care under the *Aged Care Act 1997*, with amendments, but it is not clear whether younger people residing in aged care facilities will be eligible.

ORGANISATION OF THE VOLUME

The text is organised in a similar fashion to the previous editions, as this creates an easy-to-read format and relates the information in a logical way. Three sections are organised to discuss broader issues, policy and possible future directions. The first section discusses the issues surrounding policy matters and the impact of an ageing population. The second part raises the importance of evidence-based practice and the need for ongoing research. There is still a need to explore the delivery of person-centred approaches to care and what this means to the older person. Innovations in action form the basis for the third section and the possibility of change in direction for care of older people and their families is raised. We have deliberately included the voices and opinions of people who write from their experiences and you will find few references in these chapters. We urge you to similarly value the voices, verbal or non-verbal, of the older people with whom you work. It is essential that we consider the evidence to include clinical judgment and consumer choice.

SECTION 1: CONTEXTUAL ISSUES AND INNOVATIONS

Glenn Rees provides a perspective from many years of listening to consumer viewpoints about access to, and transparency of, services for older people, especially those who have a dementia. The lack of choice and complexity of accessing what is available is daunting for older people and their families.

The issues of an ever-increasing ageing population have far-reaching impacts on the healthcare system. Swerissen and Taylor stress the importance of developing a stronger and more flexible primary healthcare focus with more community involvement.

McCormack brings us more from his longitudinal study of the 'old–old', where he found increasing numbers of people living to 100 years and older. The needs of this age group may create different issues for governments and policy development.

Greenway-Crombie, Disler and Threlkeld discuss the issues of growing old in rural communities and the provision of resources required for this group.

The younger age group residing in residential aged care is increasing in numbers. Garratt and Kelly remind us of the lifestyle gap and expectations of younger people who have limited choices in how and where they live.

Wells and Ryburn give an overview of community services available for older Australians and the need for a systems overhaul and new directions for service delivery.

SECTION 2: PRACTICE ISSUES AND INNOVATIONS

Person-centred care has become the focus for care provision. Nay, Fetherstonhaugh and Winbolt believe there is much to still be done to see this approach to care in practice. They emphasise the importance of all stakeholders being 'persons' and person-centred care being practised at all levels and in all relationships.

Ibrahim and Davis remind the reader of the difficulties in maintaining a balance between risk taking and maintaining safety while also providing quality care.

Healthcare of older Aboriginal and Torres Strait Islander people requires complex assessments based on cultural understanding and knowledge of what services are available for this group. The chapter by LoGuidice, Flicker and Smith outlines some of the issues involved in delivering care in isolated areas of the country that can be translated to city circumstances.

Bauer et al stress the importance of relationships between staff and family, staff and clients and clients and family. The continuation of these relationships is vital for quality care outcomes.

Hospitals are not good environments for older people. Reports indicate confusion, nutrition and hydration issues; falls are increased in this adverse environment. Ames and Nay indicate improved systems in community healthcare may reduce the number of hospital admissions, and improve more effective discharge.

Person-centred comprehensive geriatric assessment is an interdisciplinary team effort and is the best way to gain an insight into the care needs of older people. Garratt and Pond also highlight the importance of family or significant others in the ongoing care delivery process.

Summers offers a good overview of causation and pathological changes in the brain in dementia. His research on neuroplasticity is particularly encouraging.

Neville and Byrne raise the complexity in diagnosing older people who may have depression and who are at risk of suicide. The clinical differences between dementia and depression are very similar and require thorough investigation. Treatment for clinical depression is essential and must not be confused with loss and grief.

Gibson et al address the assessment and treatment of persistent pain in older people. The use of assessment tools and alternative methods of pain relief are raised.

Sexuality issues with older people are discussed by Bauer, Nay and Beattie. This chapter addresses one of the major taboo topics in healthcare.

Kurrle raises issues surrounding the assessment and intervention required in cases of elder abuse and neglect. The legal aspects of intervention and guardianship must be understood by caregivers, especially if family members are involved.

End-of-life decision making for older people is becoming more widely accepted, but as each state and territory in Australia has different laws and approaches to this issue it is important that the correct documentation is completed and families understand the consequences. Fetherstonhaugh and Tarzia discuss the implications of this issue.

SECTION 3: INNOVATIONS IN ACTION

Garratt and Baines explore the meaning of self, dignity and self-esteem in understanding dementia. Knowledge of the person's lifestyle and what is important to them is fundamental to explaining how these concepts affect the quality of life of people who have dementia.

Accreditation, quality and risk are factors necessary to provide positive care outcomes. Brandon describes the components involved in maintaining quality health outcomes for older people, especially those who live in residential care.

Environments that enhance dementia care can be adapted and adopted with careful planning and leadership. Fleming and Bennett address some of the ways in which the environment can be changed to become a more positive experience for older people and care staff.

Horner, Soar and Beattie discuss the future involvement of technology in care. Technology designed to assist in safety, to maintain independence and to monitor health patterns will become more acceptable and used to allow older people to remain in their homes for longer.

Nay, Katz and Murray describe the changing patterns of work in healthcare and the need for innovative change to meet the future. Flexible work hours, improved education and the use of technology will shape a new direction for the aged care workforce and lead to transparency and improved continuity in care.

Carr invites the reader to join her in understanding the family concerns when dementia is diagnosed in a parent. When both parents develop the disease the need for support from healthcare workers and community is essential. Finding out where to access this help is fraught with difficulty and often increases the carer's despair.

Daly, Jackson and Nay discuss the components of good leadership and the necessity to develop such leaders in aged care. Without sound leadership, changes to improve quality care outcomes and meaningful lifestyles for older people will not occur. The future depends on leaders who have vision, capacity for change and commitment to aged care and the workforce involved in delivery of care.

CONTRIBUTORS

David Ames
BA, MD, BS (FRCPsych), FRANZCP
Director, National Ageing Research Institute, Victoria
Professor of Ageing and Health, The University of Melbourne, Victoria

Patricia Baines
MA (Psych), MA (Art Therapy), PhD (Anthropology)
Art therapist and counsellor, Alzheimer's Australia, Tasmania

Michael Bauer
PhD, MGer, BA, DipEd
Senior Research Fellow, Australian Centre for Evidence Based Aged Care
(ACEBAC), Australian Institute for Primary Care and Ageing, La Trobe
University, Victoria

Elizabeth Beattie
PhD, RN, FGSA
Professor of Nursing and Director, Dementia Collaborative Research Centre
– Carers and Consumers, School of Nursing, Queensland University of
Technology, Queensland

Kirsty A Bennett
**BArch (Hons), GradDipGer, BD (Hons), Registered Architect (Vic),
RAIA**
Manager, Environmental Design Education Services, NSW/ACT DTSC,
University of Wollongong, New South Wales

Mark Brandon
GradDip (Employment Relations)
Chief Executive Officer, Aged Care Standards and Accreditation Agency Ltd
Vice Chair, Accreditation Council, International Society for Quality in Health
Care (ISQua)
Chair of Organising Committee and Convener, ISQua International Special
Interest Group: 'Quality in Social Care for Older Persons'

Gerard Byrne
BSc (Med), MBBS, PhD, FRANZCP
Head of Psychiatry, School of Medicine, University of Queensland,
Queensland
Director, Geriatric Psychiatry, Royal Brisbane and Women's Hospital,
Queensland

Jennifer Carr
Therapist Company Director, Montessori Rehabilitation (Dementia)

John Daly
PhD, RN, FACN
Dean & Professor of Nursing, Faculty of Health, University of Technology,
New South Wales

Marie-Claire Davis
BPsych (Hons), MPsych (ClinNeuro)
Brain Disorders Program, Austin Health, Victoria
Department of Forensic Medicine, Monash University, Victoria
Melbourne School of Psychological Sciences, The University of Melbourne,
Victoria

Peter Disler
PhD, MBBCh, FRACP, FRCP (Lond), FAFRM, DPH
Professor of Medicine, Bendigo Regional Clinical School, Monash University,
Victoria
Consultant Physician, Geriatrics and Rehabilitation Medicine, Bendigo Health,
Victoria

Deirdre Fetherstonhaugh
RN, DipApplSc (Nsg), Renal Cert, BA, MA, PhD
Director, Australian Centre for Evidence Based Aged Care (ACEBAC),
Australian Institute for Primary Care & Ageing, La Trobe University, Victoria

Richard Fleming
BTech (Hons), DipClinPsy
Director, NSW/ACT Dementia Training Study Centre, University of
Wollongong, New South Wales

Leon Flicker
MBBS, PGDip (Epid), PhD, FRACP
Western Australian Centre for Health & Ageing, Centre for Medical Research,
University of Western Australia, Western Australia
School of Medicine and Pharmacology, University of Western Australia,
Western Australia
Department of Geriatric Medicine, Royal Perth Hospital, Western Australia

Sally Garratt
DipAppSc (NsgEd), BEd, MscN, DN (Honaris Causa), DLF, CNA
Aged Care Consultant, Adjunct Associate Professor, La Trobe University, Victoria

Stephen J Gibson
BBSc (Hons), PhD, MAPsS
Professor, Department of Medicine, The University of Melbourne, Victoria
Deputy Director, National Ageing Research Institute, Victoria
Director, Caulfield Pain Management and Research Centre, Victoria

Angela Greenway-Crombie
RN, Cert IV Workplace TAA, GradDipHlthSc (Admin), MHlthSc, PhD (candidate)
Operations Manager, Collaborative Health Education and Research Centre (CHERC), Bendigo Health, Victoria

Barbara J Horner
PhD, MEd, BAppSc, RN
Senior Researcher Ageing & Dementia, Faculty of Health Sciences, Curtin University, Western Australia

Joseph E Ibrahim
MBBS, GradCertHE, PhD, FRACP, FAFPHM
Research Fellow, Department of Forensic Medicine, Victorian Institute of Forensic Medicine, School of Public Health and Preventive Medicine, Monash University, Victoria
Consultant Physician and Clinical Director, Subacute Services, Ballarat Health Services, Victoria

Debra Jackson
RN, PhD
Professor of Nursing, Faculty of Health, University of Technology, New South Wales

Benny Katz
FRACP, FFPMANZCA
Director of Geriatric Medicine, St Vincent's Hospital, Victoria
Adjunct Associate Professor, Australian Centre for Evidence Based Aged Care (ACEBAC), La Trobe University, Victoria

Anne Kelly
RN, Dementia Consultant
Montessori for Dementia Australia

Susan Kurrle
MBBS, PhD, DipGerMed
Chair, Health Care of Older People, Faculty of Medicine, University of Sydney, New South Wales
Senior Staff Specialist Geriatrician, Division of Rehabilitation and Aged Care, Hornsby Ku-ring-gai Health Service, New South Wales

Dina LoGiudice
MBBS, FRACP, PhD
Consultant Physician, Geriatric Medicine, Melbourne Health, Victoria

John McCormack
PhD
Health Sciences, La Trobe University, Victoria

Wendy Moyle
PhD, MHsc, BN, RN
Professor and Director, Griffith Health Institute, Griffith University, Queensland

Michael Murray
PhD
Director of Geriatric Medicine, St Vincent's Health, St Georges Hospital, Victoria
Adjunct Associate Professor, Australian Centre for Evidence Based Aged Care, La Trobe University, Victoria

Rhonda Nay
PhD, MLitt, BA, RN, FACN, FAAG
Emeritus Professor, La Trobe University, Victoria
Hon. Professorial Fellow, National Ageing Research Institute, Victoria

Christine Neville
RN, PhD, FACMHN
Associate Professor, School of Nursing and Midwifery, The University of Queensland, Queensland

Dimity Pond
BA, DipEd, DipSocSci, MBBS, FRACGP, PhD
Professor of General Practice, University of Newcastle, New South Wales

Glenn Rees
AM
Chief Executive Officer, Alzheimer's Australia, Australia Capital Territory

Bridget Regan
BA (Hons), DPsych (ClinNeuro), MAPS
Research Fellow, Lincoln Centre for Research on Ageing, La Trobe University, Victoria
Senior Clinical Neuropsychologist, Cognitive Dementia and Memory Service, Monash Health, Victoria

Samuel Scherer
MBBS, DGM
Senior Geriatrician, Royal Freemasons Ltd, Victoria

Kate Smith
PhD, BSc (OccTherapy)
Assistant Professor, Western Australian Centre for Health and Ageing, University of Western Australia, Western Australia

Jeffrey Soar
PhD, FACHI
Chair, Human-Centred Technology, University of Southern Queensland, Queensland

Mathew J Summers
BBSc (Hons), MPsych (ClinNeuropsych), PhD, MAPS (CCN)
Senior Lecturer, School of Psychology, University of Tasmania, Tasmania
Research Fellow, Wicking Dementia Research and Education Centre, University of Tasmania, Tasmania

Hal Swerissen
BAppSc, BA (Hons), GDipPsych, MAppPsych
Professor of Public Health, Faculty of Health Sciences, La Trobe University, Victoria

Laura Tarzia
BCA, GradDipArts (Socio), PGradDipArts (Socio), PhD
Research Officer, Australian Centre for Evidence Based Aged Care (ACEBAC), La Trobe University, Victoria

Michael Taylor
BPharm (Hons) LLB (Hons) GradDip (LegalPrac), MSc, PhD
Lecturer, Faculty of Health Sciences, La Trobe University, Victoria

Guinever Threlkeld
PhD
La Trobe Rural Health School, La Trobe University, Albury-Wodonga, Victoria

Yvonne Wells
BA, MPsych, PhD, MAPS, FAAG, FAPS
Head, Lincoln Centre for Research on Ageing, La Trobe University, Victoria
Professor of Aged Care Research and Policy Development, Faculty of Health
Sciences, School of Health Sciences Research, Australian Institute for Primary
Care and Ageing, La Trobe University, Victoria

Margaret Winbolt
RN, PhD
Senior Research Fellow, Australian Centre for Evidence Based Aged Care, La
Trobe University, Victoria

REVIEWERS

Suzanne Blume
RN, PhD
Ballarat University, Victoria

Jean Booth
DipAppSc (Nsg), BHSC (Nsg), MHSc (Nsg), PhD, MACN
Consultant, Aged Care, Jean Booth Consulting, Bendigo, Victoria

Marguerite Bramble
RN, BEc, GradCert (Strat Marketing), PhD
Adjunct Senior Lecturer, School of Nursing and Midwifery, University of
Tasmania, Tasmania

Kaye Crookes
**RN, BA, Grad DipEd, Grad Cert (Gerontology & Rehab St), MN (re-
search candidate) University of Wollongong**

Coralie J Graham
RN, BSc (Hons) Psych, PhD
Lecturer, School of Health, Nursing & Midwifery, University of Southern
Queensland, Queensland

Deborah Hatcher
RN, DipTeach (PhysEd), BHSc (N), MHPEd, PhD
Senior Lecturer, University of Western Sydney, New South Wales

Lisa Hee
PhD (candidate), MMgt, Med (Prof), GDipNsg (Ger), BN
Lecturer, Post Graduate Ageing and Dementia Studies Area Coordinator,
Queensland University of Technology, Queensland

Diana Jefferies
RN, BA, PhD
Lecturer, Clinical Leadership, School of Nursing and Midwifery, University of
Western Sydney, New South Wales

(Janie) E A Mason
RN (General, Midwifery, Infant Health) MSc
Senior Lecturer, Health/Nursing, Charles Darwin University, Northern Territory

Stephen Neville
RN, PhD, FCNA (NZ)
Senior Lecturer, Massey University, New Zealand

Natashia Scully
BA, BN, PG (DipNSc), MPH, PhD (candidate), MACN
Lecturer, Nursing, School of Health, University of New England, Armidale, New South Wales

Dean Whitehead
PhD, MSc, BEd, FCNA (NZ)
Senior Lecturer, Massey University, Palmerston North, New Zealand

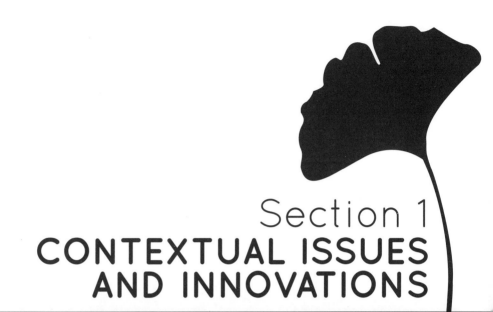

Section 1
CONTEXTUAL ISSUES
AND INNOVATIONS

CHAPTER 1

CARING FOR OLDER PEOPLE: ISSUES FOR CONSUMERS

Glenn Rees

CEO, Alzheimer's Australia

Editors' comments

This chapter is written by Glenn Rees, perhaps the most influential lobbyist for consumers this country has seen. We asked him to write about, and from, his experience so you will see it is not heavily referenced. While Glenn may not be a 'consumer' himself, he has established mechanisms to enable consultations with consumers and for consumer voices to be heard. He is listening and enabling these voices to be heard across the country and internationally, and is constantly taking the messages to governments, the media and the public. It is from his extensive experience he writes and provides a context for the book.

You can also see Glenn and hear further comments from him in Session 3 of Evolve.

INTRODUCTION

Arguably the last time there was major reform of aged care in Australia was the mid-1980s. The scene is now set for a new wave of aged care reforms. The reforms that were implemented in the 1980s, and those the Australian Government has now committed to in Living Longer Living Better (Commonwealth of Australia 2012), have two characteristics in common.

First, the policy and political rhetoric that underlies the reforms has been driven by a commitment to consumer choice. Second, the minister responsible is in cabinet and positioned to have more influence than the junior ministerial positions that have been occupied by aged care ministers in the years 1987–2011.

This chapter:
- provides an Australian consumer viewpoint on aged care services
- provides an economic view on the reform of aged care
- identifies the key drivers for change in aged care based on Australian and international evidence.

THE CONSUMER VIEW IN AUSTRALIA

The cornerstone of aged care policy in Australia has been to respond to the desire of older people to stay at home for as long as possible and to provide quality services in both residential care and the community. Unfortunately, the evidence suggests the aged care system is overwhelmingly failing older people (Alzheimer's Australia 2011a, COTA Victoria 2012). This is even more so from the perspective of people with dementia and their families, and those from diverse communities.

The recurring theme from consultations with consumers is that they are not empowered to make choices and that services are not sufficiently flexible to respond to their needs. To address these issues, consumers are looking for an aged care system that has a number of characteristics (see Alzheimer's Australia 2011a for a comprehensive report on the recent consultations including detailed notes from each consultation).

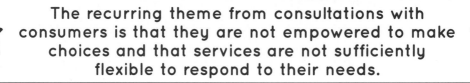

The recurring theme from consultations with consumers is that they are not empowered to make choices and that services are not sufficiently flexible to respond to their needs.

First, consumers want a more transparent system and one in which there is a single point of reference that can provide them with ongoing advice and support throughout the process of accessing services. The general view is that the current aged care system is complex, and consumers find it hard to navigate. There is no clear pathway or information on what services are available, where they are located and how best to plan for care. Often this means consumers avoid seeking services until they reach a crisis point instead of accessing lower level services that may enable them to be independent for a longer period of time.

Second, if the objective of being able to stay in the community is to be a reality, then access to community care services needs to be greatly improved. While there has undoubtedly been a strengthening of community care in Australia over the past 25 years it remains the case that community services are difficult to access for a range of reasons including the hours of care available, the inflexibility of services, and the relatively high administrative charges. These difficulties are compounded for people with dementia because there has been limited recognition of the additional costs of dementia care or the inability of staff in community services such as respite to support people with these behavioural symptoms.

Third, there is a recognition that for many older people residential care may end up being a necessity for those with high care needs. There are significant and enduring concerns about the quality of residential care, including the use of chemical and physical restraints. Consumers recognise that some of the barriers to achieving quality residential care services include inadequate staffing levels and staff who are inadequately remunerated or trained.

 There are significant and enduring concerns about the quality of residential care, including the use of chemical and physical restraints.

Fourth, consumers are looking for a health and aged care system that provides better coordinated care. For older people in hospitals, there are difficult transitions back into the community or to residential care. In addition, consumers often express concerns about long waiting periods for acute care procedures through the public hospital system. For people with dementia, quality of care in hospitals and access to timely diagnosis are areas of significant ongoing concern. A timely diagnosis and access to appropriate support and counselling has been shown to impact on the whole of the care experience, and may delay access to more formal services.

There are also concerns for people with severe behavioural and psychological symptoms of dementia and those with younger onset dementia that the interface between the aged care, mental health and disability sectors is poor. As a result, people end up falling between the gaps of the particular systems with no one taking responsibility for their care.

THE ECONOMIC VIEW

The language and analysis of economists is different from that of consumers but they end up at the same point, namely, concluding that the Australian aged care system is in need of fundamental reform.

The economic pressures of providing care to an increasing number of older people with high care needs has led many developed nations, including Australia, to rethink their strategies for providing aged care services and how to be a more sustainable and equitable system.

In Australia the Productivity Commission was tasked with a review of the aged care system in 2010 (Productivity Commission 2011). Similarly in the United Kingdom (UK), the Commissioner for Care and Funding Support in 2010 was tasked by the UK Government with reviewing the care and support system (Commission on Funding of Care and Support 2011).

Notwithstanding the differences between the health and social systems the Organisation for Economic Co-operation and Development (OECD) has been able to identify in a succession of reports the common themes that are running through the approaches to reform of aged care services in many OECD countries (OECD 2005).

The Productivity Commission's 2011 report was refreshing in its blend of economic analysis on one hand and the focus on the care needs of older people on the other. The success of the commission in balancing these considerations is perhaps the consequence of consumer views being the mirror image of the economists at the level of wanting choice, flexibility of services, a product mix that responds better to market needs and recognition of the importance of workforce issues.

THE CONSUMER VIEW

From a consumer point of view it has been important to identify the major drivers of change in achieving higher quality services that respond to the needs of consumers. Arguably the issues to address are as much cultural and attitudinal as they are system-based. The five key priorities from a consumer perspective that stand out in the Australian context, and perhaps more widely, are:
- choice
- community care
- quality of care
- evidence-based practice
- approach dementia services.

CHOICE

Over the past 10 years there has been an increased focus on providing consumers with greater choice and flexibility over the services they receive. From the consumer perspective greater choice means access to services that better meet their needs and preferences. From an economic or policy perspective choice can lead to a more efficient provision of services by matching care recipients' needs and preferences to the care they receive.

Choice is not as simple as providing consumers with a menu of services to choose from. Instead, it requires a fundamental shift in the care relationship. The consumer has to be an active partner in care and planning services, rather than passively receiving care (Alzheimer's Australia 2007). This shift in relationship with care providers can increase a sense of self-determination and empowerment for consumers (OECD 2005). Choice among providers and services also provides consumers with the ability to be more discerning about the quality of services received.

 The consumer has to be an active partner in care and planning services, rather than passively receiving care.

In Australia, and many other Western countries, 'consumer-directed care' (CDC) is the term used to describe the overarching principle of providing greater choice for consumers. The main goal of CDC is to offer consumers greater control over their own lives by providing them with the opportunity to make choices about their care, to the extent they wish to do so. In practice,

CDC describes a continuum of choice and consumer involvement on a number of dimensions of care including care planning, budget holding and service delivery (KPMG 2012).

Many developed countries have implemented care and support schemes that embrace some components of CDC. The evidence from evaluations of these approaches is that many older people prefer having greater choice in services. For many, CDC leads to greater satisfaction, feelings of greater control and less dependency when they have a say about how, when and who provides care (OECD 2005).

There seems to be broad agreement in many countries that providing greater choice in care and support is an important approach. The difficulties arise in determining how much choice is appropriate, how to balance risk and choice, and the potential workforce implications. In terms of risk, there are relatively few examples of outright abuse of the system, and the quality of care in most cases has been found to be similar to standard care or better (OECD 2005). There is of course a need to implement safeguards to reduce opportunities for abuse, particularly for clients who may be more vulnerable such as those with cognitive impairment.

There is nothing new about the principles that underpin CDC. CDC can be traced to the disability rights and self-determination movements in the UK and United States (US) in the 1970s that led to deinstitutionalisation of people with disabilities and moved towards independent living programs. Some date CDC further back to the 1950s when a home care program for polio patients was developed in the US as an alternative to more costly hospital treatments (Doty 2010).

Aged care policy in Australia since the reforms of the middle 1980s has been premised on the assumption of providing support for consumers in their choice to stay at home, as well as providing services that are responsive to their needs. Australia has taken a series of small steps towards providing greater choice for consumers. In 2010 the Commonwealth funded a trial of 500 CDC places in community care; a further 500 places were allocated in 2011. During this time they also funded 400 CDC respite packages.

Overall, the outcome of an independent evaluation (KPMG 2012) revealed that CDC led to increased satisfaction and sense of control. Although the evaluation was largely positive, the findings also revealed the different ways CDC was defined even within the same program. There was wide variation in how CDC was implemented and how much it differed from the offerings of traditional services. Some providers used a goal-based planning approach, whereas other providers had an approach that was driven more by a menu of services (KPMG 2012).

In part as a result of the successful evaluation, the Australian Government made a commitment to a CDC approach to aged care services in the 2012–13 federal budget. For consumers this is an exciting development. All new community care packages will be offered on the basis of CDC and this will eventually be rolled out to all existing packages. In addition, the government is looking to trial how CDC could be implemented within residential aged care services (Commonwealth of Australia 2012).

A number of questions still remain in terms of implementation.

Reflective questions

1. What will CDC look like and how will it differ from traditional services? How will the provision of choice be monitored to ensure a new approach to services?

2. What will be the boundaries of choice? Will consumers be given options to cash out services and employ family/friends?

3. How will consumers be supported in adopting this new model of care?

4. How will the government support the cultural shift required for providers to work with consumers as partners in care?

COMMUNITY CARE

There is overwhelming evidence that most older adults in developed nations would prefer to receive care within their own home rather than enter a residential facility. The majority of care provided in the community is informal care provided by family members and friends. In Australia in 2010, an estimated 2.9 million informal carers provided 1.3 billion hours of care (Access Economics 2010).

Over the past 10 years, care systems in most developed nations have moved away from a dichotomous choice of receiving unsupported care at home from a relative to receiving formal services in a nursing home. Instead, many countries are now providing at least some health and support services in the community, most often supplemented by the work of informal carers (OECD 2005).

In Australia since the 1980s, care in the community has been supported through a variety of community care packages and services. Yet in the past 10 years there has been little change in the proportion of people receiving care at home compared with residential care. The figure has remained relatively constant at 54% (compared with an average for OECD of 64.5% in 2009) (OECD 2011).

The Australian Government currently funds almost 60,000 community care packages that range in the level of services they provide from an average of 6.5 hours of direct care per week to an average of 17.5 hours of care per week. The funding for the highest level of package is equivalent to the care subsidy received by residential aged care providers for the highest level of care (Department of Health and Ageing 2010).

The majority of people receiving government-funded community care packages in Australia are also receiving significant support from an informal carer in the community. For those receiving the highest level of care package, 87% have an informal primary carer. It is likely that many of these people would not be able to remain in the community without this additional support care (Department of Health and Ageing 2010). At the same time the availability of informal carers in the future is likely to decrease due to the ageing of the population, changing family structures and increased female workforce participation (Access Economics 2010).

The majority of people receiving government-funded community care packages in Australia are also receiving significant support from an informal carer in the community.

In addition to affecting the ability of older people to access adequate support, decreasing numbers of informal carers may lead to increased loneliness and risk of social isolation. Research has consistently demonstrated the importance of social and family relationships in achieving a high quality of life for older people and the connection between social isolation and depression (Victor et al 2000). A wellness approach to community care in which issues of social engagement are considered as part of the range of services will be vital to supporting a high quality of life.

The recent reforms announced in the 2012–13 federal budget include an expansion of community care from 27 community care packages per 1000 people aged 70 years or older to 45 places per 1000 people aged 70 years or older over a period of 10 years. The reforms have also created two new types of community care packages to provide a greater continuum of care options (Commonwealth of Australia 2012).

The focus on increased community care is welcomed by consumers. But questions still remain in implementing the reforms.

Reflective questions

1. Community care was only increased by approximately 10% in 2012–13. Is this sufficient to rebalance community and residential care according to consumer demand?

2. Should government designate the split between residential and community care or should the split be based on consumer demand?

3. How will reductions in the availability of informal carers impact on the demand for community care? How can people living alone be adequately supported?

QUALITY OF CARE

Despite a high level of regulation in the Australian aged care sector, quality of care remains a concern. One of the challenges faced by consumers is difficulty in assessing quality before choosing a service. The current Residential Aged Care Accreditation Standards offer a process of monitoring care and providing a safeguard for a minimal level of quality. The standards, however, do not provide meaningful information for consumers who are trying to select between different services.

Other countries face similar difficulties with providing transparent information on quality. A recent European project, Quality Management by Result-oriented Indicators—Towards Benchmarking in Residential Care for Older People, was conducted to develop and validate result-oriented quality indicators (European Centre for Social Welfare Policy and Research 2010). The European consortium finalised 94 quality indicators, clustered in five domains: quality of care, quality of life, leadership, economic performance and context.

Other countries face similar difficulties with providing transparent information on quality.

In the US, the Centers for Medicare and Medicaid Services (CMS) began developing the Nursing Home Quality Initiative (NHQI) in 2002. The NHQI provides a framework for public reporting on quality measures indicating the care quality provided in aged care homes. The quality indicators are reported on a publicly accessible website, providing consumers with a source of information on how well residential aged care services meet their residents' physical and clinical needs.

In Australia the government has committed to developing the 'My Aged Care' website in 2013 to provide comprehensive information about aged care. National aged care quality indicators will be developed in consultation with stakeholders and will be operational in residential care from 2014. These indicators will provide the basis for establishing a rating system for aged care providers that will be published on the My Aged Care website. The goal is to create a system that will empower consumers to make informed decisions and assist in comparing services (Commonwealth of Australia 2012).

The focus of the reforms on improving the quality of aged care services is welcomed. But again the question remains about the implementation of the reforms.

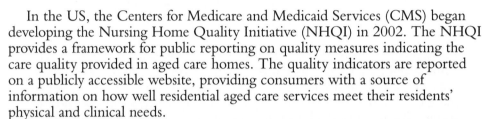

Reflective questions

1. What outcome indicators will be both meaningful for consumers but not result in disincentives for providers to take on high-need individuals who may be at greater risk for complications?

2. How can government make better links between financing/costing aged care and the quality of care provided?

3. How can outcome indicators be developed and measured in community care settings?

EVIDENCE-BASED PRACTICE

There are significant gaps between existing evidence and mainstream practice in many areas of medicine, health and aged care. As a result, many care recipients receive suboptimal, and sometimes even detrimental, care. It is estimated in Australia that 30–40% of healthcare is inconsistent with clinical guidelines; this is consistent with estimates from other developed countries (Runciman et al 2012). The gulf between what is known and accepted by researchers about best practice care, and the mainstream care provided by health and aged care workers, has a significant negative impact on the quality of care received.

In Australia an estimated 30–40% of healthcare is inconsistent with clinical guidelines.

In Australia there has been an increasing recognition of the need to ensure investment in research leads to systems change. For example, the National Health and Medical Research Council has recently funded a $25 million Partnership Centre called Dealing with Cognitive Decline and Related Functional Decline in Older People. The goal of the Partnership Centre program is to bring teams of researchers and decision makers together to create better health services through collaborative work that focuses on systems change.

Perhaps one of the more exciting developments in Australia is a new focus on giving consumers a voice in research and knowledge translation. Through the Alzheimer's Australia Consumer Dementia Research Network (CDRN), consumers are for the first time setting funding priorities, commenting on research proposals, making funding decisions and collaborating with researchers. The CDRN is closely involved in the new Partnership Centre and there is beginning to be a recognition that for research to lead to meaningful outcomes it must be informed by the priorities of consumers.

Concerns remain that both dementia research and knowledge translation are significantly underfunded compared with other chronic diseases. It is clear that greater investment in research is needed to develop evidence-based approaches to quality care.

Perhaps one of the more exciting developments in Australia is a new focus on giving consumers a voice in research and knowledge translation.

DEMENTIA SERVICES ACROSS HEALTH AND AGED CARE

Dementia has for many years been primarily seen as an issue of ageing. This has meant it has been difficult to get traction in health policy on important issues such as timely diagnosis, quality care in hospitals and appropriate management of dementia. These issues are of great concern to consumers, and initial experiences with the healthcare system can often have long-term impacts on how a person lives with dementia (Alzheimer's Australia 2011a).

There is now good evidence both in Australia and overseas of the difficulty faced by people seeking a diagnosis of dementia. In Australia it takes an average of 3.1 years between first noticing symptoms of dementia and getting a diagnosis (Alzheimer's Australia 2011b). This is consistent with worldwide estimates (Alzheimer's Disease International 2011).

Similarly, there is good evidence from both Australia and overseas that hospital services for people with cognitive impairment are generally poor and that hospitals are dangerous and confusing places for people with dementia (Alzheimer's Society 2009). People with dementia stay longer in hospitals than people without dementia, even after accounting for their principal reason for admission and the procedure received (Alzheimer's Society 2009, Australian Institute of Health and Welfare 2011), and are at greater risk of hazards and poor outcomes (Balance of Care Group in association with the National Audit Office 2006).

The recent aged care reforms in Australia have acknowledged the impact of dementia across both the health and aged care systems. Dementia has been acknowledged for the first time as a national health priority area that provides opportunities for coordinated action between the Commonwealth and states/territories to address dementia. In addition, the Living Longer Living Better reforms include funding to address primary care and quality of dementia care in hospitals.

For consumers there is still a number of challenges that remain.

Reflective questions

1. How can messages of dementia risk reduction be incorporated into primary care?

2. What systems need to be developed to provide better management of dementia in the community and reduce hospitalisations?

3. As clinicians become better at diagnosing dementia, will the service system be able to respond to the large increase in numbers of people seeking services?

CONCLUSION

Acknowledging the economic and social impacts of our ageing population has led many developed countries to begin to rethink their system of aged care and support. In Australia this has led to the start of significant reforms of aged care that have begun to address issues that are of key importance to consumers. Although there is a focus on developing a program that is sustainable and financially viable, there has also been an acknowledgment of the need to address consumer priorities including choice, community care and improved quality and care across the health and aged care systems. There is a need to ensure that consumers are involved in implementing these reforms and that the reforms lead to beneficial outcomes to consumers.

References

Access Economics, 2010. Caring places: planning for aged care and dementia: 2010–2050. Deloitte, Barton, ACT.

Australian Institute of Health and Welfare, 2011. Australian hospital statistics 2009–2010. AIHW, Canberra.

Alzheimer's Australia, 2007. Consumer directed care: a way to empower consumers? Alzheimer's Australia, Scullin, ACT.

Alzheimer's Australia, 2011a. Consumer engagement in the aged care reform process. Alzheimer's Australia, Scullin, ACT.

Alzheimer's Australia, 2011b. Timely diagnosis of dementia: can we do better? Alzheimer's Australia, Scullin, ACT.

Alzheimer's Disease International, 2011. World Alzheimer's report 2011: the benefits of early diagnosis and intervention. ADI, London.

Alzheimer's Society, 2009. Counting the cost. Alzheimer's Society, London.

Balance of Care Group in association with the National Audit Office, 2006. Identifying alternatives to hospitals for people with dementia: report of findings. London.

Commission on Funding of Care and Support, 2011. Fairer care funding: the report of the Commission on Funding of Care and Support. London.

Commonwealth of Australia, 2012. Living longer. Living better. Australian Government, Canberra.

COTA Victoria, 2012. Aged Care reform consultations summary. Online. Available: http://www.cotavic.org.au/wp-content/uploads/2012/08/Aged-Care-Reform-SessionsSummary-Report.pdf, 22 Aug 2012.

Department of Health and Ageing, 2010. The 2008 community care census. Australian Government, Canberra.

Doty, P., 2010. History of self direction. Developing and implementing self direction programs: a handbook. Robert Wood Johnson Foundation, Princeton.

European Centre for Social Welfare Policy and Research, 2010. Measuring progress: indicators for care homes. Online. Available: www.euro.centre.org, 22 Aug 2012.

KPMG, 2012. Evaluation of the consumer directed care initiative: final report. Department of Health, Melbourne.

Organisation for Economic Co-operation and Development, 2005. Ensuring quality long-term care for older people. OECD Publishing.

Organisation for Economic Co-operation and Development, 2011. Health at a glance 2011: OECD indicators. OECD Publishing.

Productivity Commission, 2011. Caring for older Australians, Report No. 53. Final Inquiry Report, Canberra.

Runciman, W.B., Hunt, T.D., Hannaford, N.A., et al., 2012. Care track: assessing the appropriateness of health delivery in Australia. Medical Journal of Australia 197 (2), 100–105.

Victor, C., Scambler, S., Bond, J., et al., 2000. Being alone in later life: loneliness, social isolation and living alone. Reviews in Clinical Gerontology 10 (4), 407–417.

CHAPTER 2

PUBLIC HEALTH FOR AN AGEING SOCIETY

Hal Swerissen and Michael Taylor

Editors' comments

Will we have longer life expectancy with less quality of life? Or will morbidity be compressed in the last few years of life, and thus we experience more years of quality life? What role can public health play in giving us opportunities for 'living longer, living better'? Is old age a burden on the health system or a marker of its success? These are some of the questions addressed in this chapter. While the drive towards increased primary and community healthcare is a worthy ideal and is less expensive than hospital-based care, it will incur other indirect costs, such as those borne by families providing informal care to older people.

INTRODUCTION

> *... as a result of our success in conquering infections and some of the most deadly diseases of childhood, we now have an adult population that is larger in proportion that it has ever been before. It promises to grow even greater as the years roll by. This poses new public health problems, and hitherto neglected diseases assume compelling importance. The care of the aged and chronically ill must not be left to the old man with the long white beard and the scythe.*

Theodore G Klumpp, MD
President, Winthrop Chemical Company
(Klumpp 1947)

The choice of opening quotation was deliberate. Like an increasing proportion of our global population in 2013, the quotation is more than 65 years old. It reflects public health's view of population ageing at the time and remains relevant even today, although the 'hitherto neglected diseases' (such as diabetes and cancer) are no longer 'neglected'. While indeed correct in that population ageing poses 'new public health problems', it should also be borne in mind that population ageing, as a result of improved prevention of disease, also represents 'a major successful outcome of public health interventions of the past 100 years' (Fried 2012).

Public health endeavours to promote, protect and restore people's health. Historically, public health was largely focused on preventing disease and death, particularly that caused by communicable diseases. Public health's aforementioned 'success in conquering infections' was the result of identifying specific factors associated with infectious diseases and developing interventions designed to prevent—or at least minimise—their impact on the population.

As successful models of prevention and treatment of infectious diseases developed, public health's post–World War II emphasis began to shift towards those 'hitherto neglected diseases' such as cancer, diabetes and other chronic diseases (Lombard 1947, Wilkerson 1947). Given the increased prevalence of these non-communicable diseases with age, public health will play as critical a role to today's ageing society as it did in the past with communicable diseases. This chapter will outline that role and the scope for public health in an ageing society.

PUBLIC HEALTH AND THE CHANGING PATTERN OF LIFE EXPECTANCY

Public health's traditional focus on infectious diseases, and the development of interventions to prevent or minimise their transmission, resulted in a substantial reduction of infant mortality due to infectious diseases. Using Australian data to illustrate, in 1907 the mortality rate from infectious diseases among children aged birth to four years was 808.3 per 100,000 population; by 2003, this rate was 4.9 per 100,000 population (Australian Institute of Health and Welfare (AIHW) 2006b). Improvements in infectious disease mortality were not confined to the early years of life; for people aged 45–64 years, the rate has decreased from 439.6 deaths per 100,000 population in 1907 to 10.8 per 100,000 in 2003 (AIHW 2006b).

Such shifts in mortality over the course of the 20th century, in conjunction with other improvements in social, environmental and economic circumstances, resulted in profound increases in life expectancy. Figure 2.1 shows that, in Organisation for Economic Co-operation and Development (OECD) countries since the 1960s, there have been considerable gains in life expectancy at birth (OECD 2012).

Overall, average life expectancy across the OECD countries increased from 68.1 years in 1960 to 79.7 years in 2010. As shown in Figure 2.1, Australian life expectancy at birth has historically been above the OECD average: 70.9 years in 1960, increasing to 81.8 years in 2010. Japan, where life expectancy at birth was comparable to the OECD average in 1960, had the longest life expectancy (83.0 years) in the OECD in 2010. Figure 2.1 also gives an example

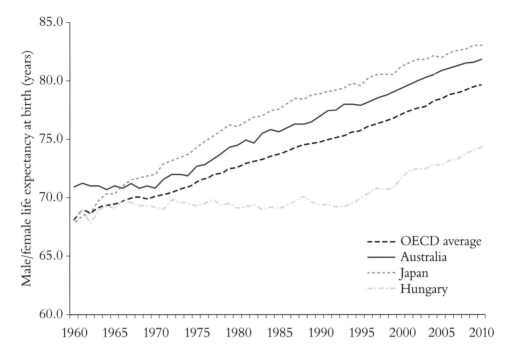

Figure 2.1

Life expectancy at birth (males and females) for selected OECD countries, 1960–2010

Source: OECD 2012

of Hungary, an OECD country where historical shifts in life expectancy have been somewhat different. In 1960 Hungary had a life expectancy at birth comparable to the OECD average (68.0 years), but unlike Japan there was no appreciable increase in life expectancy until after the year 2000. As a result, life expectancy at birth in 2010 in Hungary was 74.3 years, among the lowest within the OECD.

While public health has contributed substantially to these increases in life expectancy *at birth*, it should be borne in mind that increases in life expectancy at other ages have been less pronounced (AIHW 2006b). As shown in Figure 2.2, although life expectancy at age 30 for Australian females increased over the course of the 20th century, the change was far less pronounced than that observed for females at birth. For females aged 65, life expectancy remained relatively unchanged until the 1970s: from 77.8 years in 1900, to 80.7 years in 1961 and to 85.8 in 2001. An almost imperceptible change occurred in life expectancy for females aged 85 years; from 89.2 years in 1900 to 91.8 years in 2001.

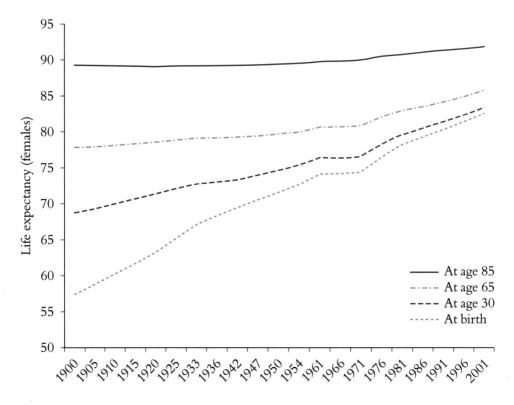

Figure 2.2

Female life expectancy by age Australia, 1900–2001
Source: AIHW 2006b

While public health has contributed substantially to increases in life expectancy *at birth*, it should be borne in mind that increases in life expectancy at other ages have been less pronounced.

Although life expectancy at birth is a major indicator of a society's health, behind this statistic are patterns of mortality rates. Mortality rates have declined over the course of the 20th century, and the underlying causes of mortality have undergone considerable transition throughout the life span. Using three major causes of death—infectious diseases, cardiovascular diseases and cancers—as markers, it is clear that the changing focus of public health, from infectious diseases to those 'hitherto neglected' diseases, has made a substantial contribution to the ageing of our society.

Figure 2.3 shows each marker disease's proportional share of Australia's overall (and declining) mortality rate since World War II (AIHW 2006b). Again reflecting public health's efforts in reducing infectious disease mortality, for those

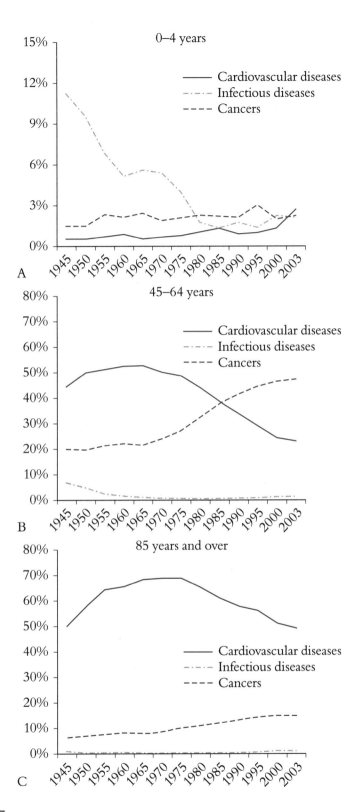

Figure 2.3

Proportional causes of mortality, Australia, 1945–2003

Source: AIHW 2006b

aged between birth and four years the proportion of mortality due to infectious diseases has declined from 11.2% in 1945 to 2.1% by 2003 (Figure 2.3, panel A). The proportion of the overall mortality rate due to cancer and cardiovascular disease in this age bracket has remained relatively constant (less than 3%).

For adults aged 45–64, a transition between cardiovascular disease and cancer being responsible for a major proportion of the mortality rate is observed (Figure 2.3, panel B). From the 1950s to 1970s, cardiovascular disease represented as many as half of all mortality in this age group; improved prevention and treatment of cardiovascular disease substantially reduced this. The proportion of mortality due to cancer has more than doubled over this time (20.0% in 1945 compared with 47.3% in 2003). The contribution of infectious diseases to mortality in this group also declined; since the 1960s, infectious diseases have been responsible for less than 2% of the overall death rate in this age group.

In the oldest age group—those aged 85 and older—a somewhat similar pattern is observed for cardiovascular disease in terms of its plateau: a peak period during the 1950s to 1970s (Figure 2.3, panel C). On a proportional basis, cardiovascular disease contributes the same in 2003 as it did in 1945; however, the decline in the *overall* mortality rate means than in absolute rate terms, cardiovascular disease mortality has still substantially declined among those aged 85 years and older (27,709 deaths per 100,000 population in 1945 to 14,407 per 100,000 in 2003).

PUBLIC HEALTH'S SHIFT TOWARDS CHRONIC DISEASE

As infectious diseases declined, particularly in children and younger adults, life expectancy consequentially increased and a new 'epidemic' of chronic disease emerged. Initially, the focus was on cancer and cardiovascular disease but expanded to include chronic obstructive pulmonary disease, renal disease, diabetes, mental illness and musculoskeletal conditions. In recent times, attention has centred on the ever-increasing prevalence of dementia and the importance of providing dementia care.

Chronic diseases are complex systemic conditions, often influenced by social and environmental influences as well as underlying genetic variability. The incidence and prevalence of these chronic diseases is higher for more disadvantaged populations and strongly associated with particular behaviours such as smoking and physical activity. Reflecting this change in need, public health and health systems have shifted their focus. The 'new public health' focuses on the social determinants of health and chronic disease prevention, and the health system is (gradually) reorienting itself to provide better management of chronic disease.

For public health, contemporary interventions have focused on social and behavioural influences on cancer and cardiovascular disease. The changes shown in Figure 2.3 post-1970 were primarily associated with declining smoking rates, improved diet, improved early intervention where disease occurs, introduction of effective antihypertensive drugs and more effective interventions for acute myocardial infarction.

For the health system, the rise in chronic disease has necessitated the development of more complex models of health that focus on the interaction of social, cultural, environmental and behavioural influences on disease, as well as ageing. Such management, and the influence of ageing, is dramatically played out through the increasing tendency for *multimorbidity*, where chronic diseases overlap, complicating the clinical management of individual patients.

As infectious diseases declined, particularly in children and younger adults, life expectancy consequentially increased and a new 'epidemic' of chronic disease emerged.

POPULATION AGEING AND SOCIETY

Population ageing is the product of increased life expectancy and declining fertility rates. Throughout the developed world, declining fertility rates characterised the latter half of the 20th century, and currently stands at (or below) 'replacement level', contributing to the ageing nature of the population (UN Department of Economic and Social Affairs 2002).

According to the United Nations' *World Population Ageing: 1950–2050* report (UN Department of Economic and Social Affairs 2002), the worldwide population of people aged older than 60 years almost tripled between 1950 and 2000, from 205 million to 606 million people. Projections indicate that another tripling of the population aged over 60 will occur by 2050, to approximately two billion people.

This changing proportion of older people within the population is often illustrated in public policy discussions using the dependency ratio (DR). At its most basic, it is the ratio between 'dependants' and those within the population supporting (or capable of supporting) them. For the purposes of the DR, the dependent population consists of those aged 0–15 years and all those aged 65 years or older; this is expressed relative to those aged 16–64 years (the working-aged population). Two sub-ratios are also used: the child dependency ratio (CDR, the ratio of the population aged 0–15 years to the working-aged population) and the aged dependency ratio (ADR, the ratio of the population 65 years and older to the working-aged population). Figure 2.4 shows all three types of DRs for Australia through to 2030, based on the most likely projections of fertility, mortality and migration rates (Australian Bureau of Statistics (ABS) 2008).

In 2010 the DR was 0.515, translating to approximately one dependent person for every two working-aged people. By 2020 the value of the DR increases to 0.573—an 11% increase on the 2010 value. Change in the ADR is the most pronounced—from a value of 0.208 in 2010 (approximately one person aged 65 or over for every five working-aged persons) to 0.265 in 2020 and 0.321 in 2030, increases of 27% and 54% on the 2010 ADR value, respectively. Reflective of the low fertility rate used in the projections, the CDR remains virtually stagnant over time; in 2010, the value of the CDR was 0.307 (almost one child for every three working-aged people).

Longer life expectancy, and the increasing proportion of older people in the population, are changing perceptions and expectations about ageing. As the

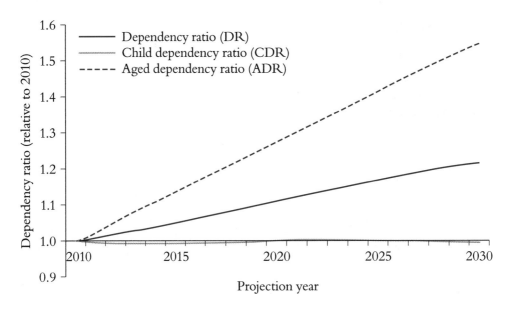

Figure 2.4

Dependency ratios for Australia, 2010–2030
Source: ABS 2008

length of healthy life and the proportion (and expectations) of older people increase, a range of new social and economic policy responses are required to address retirement incomes, housing options, social participation and—of greatest relevance here—health.

While it is generally true that most people aged over 65 years will continue to be healthy and active for a significant period, it is also true that ageing is inevitably associated with increased disease, disability and (ultimately) death. Chronic disease multimorbidity (i.e. having at least two chronic diseases) is also a prominent feature of ageing, where advancing age typically results in an accumulation of chronic diseases over time (Schafer et al 2012).

Ageing therefore becomes an issue as understandable concerns that greater population ageing will lead to increased demand for health and aged care services emerge. Not surprisingly, public health is (and will increasingly be) tasked with trying to prevent chronic disease and of finding ways of managing these diseases as efficiently as possible when they occur.

> While it is generally true that most people aged over 65 years will continue to be healthy and active for a significant period; it is also true that ageing is inevitably associated with increased disease, disability and (ultimately) death.

THE IMPACT OF AGEING ON DEMAND FOR HEALTH AND AGED CARE

Estimates of the impact of population ageing on demand for health services are complex and contested. However, in part, projections depend on the extent to which increased life expectancy is associated with more or less disability, and the impact of population ageing in general. Healthcare service demand (and costs) rise dramatically with age, and a significant proportion of lifetime healthcare costs are borne in the period immediately prior to death. Across population age groups, aggregate healthcare costs generally peak at around 85 years of age, after which they decrease due to mortality rates.

Vignette

Age, healthcare demand and costs in Medicare

In terms of how healthcare demand and costs increase throughout the life span, the Australian Medicare program is instructive. Figure 2.5 shows the service delivery rates for each age–sex category receiving medical services (e.g. professional attendances and pathology tests) subsidised by the Australian Medicare program (Medicare Australia 2013).

As a case study for age and service demand and spending, consider Australian males aged 35–44 years as the 'base case', receiving (on average) 9.2 services per person in 2012 at a cost of $478. Compared to this base case, males aged 75–84 years received four times as many services (and at four times the cost). These figures are expressed as a rate (i.e. services delivered per person); the increasing proportion of the population within the older age brackets will therefore increase the total volume of services required. This in turn has other consequences, for example, with professional attendances, the extra numbers of general practitioners (GPs) required to meet this increased demand for consultations.

Reflective question

As shown in the vignette, the ageing of the population will create greater demand for healthcare services, such as face-to-face consultations with GPs. How might 'medical delegation' or 'medical substitution' to nurses assist with meeting that demand?

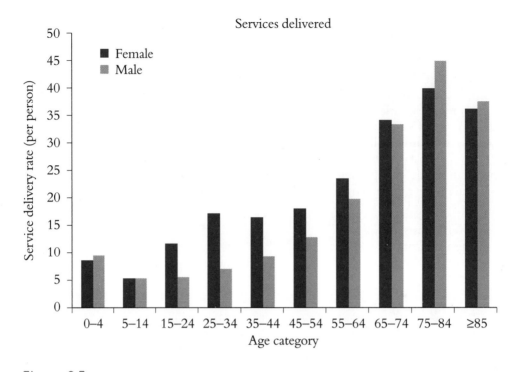

Figure 2.5

Medicare service delivery rates by age–sex category
Source: Medicare Australia 2013

If disease and injury are prevented, it is arguable that healthy life years will be gained. On the other hand, if disease and injury are treated to prolong life, then it is possible that years of life will be gained at the expense of quality of life. There are two main hypotheses that have been developed to predict the impact of increased life expectancy on healthcare costs. The *expansion of morbidity* hypothesis predicts we will live longer but with greater levels of disease and disability and therefore greater costs (Gruenberg 1977). The *compression of morbidity* hypothesis suggests we will live longer and that our increased life expectancy will be associated with a decreased period of disease and disability (Fries 1980, 1989).

To understand the debate about the compression or expansion of morbidity, it is important to understand the relationship between average life expectancy and maximum life span. Despite the significant increase in life expectancy over the past century, there has been little change in maximum life span, which remains at about 120 years. In effect, life expectancy has increased by reducing the incidence and prevalence of disease and injury earlier in life, and reflects Figure 2.2 where life expectancy for those aged 85 years has changed little over time. As morbidity and mortality has declined for younger age groups, morbidity and mortality have been compressed into a narrower range for older age groups.

How long can this trend continue? The compression of morbidity hypothesis proposes that maximum life span is set by biological limits that are difficult to alter. Progressive prevention of diseases and injury will result in longer disability-free life expectancy until average life expectancy approaches this limit. As it does, morbidity will increasingly be compressed within a narrower age range.

On the other hand, the expansion of morbidity hypothesis suggests that treatment and intervention will reduce mortality but not the morbidity associated with disease. As a result, life expectancy will increase, but we will live for longer periods with more disease and disability. If this were true, there would be a trade-off between increased duration of life and decreased quality. This hypothesis also implies that maximum life span may shift upwards as well.

The implications for healthcare costs are significant. If morbidity is compressed, there is little impact on healthcare costs associated with increased life expectancy. Effectively, costs are deferred until later in life. On the other hand, if morbidity expands, healthcare costs will increase as life expectancy increases. If this occurs, it is likely that each year of healthy life would become increasingly costly. As the average quality of additional years declines, it would also be necessary to make judgments about the relative merit of the increasingly marginal trade-off between the quality and the length of life.

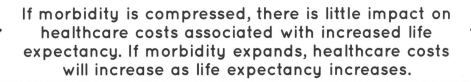

If morbidity is compressed, there is little impact on healthcare costs associated with increased life expectancy. If morbidity expands, healthcare costs will increase as life expectancy increases.

Over the past 40 years, during which life expectancy has increased, there has been some expansion of morbidity (Mathers 2007). However, it appears this expansion has been confined to less severe disability. This suggests that the period of more severe morbidity in the period immediately preceding death may not be expanding as average life expectancy increases.

Some commentators (e.g. Richardson & Robertson 1999) conclude that increased life expectancy will have little impact on ageing. Other factors such as improved technology and economic growth are seen as more significant in general.

However, where there is a significant demographic change that increases the proportion of older people in society, this impact needs to be taken into account. Even if continuing increases in life expectancy do not result in increased costs, health and aged care costs will increase significantly as the proportion (and absolute number) of older people in the population increases, particularly as the number of people aged over 80 years increases (Productivity Commission 2005).

It should also be noted that this increased expenditure due to population ageing will differ according to chronic disease. For example, almost half of the projected increase in health and aged care expenditure due to cardiovascular and neurological diseases in Australia by 2033 will be due to population ageing (AIHW 2008). In addition, increased 'volume per case'—that is, the amount of health services needed to treat an individual—will account for approximately 31% of this expenditure on cardiovascular disease. Secondary prevention and early intervention strategies have the potential to reduce future volume per case and therefore contain this additional expenditure.

Such projections also demonstrate the importance of public health's role in providing primary prevention. While population ageing and volume per case add substantially to future expenditure on cardiovascular disease, decreased rates of cardiovascular disease will prevent this expenditure from being approximately 24% higher than it is already expected to be.

Not surprisingly, governments and the community more generally have become concerned about these costs. In response, they have begun to explore new strategies to prevent and manage the emerging problem of chronic disease.

ROLE OF PUBLIC HEALTH IN AN AGEING SOCIETY

Chronic diseases are largely age-related in their onset and effects, and almost all older people report having one (or more) long-term health condition(s). Sensory conditions, arthritis and other musculoskeletal conditions are common, and other prevalent conditions include cardiovascular disease, stroke, cancer, diabetes, chronic respiratory disease, mental/behavioural problems and dementia. As life expectancy continues to increase, it is predicted these conditions will become more prevalent (AIHW 2006a).

Chronic diseases are difficult to manage successfully; once established, intervention often focuses on supportive treatment and care to prevent disease progression and reduce pain, discomfort and activity limitation. Many chronic diseases progressively result in increased pain, discomfort and disability over time and require increasingly more complex and intensive interventions.

Ideally, the onset of chronic disease should be prevented or, at the very least, delayed, and public health has a critical role in achieving this. The age-standardised decline in cardiovascular disease over the past 30 years is a clear example of successful prevention of chronic disease. In particular, this success goes to: the dramatic decline in smoking rates; the improvement in managing hypertension, hypercholesterolemia and coronary artery disease; and the use of thrombolysis, which have had a major influence on this improvement (Mathers 2007).

Prevention can be thought of as occurring across a continuum, from 'upstream' social and environmental factors that affect health (e.g. employment, housing and urban design) to 'downstream' behavioural risks (e.g. smoking, nutrition and physical activity). Primary prevention focuses on improving health by optimising upstream social determinants and reduces the likelihood that risk factors will occur. Secondary prevention focuses on reductions in risk factors once they are evident and early intervention with disease to reduce the potential for adverse outcomes. Secondary prevention is more concerned with behavioural and healthcare interventions for people already at risk.

Successful primary and secondary prevention strategies, like those that have produced improvements in cardiovascular disease, combine social, environmental and behavioural change strategies systematically over the long term. Over time, they can produce significant population shifts in critical risk factors such as smoking and nutrition.

The primary prevention strategies that apply generally for the population also apply for older people. Older people with better income and housing, who live in well-integrated communities and who have higher levels of social participation, will have better health outcomes. Public health will play a significant role in this respect, with enormous scope to improve the health and wellbeing of older people by reversing current trends towards underutilisation of effective interventions for common chronic diseases such as arthritis (Hootman et al 2012). Substantial gains can potentially be made through increasing the physical activity of older people generally (King & King 2010).

While the health and aged care systems have an important role to play in supporting primary prevention, gains are more likely to be made through interventions outside the health system. Population shifts in risk factors such as smoking, nutrition, alcohol use and physical activity, or protective factors such as social participation, require changes to regulation, taxation, environmental design and broader social policy.

Public health must also consider the role of socioeconomic disadvantage, given that those considered most disadvantaged are more at risk from factors such as smoking, low physical activity and poor nutrition, and have more avoidable hospital admissions. To return to mortality data, clear differentials in mortality exist across levels of disadvantage. A classic Australian study of socioeconomic status and mortality demonstrated that, for adults, the age-standardised mortality rate from coronary heart disease was 43.0 people per 100,000 population in those areas considered the *least* disadvantaged, compared with 80.7 per 100,000 in areas considered *most* disadvantaged (Turrell & Mathers 2001). 'Equalising' these inequalities—that is, if the mortality rates of the least disadvantaged applied to the most disadvantaged—would result in substantial decreases in mortality and, as a consequence, increased life expectancy for disadvantaged people.

However, greater focus on prevention is not simply about increasing life expectancy. While much of the measurement of health and wellbeing has centred on mortality and morbidity, health is not simply the absence of disease. It is an instrumental value. People value health because good health allows them to participate in society. The quality of life people experience and their capacity to continue to participate in activities that they value are, therefore, more important measures of success for prevention programs (and healthcare) than simple indices of life expectancy and the incidence and prevalence of disease.

In summary, where the earlier and very successful focus of public health interventions were on underpinning environmental circumstances of disease transmission, now the emphasis has moved to broader consideration of the social determinants of health. Health and wellbeing are now increasingly seen as produced by social and environmental circumstances in which people live.

REORIENTING HEALTH AND AGED CARE

As chronic and complex conditions become more prevalent with ageing, there is pressure to reorient the care system. Current models of healthcare remain heavily focused on episodic, often medicalised, service delivery and acute care. Practices were designed for a different time when complex and intensive care was provided in hospital and institutional settings.

Chronic and complex problems cannot be resolved through acute medical interventions, although they often play a part in the overall management of care. Contemporary public health models suggest a shift to secondary prevention, early intervention and ongoing management and support in primary and community care settings, often over extended periods of time to assist people to live independently at home and in the community.

This reorientation towards prevention is not simply about trying to increase life expectancy by preventing the occurrence of disease. It is a more fundamental shift to both understanding that health and wellbeing are determined by social circumstances and also understanding that the purpose of being healthy is to be able to participate in valued activities. The shift to a social model of health has not only influenced the approach to prevention of chronic disease, it is also changing the way health and aged care services are delivered.

Aged care services have often been heavily focused on providing personal assistance and care in institutional settings. The increased prevalence of chronic and complex conditions drives a much greater emphasis on models of care that integrate services around needs of the users at home and in the community.

The next generation of health and aged care consumers are unlikely to accept the options that are currently available. There are increasing expectations that health and aged care programs and services are much more focused on enabling older people to continue to live independently at home and in their community for as long as possible (Productivity Commission 2011).

This ongoing reorientation of healthcare highlights the importance of primary and community care within the health system. In the past, the service system used by older people comprised acute hospital care, subacute care focused on rehabilitation and long-term residential care for those who could not return home. Community care was largely provided by primary care clinicians supported by domiciliary nursing, personal care and home support.

More recently, managing chronic disease in primary and community settings has focused on preventing unnecessary use of acute and subacute hospital services. This has included an increased emphasis on post–acute care and community rehabilitation services, more intensive home-based care and support, and palliative care.

In part, the substitution of community-based for institutional services has been driven by pressure to reduce the costs of more intensive, bed–based services. Community-based care is less expensive because much of it is provided by family, friends and neighbours.

Community-based care is less expensive because much of it is provided by family, friends and neighbours.

However, the evidence also suggests that stronger primary care services result in better health outcomes. Countries and regions that have greater access to primary care services have lower mortality rates (Starfield et al 2005). More detailed research has demonstrated that integrated primary and community care significantly improves the prevention and management of chronic and complex disease while at the same time reducing the overall costs of managing these conditions (Wagner 2000, Wagner et al 2001).

Historically, primary and community care have often developed in piecemeal fashion as an adjunct to institutional and family care. As a result, the organisation and capacity of community care is often underdeveloped.

Increasingly, more complex healthcare is being provided by the formal care system at home and in community settings than was previously the case. Length of stay in hospitals has reduced, same-day procedures have increased, rehabilitation and treatment have transferred from hospital to community settings, institutions for people with disabilities and mental illness have been closed, and older people stay at home for longer while frail, ill and disabled. At the same time, the availability of informal care and support provided by family, friends and neighbours has lessened. The boundaries are blurring.

Primary and community care is better thought of as a setting for providing care rather than a separate functional tier of the healthcare system (i.e. primary, secondary, tertiary). The main health and care functions provided in this setting can be described on a continuum that includes:

- secondary prevention for those with behavioural, social and psychological risks
- identification and treatment of straightforward acute conditions across a range of modalities (e.g. medical, dental, psychological)
- identification and referral of complex and acute conditions for specialist assessment and intervention (e.g. diagnostics, surgery, acute hospital admission)
- identification and early intervention for chronic and potentially complex conditions
- community and home-based rehabilitation for post-acute and subacute conditions (including post-acute care)
- ongoing treatment and support of people with chronic and complex conditions in the community and at home (including palliative care).

The challenge for governments in developed countries faced with increasing prevalence of chronic and complex conditions for ageing populations is to reorient their health systems away from institutional and acute care to integrated primary and community care and support services.

The evidence suggests that more effective management of chronic disease requires concentration on systemic factors including (Swerissen & Taylor 2008, Taylor & Swerissen 2010):

- healthcare organisations that ensure governance and management of healthcare providers around the needs of consumers for enrolled or catchment populations
- partnerships between consumers and providers to ensure consumers are able to effectively self-manage risks and chronic disease
- consistent application of practice guidelines and decision support for preventing and managing specific conditions such as diabetes, chronic obstructive pulmonary disease and renal disease
- care pathways for preventing and managing chronic disease where consumers access programs and services on the basis of systematic assessment and care planning
- coordinated, team-based, multidisciplinary care across a service continuum ranging from risk prevention to complex care
- integrated information systems for transferring client/patient information across providers, the provision of practice guidance and the coordination of care
- payment models that promote best practice and effective outcomes for consumers.

Primary and community care have a critical role in keeping people well and providing them with the interventions, care and support they need so they can continue to participate in their family and community life when they develop longer term illness and disability. They should complement and integrate with the informal care that is provided by family and friends, and coordinate services that are required from more complex and specialised providers in the health and aged care service system.

In many cases this will require significant reorganisation and investment in primary and community services. Primary and community care often includes relatively small scale, individual primary medical practices that are organisationally separate from more specialised long-term care agencies, which focus on: older people; people with a mental illness and alcohol and drug problems; people with disabilities; and sometimes people with chronic illness or those who have post-acute care needs. Similarly, the service system often separates out specialist services, home support, personal care and nursing.

In addition to reorienting the system, the greater focus on health and wellbeing has consequently increased the emphasis on the extent to which health and social care improve the quality of life—an important shift in thinking. The outcomes for treating acute illness are relatively straightforward: improvements in clinical indicators are usually associated with equally dramatic improvements in perceptions of health and wellbeing, improvements in function, and a return to participation in everyday life. For treatment and care of chronic and complex conditions, this is less clear. Often medical interventions are relatively ineffective; pain, distress and disability progressively increase; more personal care and support are required; and participation in valued relationships and activities at home and in the community decline.

When the very successful acute care model of intervention is inappropriately applied to chronic and complex conditions, health and aged care can easily become focused on clinical outcomes, rather than the quality of life actually experienced.

CONCLUSION

The prevention, promotion and restoration of health for older people is an important public health goal. The recent reorientation towards a social model of public health is critical to preventing and managing chronic and complex disease.

It is not yet clear whether increased life expectancy will be associated with greater levels of dependency and disability, although there appears to be some increase in mild and moderate disability. However, there will certainly be a significant increase in demand for health and aged care services associated with demographic ageing.

Changing consumer preferences and increased demand will drive a greater focus on developing comprehensive and integrated primary and community care services focused on supporting individuals at home and in the community so they can continue to participate in valued activities and relationships for as long as possible. This will require a significant reform of the primary and community care service system and, alongside effective public health interventions, will greatly improve the health and wellbeing of older people.

Reflective questions

1. How can the system be changed to provide a flexible service delivery that makes transition between services more effective for older people, for example, the acute sector and the aged care sector managing transition more effectively?

2. If primary healthcare is better community based, how can this sector be strengthened to offer improved health, social and psychological support for older people?

3. Using a particular example of a contemporary public health intervention, campaign or strategy, what is necessary to adapt it to an ageing population?

4. How can the partnership between the consumer and the provider be strengthened so older people are empowered to self-manage their health and take risks?

References

Australian Bureau of Statistics, 2008. Population Projections: Australia, 2006 to 2101. Online. Available: http://www.abs.gov.au/ausstats/abs@.nsf/detailspage/3222.02006%20to%202101?opendocument, 16 Sep 2012.

Australian Institute of Health and Welfare, 2006a. Chronic diseases and associated risk factors in Australia. Australian Government, Canberra.

Australian Institute of Health and Welfare, 2006b. Mortality over the twentieth century in Australia: trends and patterns in major causes of death. Australian Government, Canberra.

Australian Institute of Health and Welfare, 2008. Projection of Australian health care expenditure by disease: 2003 to 2033. Australian Government, Canberra.

Fried, L.P., 2012. What are the roles of public health in an aging society? In: Proshaska, T.R., Anderson, L.A., Binstock, R.H. (Eds.), Public Health for an Ageing Society. The Johns Hopkins University Press, Baltimore.

Fries, J.F., 1980. Aging, natural death, and the compression of morbidity. N Engl J Med 303 (3), 130–135.

Fries, J.F., 1989. The compression of morbidity: near or Far? Milbank Q 67 (2), 208–232.

Gruenberg, E.M., 1977. The failures of success. Milbank Mem Fund Q Health Soc 55 (1), 3–24.

Hootman, J.M., Helmick, C.G., Brady, T.J., 2012. A public health approach to addressing arthritis in older adults: the most common cause of disability. Am J Public Health 102 (3), 426–433.

King, A.C., King, D.K., 2010. Physical activity for an aging population. Pub Health Rev 32 (2), 401–426.

Klumpp, T.G., 1947. Problems of an aging population: care of the aged and chronically ill. Am J Public Health 37 (2), 156–162.

Lombard, H.L., 1947. Problems of an aging population: preventive aspects of cancer control. Am J Public Health 37 (2), 170–176.

Mathers, C.D., 2007. The health of older Australians. In: Borowski, A., Encel, S., Ozanne, E. (Eds.), Longevity and social change: australia in the 21st century. University of New South Wales Press, Sydney.

Medicare Australia, 2013. Medicare Australia Statistics. Online. Available: https://www.medicareaustralia.gov.au/statistics/mbs_group.shtml, 8 Feb 2013.

Organisation for Economic Co-operation and Development (OECD), 2012. OECD Health Data 2012. Online. Available: http://www.oecd.org/health/healthpoliciesanddata/oecdhealthdata2012-frequentlyrequesteddata.htm, 21 Sep 2012.

Productivity Commission, 2005. Economic implications of an ageing Australia. Australian Government, Canberra.

Productivity Commission, 2011. Caring for older Australians. Australian Government, Canberra.

Richardson, J., Robertson, I., 1999. Ageing and the cost of health services. In: Policy Implications of the Ageing of Australia's Population. Productivity Commission & Melbourne Institute of Applied Economic and Social Research, Canberra. pp. 329–356.

Schafer, I., Hansen, H., Schon, G., et al., 2012. The influence of age, gender and socio-economic status on multimorbidity patterns in primary care. First Results from the Multicare Cohort Study. BMC Health Serv Res 12, 89.

Starfield, B., Shi, L., Macinko, J., 2005. Contribution of primary care to health systems and health. Milbank Q 83 (3), 457–502.

Swerissen, H., Taylor, M.J., 2008. Reforming funding for chronic illness: Medicare-CDM. Aust Health Rev 32 (1), 76–85.

Taylor, M.J., Swerissen, H., 2010. Medicare and chronic disease management: integrated care as an exceptional circumstance? Aust Health Rev 34 (2), 152–161.

Turrell, G., Mathers, C., 2001. Socioeconomic inequalities in all-cause and specific-cause mortality in Australia: 1985–1987 and 1995–1997. Int J Epidemiol 30 (2), 231–239.

UN Department of Economic and Social Affairs, 2002. World population ageing: 1950–2050. United Nations, New York.

Wagner, E.H., 2000. The role of patient care teams in chronic disease management. BMJ 320 (7234), 569–572.

Wagner, E.H., Austin, B.T., Davis, C., et al., 2001. Improving chronic illness care: translating evidence into action. Health Aff (Millwood) 20 (6), 64–78.

Wilkerson, H.L., 1947. Problems of an aging population: public health aspects of diabetes. Am J Public Health 37 (2), 177–188.

CHAPTER 3

REDEFINING 'OLD AGE': THE CENTENARIANS

John McCormack

Editors' comments

There was a time when reaching 100 years of age was considered extraordinary. McCormack's research raises the possibility that this may be, within the lifetime of some readers, not at all unusual. You might imagine centenarians being very ill, frail and experiencing a poor quality of life. Not so. It seems people who live this long are reporting their health and quality of life as generally good to very good. What will this mean for future policy and practice?

INTRODUCTION

When Peggy Ashburn turned 80 years of age a few years ago, she recounted to me how her friends were often quite shocked when she told them she was about to take her father, Jack Ross, then aged 109 years, out for a meal. She told this author, who keeps the list of the oldest age-validated Australians, that she thinks people are surprised for a number of reasons. First, that at her own advanced age she still had a living parent; second, that her father had lived such a long life; and third, being an enlisted veteran of both world wars, that he had survived the trauma of war and lived for such a long time. Mr Ross lived at home until 104 and then entered residential care after a fall, but he remained relatively active and interested in the world around him. He has since died but did reach the age of 110 years. He is remembered as a national treasure because he was one of the few remaining First World War veterans in the world. All those veterans have now died; however, Mr Ross' story is not unique.

When French woman Jeanne Calment died in August 1997 aged 122 years and five months, she had achieved the remarkable feat of extending the human life span. Previously, the maximum life potential (i.e. the verifiable age at death of the longest-lived member of the species) was thought to be biologically limited to 120 years (Moody 1998). This ultimate limit to length of life has itself had a durable longevity until the unique Ms Calment challenged its intractability. Similarly in Australia, Christina Cock, who died aged 114 years, was most likely the oldest ever woman in Australia, and the oldest person ever in Australia. At the time of her death in 2002 she was the third-oldest age-validated person alive in the world.

There is no doubt that these people have lived to an extraordinary age—validated ages never before observed or experienced in human civilisation. In addition to this group of people, however, is another almost equally exceptional group. This is the growing number of people reaching the milestone of 100 years of age. Japan exceeded 44,450 centenarians by the year 2010 (up from 13,000 in 2000), and despite the affects of the 2011 earthquake/tsunami on older people, is expected to reach almost one million centenarians by 2050 (United Nations 2010). One American estimate of centenarians was more than 72,000 in the early decades of the 21st century (Administration on Aging 1996, Medserve 1998); and the United Nations predicts there will be more than three million centenarians alive in 2050, with very large numbers of centenarians in China and India (United Nations 2006).

In recognition of the importance of this new extreme ageing phenomenon that is redefining 'old age', there is an increasing number of centenarian studies underway, looking predominantly at the biomedical aspects of extreme ageing in terms of how and why more people are reaching this very old age. Only a few studies, such as The Georgia Centenarian Study (Poon 2006), The New England Centenarian Study (Perls et al 1999), The Berlin Aging Study (Baltes & Smith 2003) and more recently the newly initiated, but yet to be published, Sydney Centenarian Study (Sachdev 2012), have included the psychosocial aspects of survivorship. All these latter studies have used multidisciplinary teams to comprehensively assess centenarians. None, however, take this forward to the next step of intervention approaches. While it is essential that we understand why so many more people are reaching very old age, we also need to know the quality of their life at this milestone age. Does this demographic transition add life to years or just years to life? Also, we need to start understanding what the healthcare implications of this new longevity regime might be, and how we might prepare for it. No one researcher or country has fully clarified the impact of this new ageing phenomenon to date.

 While it is essential that we understand why so many more people are reaching very old age, we also need to know the quality of their life at this milestone age.

In Australia until recently very little work has been undertaken with this group (McCormack 2000, 2002). There are many publications on 'the aged' (i.e. those aged 65 years or older), but these works often present findings at such a highly aggregated age level that it can be difficult to detect differences within the group. Similarly, while we know that it is the ageing of the oldest-old who will increase at the fastest rate (Australian Bureau of Statistics (ABS)

2003), and that this group may be more vulnerable to the stresses of time (Baltes & Smith 2003), there is no specific social or financial estimates of the impact of, or on, the very old that have been developed in Australia. Vaupel and Oeppen (2002) estimate that females born today in low-mortality, high-longevity countries like France and Japan already have a 50% chance of living to 100 years. Australia is also in that group of high-longevity countries (see Fig 3.2) and recent estimates claim the official population projections underestimate our future aged population, and this can be clearly seen among the oldest-old where, for example, the number of females aged 95–99 years will increase over the next 25 years by a factor of 5.8 compared with a factor of 2.0 for females aged 65–69 years (Booth 2003, Booth & Tickle 2004). These demographic imperatives emphasise the importance of us knowing and understanding the health and welfare implications of increasing longevity, especially with this growing group of remarkable people who survive to very old age.

These demographic imperatives emphasise the importance of us knowing and understanding the health and welfare implications of increasing longevity, especially with this growing group of remarkable people who survive to very old age.

This chapter presents some preliminary descriptive findings for Australia on what Belle Boone Beard (1991) called this 'new' generation of people aged around 100 years and older. The chapter first draws on historical census data to illustrate the emergence of centenarians in Australia, and then highlights some of the technical difficulties associated with actually identifying centenarians. After that, their sociodemographic details are reported, as well as some health data, before moving on to provide a more personal perspective on the life of centenarians as reported in the Quality of Life (QoL) survey.

HOW MANY AUSTRALIAN CENTENARIANS ARE THERE?

It needs to be stated at the outset that there are no exact or validated figures on the number of centenarians in Australia. Nor are there any exact figures on single year of age, such as the number aged exactly 100 years, 101 years, 102 years and so on; the recent Australian censuses provide mainly a single aggregated number for 'aged 100 years or more'. Some estimates for those single years of age were provided from the 2006 census, but they are still under revision due to great variability in the census self-reported 100-plus ages. Presumably in the past, and still now to some extent, the relatively small number of people achieving this remarkable chronological milestone was not cause for detailed reporting. Unfortunately, despite the rapid increase in centenarians in Australia, our national statistics still do not collect or report this age disaggregation in any great detail or publication. Use of the word 'centenarians' here therefore usually refers to the sum of those aged 100 years

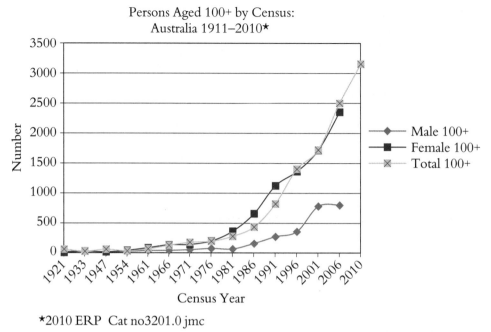

Persons Aged 100+ by Census:
Australia 1911–2010★

★2010 ERP Cat no3201.0 jmc

Figure 3.1

Centenarians in Australia
Source: ABS Census 2006

or older, and we need to look back in time over these reported aggregates to observe the growth in this demographic group.[1]

While life expectancy at all ages has continued to increase, the Australian census, from the early 1900s, consistently reported people living to very old ages (see Fig 3.1). The census records show there were 64 living centenarians recorded at the 1911 census, and that 27 centenarians had died in that year. Information on their deaths was provided in the 1911 Commonwealth Year Book (ABS 2001). However, the Statistical Registrar-General commented in relation to 'abnormally high ages' that 'no absolute reliance can be placed on the accuracy of the ages [shown], owing to the well-known tendency of very old people to overstate their ages' (ABS 2001 p 192). Not only was he making reference to the important issue of age-validation or age-misreporting but also to the poor record-keeping of registration of births in other countries of origin.

For example, only two of the 14 centenarians who died in 1911 were born in Australia. The majority were born in England, and two were born in China. Ten of the 14 were more than 100 years of age, the oldest being 108 years. Only three were on the public old age pension, whereas the rest were listed as having an occupation. Similarly, of the 13 female centenarians who had died in 1911, seven were aged older than 100 years, with the oldest being 105 years.

....
[1]Note that much of the data used in this chapter are unpublished data purchased by the author.

The most frequent cause of death was listed as 'senility', although 'rodent ulcers', 'gangrene', 'diarrhoea', 'heart disease' and 'influenza' were also cited.

There were low numbers of centenarians until the 1970s, after which the number of centenarians and their growth rate increased substantially. There was then a 47% average five-yearly increase for people in this age group during the years 1971 to 2006 (ABS 2006). The increase in females is greater than the increase in males, with females representing 79% of people aged 99 years or older in the 1996 census, but this had dropped slightly to 75% (ABS 1996) by the 2006 census (ABS 2006). Similarly, the gender ratio for this group at that 1996 census was 27 males per 100 females, but this increased to 34 males per hundred females for 2006. As above, and as can be seen from Figure 3.1, the reported increase in male centenarians over the past 10-year period may need further investigation to substantiate this rapid increase. Overall, however, despite these data difficulties, it is clear that there is a very marked increase in numbers of people aged 100 years or older in Australia.

It is clear that there is a very marked increase in the number of people aged 100 years or older in Australia.

The Australian census for 2006 is the most recent count of centenarians and the ABS used those census figures (which on the census form was a box tick if aged 100 years or older), along with birth, death and migration data, to develop the estimated resident population (ERP) of Australia. According to the ABS, the census tends to under-enumerate (ABS 2002), although it is not clear how much this impacts on centenarians. However, the 2006 census count of 3157 centenarians (802 males and 2355 (75%) females) is in accord with the numbers one would expect in an advanced industrial economy of about 100 centenarians per million of the total population. The actual rate of 133 would, using Ruisdael's survey data (2003), mean Australia is about sixth in the top 10 countries for the centenarians per million index figure but just outside (11th) the top 10 developed countries for number of centenarians. Ruisdael's data in Figure 3.2 shows only France, the United States, the United Kingdom, Japan and Italy rate above Australia on the index.

In trying to understand what is behind this apparent increase in Australian centenarians, the author applied Thatcher's (1999) methodology to current and historical ABS data and life tables to identify relevant individual factors (see Table 3.1).

Applying this to the period up to 2001, the product of the factors shown accounts for the approximately 40-fold increase in Australian centenarians, from 64 in 1911 to about 2500 in 2001. Among the individual factors, improved survival from age 80 to 100 years accounts for about half of the total increase, and females play a larger role in this. However, in the overall product of factors, males account for a higher proportion of the overall increase than do females. As Poon (2006) says, there is no single magic bullet to explain this late-life survival but more likely a constellation of factors, including Australia's pervasive and effective healthcare system. Changes among those aged older than 100 years so far account for only a small component of the overall increase

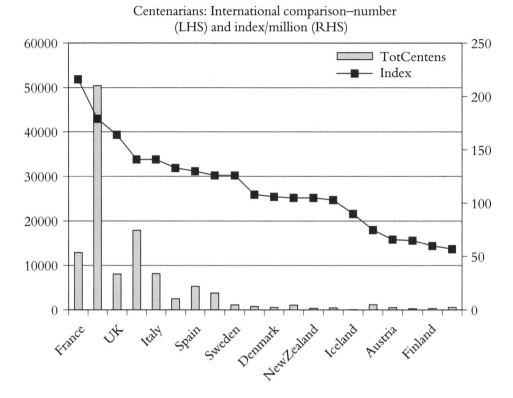

Centenarians: International comparison–number
(LHS) and index/million (RHS)

Figure 3.2

International centenarian comparison
Source: Ruisdael 2003

Table 3.1

Decomposing Australian centenarian increase

CAUSE	MALE	FEMALE
Increase in births, 1860–1899	2.14	2.14
Improved survival from birth to age 80 years	3.96	3.92
Improved survival from age 80–100 years	7.14	13.1
Changes above age 100 (ratio 100+:100, 1985–1995)	.2	.1
Reduced probability of death at age 100: 1953–1995	1.8	1.6
Product of above factors	21.8	17.6

in centenarians. However, not a lot is known about these older centenarian age groups, as detailed below. Before moving to look briefly at them, we will look at other data from another older census (2001) when greater detail data was available, in terms of what it can tell us about very old age in Australia. (Note that this is unpublished data that had to be purchased from the ABS because the ABS does not produce detailed figures for this age group.)

MARITAL STATUS AND LIVING ARRANGEMENTS

The census data provide some information about the number of centenarians still living in Australia. For example, there is a statistically significant difference in marital status between male and female centenarians (χ^2 321.7, 4df, p < 0.001) (see Table 3.2). There is a much greater proportion of males never married (32%) than females (14%), and an even greater proportion of males still married (19%) than females (6%). Females, on the other hand, are far more likely to be widowed (76%).

Only 6.4% of males aged 65 years or more at the previous census reported never being married and 72% were currently married. The corresponding figures for females were 5% never married and 42% currently married. Compared with the larger 65-years-plus group, centenarians therefore have a much higher proportion of 'never married' (males 32% and females 14%) but lower proportion of 'currently married' (males 19% and females 6%). In living to very old age, being a 'never married' male or female may not necessarily be a disadvantage.

Amazingly, more than half (51%) of all centenarians live in the community in private dwellings while only 49% are in health- and retirement-related accommodation (see Table 3.3).

Table 3.2

All centenarians by gender and marital status, Australia

MARITAL STATUS	MALE (PROP)	FEMALE (PROP)	TOTAL (PROP)
Never married	251	232	483 (0.19)
Widowed	265	1312	1577 (0.63)
Divorced	74	53	127 (0.05)
Separated	43	24	67 (0.03)
Married	151	97	248 (0.10)
Total	784 (0.31)	1718 (0.69)	2502

Source: ABS Census 2001, unpublished

Table 3.3

All centenarians by gender and living arrangements, Australia

LIVING ARRANGEMENTS	MALE	FEMALE	TOTAL (PROP)
Total in private dwelling	617	661	1278 (0.51)
With partner only	111	111	222 (0.9)
With other family	155	237	392 (0.16)
Lone person	211	239	450 (0.18)
Other household/unrelated	140	74	214 (0.8)
Total in non-private dwelling	164	1058	1222 (0.49)
Nursing home	44	627	671 (0.27)
Other (e.g. health/aged accom)	120	431	551 (0.22)
Total	781 (.31)	1719 (.69)	2500

Source: ABS Census 2001, unpublished

The fact that five in 10 (51%) live in the community, with nearly two in 10 living alone (18%), hardly depicts these very old people as all totally frail and dependent. These figures at the 1996 census (ABS 1996) for Australia were fairly similar to those found by Wilkinson and Sainsbury (1998) in New Zealand where 34% lived at home with others and 66% lived in institutions for the elderly, but the 2001 Australian census has moved further away from this (McCormack 2000). This has probably happened in New Zealand as well because their centenarian population has increased similar to that in Australia (see Fig 3.2). The 2001 Australian census report of 18% living alone in a private dwelling is the same as recorded for New Zealand (18%).

 The fact that five in 10 (51%) live in the community, with nearly two in 10 living alone (18%), hardly depicts these very old people as all totally frail and dependent.

BIRTHPLACE

In 2001 only 56% of centenarians reported being born in Australia (see Table 3.4), but information is unavailable for a sizeable number. The 32% born in

Table 3.4

All centenarians by place born, Australia

BORN	MALE	FEMALE	TOTAL (PROP)
Australia	360	1040	1400 (.56)
Elsewhere	318	474	792 (.32)
Not stated	106	204	310 (.12)
Total	784 (0.33)	1718 (0.67)	2502

Source: ABS Census 2001, unpublished

other countries is considerably higher than the birthplace composition of the total Australian population, which recorded 21.9% of people born overseas in the 2001 census. Further investigation of the 'not stated' group is needed, however, because one would expect, with the health selectivity of the migration process, that there would be a higher percentage of centenarians born overseas. On the other hand, the recent increase in centenarians, shown in Figure 3.1, suggests health and living conditions have improved and that just as many born in Australia can now reach age 100 years.

Overall, this census centenarian data reveal both similarities to and differences from the general aged population. Their marital status, living arrangements and birthplace reveal a diversity not dissimilar to those aged 65 years or older. However, there are differences in place of domicile. For example, proportionately more centenarians live in health and retirement accommodation, and fewer live alone. The centenarian diversity nevertheless has endured, and this is an important facet of this population. Very old people, like all other age groups in society, are not all the same. In fact the growth of centenarians worldwide has led to further disaggregation of the centenarian generation itself.

SEMI-SUPERCENTENARIANS AND SUPERCENTENARIANS IN AUSTRALIA

As stated above, in Australia there are major difficulties disaggregating centenarians (in this section referring to age 100–104 years) into a single-year age. Similarly, for other five-year age groupings such as the semi-supercentenarians (SSCs) aged 105–109 years or the supercentenarians (SCs) aged 110 years or older, because the officially collected ABS data has not, until the most recent census, asked centenarians their actual age last birthday (nor does it require a birth date). So again, estimates need to be made and other data is used for this, as shown in Table 3.5. The Japanese data is from the Ministry of Health, Labor and Welfare (2003), while the European data ('Euro 9') is from Ruisdael (2003), and is aggregated data for nine European countries

Table 3.5

Distribution of age groups of centenarians (%)

AGE GROUP	JAPAN	EURO9	AUS ACAS	AUS RES CARE
100–104	95	95.9	95.9	93
105–109	4.6	3.6	3.6	6.3
110+	0.4	0.5	0.5	0.3

with a sample size of 6109. The 'Aus ACAS' data is Australian health data from Aged Care Assessment Services in the state of Victoria for 2002 and the number of centenarians is 218. The 'Aus Res Care' data is from the rolls of the Australian Government Residential Care register of centenarians ($n = 1216$) in what used to be known as nursing homes and lower level hostels, for the year 2001. None of the people in the Australian data have had their ages validated because the service they received is based on health need rather than age.

Table 3.5 shows that, overall, the distributions for centenarians, SSCs and SCs are not that different for Australia and other countries. The 'Aus Res Care' data is weighted more to the older groups and this may be because the population in Australia is more unwell or less able to care for themselves, which may be a function of age. Similar health populations for Japan and Europe would be needed to present a better comparison.

This comparison is taken further in Figure 3.3 where the same Japanese and European data is compared with an estimated distribution of the Australian 2001 census figure of 2503 centenarians distributed across the single-year ages based on an average distribution derived from 13 countries' data presented in Ruisdael's survey (2003). This latter estimate for Australia should be more comparable for Japan and Europe because it includes the total centenarian population rather than a specialised health component sample.

As can be seen from the chart, the general estimate ('EstAus01') is similar to the European distribution, whereas the Japanese distribution has an older profile, with fewer 100-year-olds and more aged 101 and older. Another feature of this age distribution (not shown here) is the gender difference. Analysis by gender shows that, like Kannisto (1994), female centenarians in Australia compared with males have a lower proportion of 100-year-olds (average 44% females and 47% males) and greater proportions aged 102 or older than males. While there are more female centenarians living longer, this older age profile of female centenarians may have an impact on the higher female death rates seen in Australian mortality data. Therefore, there is a need for more gender analysis of this older female age profile and its impact on the Australian data, just as we need further investigation right up to the SC group, to start understanding the social and economic implications of people living to these extreme ages. Health is just one of the key areas for further investigation, so we now turn to consider some health data.

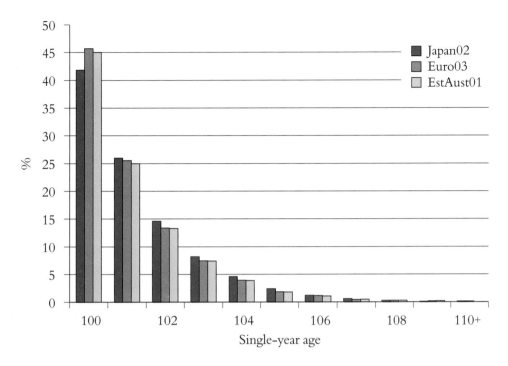

Figure 3.3

Age older than 100 years

Source: Ministry of Health, Labor and Welfare 2003, Ruisdael 2003

HEALTH OF CENTENARIANS

How we are physically can have a significant impact on how we cope in other aspects of our life, as well as the social interaction we engage in; healthcare, of course, has serious financial implications for individuals and governments. Apart from an accepted wisdom that we are likely to need more healthcare assistance with age, we actually have limited specific information on the health or healthcare needs of the very old. At very old age no one escapes some serious aches and pains, arthritis being a common disease, or indeed something even more life-threatening such as some degree of cardiovascular disease, which nevertheless might be controlled with medication and lifestyle changes (Andersen-Ranberg et al 2001). Figure 3.4 shows some comparative age-group data from Australian Aged Care Assessment Teams (ACATs) over one six-month period as an example of the information that might be useful in enhancing our understanding of health needs in very old age. The key areas of orientation (to time, place and person), mobility and continence are shown by comparing three age cohorts.

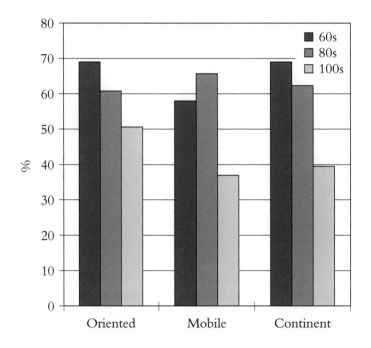

Figure 3.4

Age group health comparison

As expected, the centenarians, compared with a cohort of those in their sixties and a group in their eighties, tend to have a smaller proportion in each functional health domain. That is, on average, the centenarians generally are less oriented, less mobile and a smaller proportion fully continent. However, this is a highly selected assessment group and to this extent may well be unrepresentative of the total population of each of these cohorts. The figures also show, however, that by default not all centenarians (or indeed sexagenarians or octogenarians) who have particular health needs will be disoriented or immobile and so on. This similarity in experiencing these important problems, yet seeing differences between the cohorts in terms of rates and also within each cohort, illustrates the impact of differential ageing and warns us against generalising just on chronological grounds.

Taking this health analysis further the author has assembled some hospital data on centenarians, as hospital costs can be a major concern of governments in the light of an ageing population. (Note again, this is unpublished data specifically purchased by the author.) What is strange, however, is that the hospitalisation rates, as shown in Figure 3.5, increase with age as expected, but then there is a turning point around age 94 where hospitalisation rates decline with older age.

This counterintuitive decline may, however, also just be a reflection of the previously mentioned health/selection effect. As stated above, there is an overrepresentation of people born overseas among Australian centenarians and

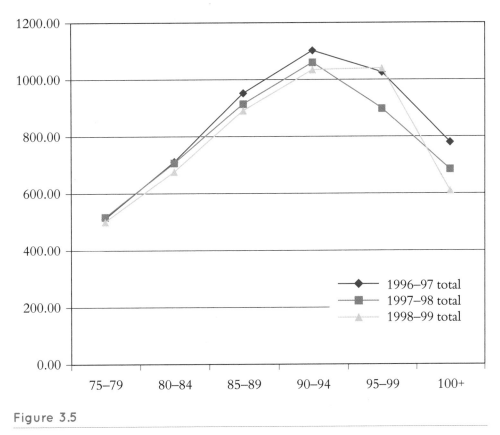

Figure 3.5

Hospitalisation rates of older age groups

this lower hospitalisation rate may reflect their high level of personal health that enabled them to pass the migration health test many years ago. That is, there is again the possibility of a health/selection effect that explains the turndown in rates. On the other hand, anecdotal information sources point out that there are other factors such as the centenarians themselves may not wish to go to hospital, and sometimes this might also be the wish of families and even a treating doctor's desire as well. These are complicated interacting factors that need to be further teased out to disentangle what this interesting data is telling us.

> **What is strange, however, is that the hospitalisation rates increase with age as expected, but then there is a turning point around age 94 where hospitalisation rates decline with older age.**

The author has also collected other hospital data by clinical specialty that shows this turndown for various specialties such as orthopaedics, gastroenterology, urology and so on. The clinical exception is psychiatry, which shows a substantial increase for centenarians. This mental health utilisation is usually in reference to dementia but does not mean, however, that all centenarians have significant dementia. The estimates derived from meta-analyses for significant dementia in centenarians ranges between 30% and 70 %. That is, at least a third do not have dementia at interview/assessment (Perls & Silver 1999). The common finding here of low hospitalisation rates is further reinforced by the author's centenarian survey, finding where very few of the 65 centenarians in the sample had had a hospital admission in the preceding 12 months. On the other hand there was a standard response to use of medications where virtually all centenarians in the survey were using at least one prescribed medication. These health findings tends to reinforce Perl's statement that the older you are the healthier you have been (Perls & Silver 1999). Many centenarians in this study had lived at home for most of their 100 years and it was only after some significant adverse health event, such as a fall leading to a broken bone, that a move to residential care occurred.

Consequently, the low hospitalisation rate results in the counterintuitive cost figures shown in Figure 3.6 where costs, at very old age, actually decline with age.

Therefore, we can see that by investigating health needs and costs at very old age there are significant findings arising, which give us much more to ponder in relation to ageing than bland assumptions that all things have an

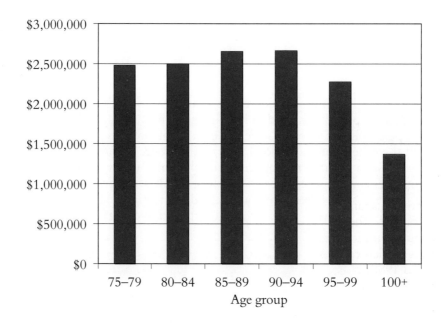

Figure 3.6

Comparative age-group healthcare costs
Source: AIHW 1999

inverse relationship with chronological age. This health data also shows that different age groups use and need health resources differentially (McCormack 2002), and therefore it is on the basis of need that we should allocate resources, rather than again assuming a negative or high-use requirement based just in chronological age.

QUALITY OF LIFE

While part of the above discussion has looked sociodemographically (as distinct from biomedically) at how and why we have this increase in numbers of people reaching very old age, we also need to know the quality of their life at this milestone age. Does this demographic transition add life to years or just years to life? The author has an exploratory study underway that addresses QoL issues for people aged around 100 years and older in Australia, and some preliminary findings are presented here.

THEORETICAL PERSPECTIVES AND DEFINING CENTENARIAN QUALITY OF LIFE

As stated earlier, the sociodemographic data illustrate some social and health diversity among centenarians, but at the same time it is unlikely that anyone reaches this age without any health problems. People have reached this age because they have avoided or delayed the serious onset of the major fatal diseases such as cancer and diseases of the circulatory system. However, all the centenarians interviewed reported some health problems ranging from chronic arthritis and diabetes to constipation. More than 80% were taking some medication, although the number of hospitalisations in the preceding 12 months was very low. We might expect, therefore, that centenarians would report low QoL due to this physical deterioration. As well, by the fact of their longevity, centenarians have experienced considerable loss over their lives. This can extend to partners, friends and even their own children. Given this, again, one might expect that centenarians would report low QoL as their social relationships may have decreased considerably.

Further, according to Cumming and Henry's (1961) disengagement theory, with increasing age centenarians would have gradually withdrawn from life and therefore again we might expect low QoL. Continuity theory (Neugarten 1969), on the other hand, predicts that people's attitudes to life and their behaviours tend to remain stable over time. Therefore, there is no reason to expect a sudden change at 100 years of age. Differential ageing (Birren & Bengston 1988) is another perspective informing us that, as with other age groups in society, there may be considerable differences among individuals within this age group, and therefore we might expect some variation across individuals, although for QoL ratings this will be within a limited range (Maher & Cummins 2001). Overall, then, we have a mixed bag of expectations to investigate in terms of QoL.

While these theoretical perspectives provide some guidance for what we might observe in relation to QoL, they do not present us with a clear definition of QoL for this group. For example, although more than half of those in this survey aged 100–102 years were mobile and alert, around a quarter of centenarians in the sample were quite physically disabled (bed-bound) and dependent, and not oriented to time or place, although not exhibiting severe dementia. How does one assess QoL for people in this state? They did respond to physical touch, had good appetites, often sang, generally looked content, and did not appear to be uncomfortable or in pain. These people obviously scored low on ability to do things for themselves and might be considered to have low QoL by external standards. By their own, or family members' standards, however, they could be considered relatively happy and having a high QoL. Who decides, therefore, what QoL is, and what the rating should be, is an area needing more research with this group (Baltes 1996).

For present purposes, as stated above, the definition of QoL relates to the individual's perception of their current physical health, memory, social relationships, ability to do things for themselves and so on. This is not unlike Rowe and Kahn's (1987) classic definition of 'successful ageing' to the extent that they define it as maintaining physical and cognitive functioning and engagement with life. However, more detailed investigation, particularly on disability at very old age, needs to occur for fear that people automatically equate successful ageing or QoL with longevity.

QUALITY OF LIFE SURVEY FINDINGS

Basic descriptive scores for the QoL-type variables are presented in Table 3.6. All mean scores are expressed using the percentage of scale maximum (written here as %MS) methodology (Maher & Cummins 2001).

This approach, when applied to large population surveys, predicts mean subjective QoL to lie within the range 70–80%MS (Maher & Cummins 2001). The mean scores in Table 3.6 approach this level on several of the items (e.g. life satisfaction) but are considerably below it on the other items (e.g. self-ability), and the standard deviations are large. The small non-representative sample of a fairly marginal and unexplored group may account for some of this normative gap. It could also be that this group, due to their longevity, experiences lower QoL. Alternatively, there may be limitations to the way QoL has been operationalised in the present investigation.

Looking at more specific domains of QoL, it can be seen that self-rated health has a considerable spread of responses (see Fig 3.7), possibly highlighting the individual variation present in the sample.

Table 3.6

Mean score on QoL variables (%MS)

	HEALTH	MEMORY	SELF-ABILITY	SOCIAL RELATIONSHIPS	LIFE SATISFACTION	LIVE TO 100	QOL SCORE
MEAN	52.9	50.8	39.7	65.3	69.7	57.5	67.5
SD	28.7	30.9	38.5	23.3	20.2	25.3	15.3

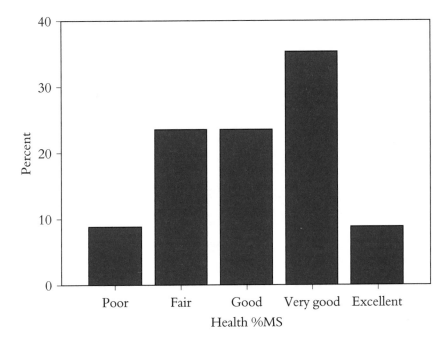

Figure 3.7

Health rating of centenarians

While the modal response is the category 'very good', about one-third (32.3%) rate their health as 'poor' or 'fair', and less than 10% rate it as 'excellent'. The mean %MS of 52.9 is therefore low by general population standards. As stated above, however, it would be surprising if individuals survived to this age without some health problems. This decline in physical health may also be seen in the item 'ability to do things for oneself' (see Fig 3.8).

More than 40% rated themselves 'fair/poor' on this item, and the %MS at 39.7 was the lowest score for any item. About 50% of centenarians live in nursing homes or cared accommodation (McCormack 2000), and this may well explain the score here as entry to those institutions is based on the need for assistance with activities of daily living. In contrast to the somewhat negative response on the above two items, when asked to rate overall life satisfaction, the %MS is much higher at 69.7, and closer to the population norm (see Fig 3.9).

Only 6% were 'not satisfied' with life, 48% were 'satisfied', and nearly half were 'very satisfied'. Therefore, despite physical limitations, centenarians may still have a positive view on life. It is after all quite an achievement to live to this age, and the personality characteristics, coping skills and adaptiveness developed over this long life may support a positive disposition to life. This is further exemplified with respondents' rating on what it is like to live to 100 years of age (see Fig 3.10).

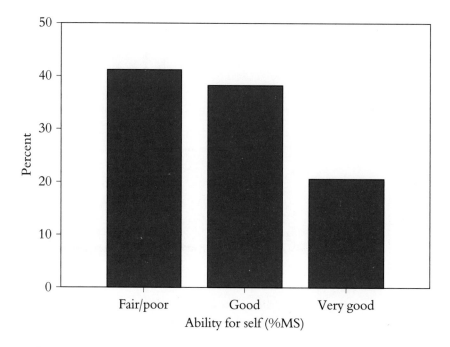

Figure 3.8

Centenarians' rating of ability to do things for themselves

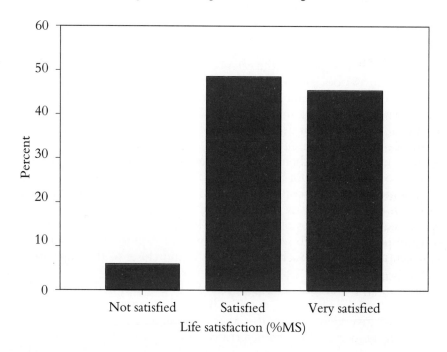

Figure 3.9

Centenarians' self-rated life satisfaction

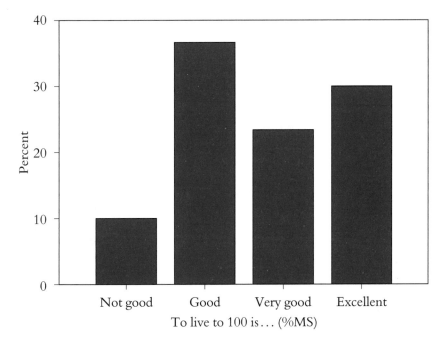

Figure 3.10

Centenarians' rating on living to 100 years

 Despite physical limitations, centenarians may still have a positive view on life.

Only 10% of the sample thought it was 'not good' to live to 100 years, while almost two-thirds thought it was 'good' or 'very good'. From interviews, there was a small group who clearly had 'had enough'. For example, two respondents said they prayed each night that God would 'take me', only to wake the next morning. Surviving to extreme age is therefore more complex than just having a will to live. This leads on to what emerged as the most significant item in these QoL domains—that of memory. As can be observed, the distribution of self-rated responses was bi-modal around either 'fair' or 'very good' (see Fig 3.11).

The %MS score for memory was the second lowest scoring item at just 50.8. A substantial 42.4% rated their memory as 'poor' or 'fair'. On the other hand, 30% rated their memory as 'very good', and 12% as 'excellent'. This latter finding is quite interesting because it emphasises the now clear position that not everybody who lives to very old age will develop dementia or similar symptoms. However, the finding here may be overstated because some respondents commented in addition to the rating that their long-term memory was excellent. This could mean their short-term memory is deficient and that they in fact may be experiencing some degree of memory loss. Further

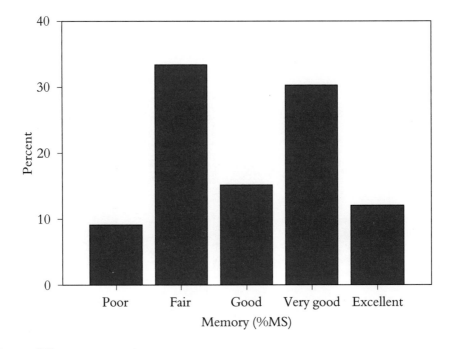

Figure 3.11

Centenarians' self-rated memory

specification of long- and short-term memory in the questionnaire is required for future sampling.

> **A substantial 42.4% rated their memory as 'poor' or 'fair'. On the other hand, 30% rated their memory as 'very good', and 12% as 'excellent'.**

When looking for associations between the items, memory stood out as the only item with significant correlations with most other variables, as shown in Table 3.7.

Age was found to be negatively correlated with memory ($r = -0.11$), which accords with prevalence studies showing that the risk of dementia increases with age. However, memory was significantly associated with all other items except life satisfaction. It seems the perception that self-memory is good is associated with the perception that one's health, social relationships, ability to do things and how one feels about living to 100 years of age are more likely to be positively rated. If one can't remember their life, or does not know how old they are now, then this difficulty in rating could carry across to other QoL domains. On the other hand, in a non-agitated mood, people with memory loss can appear quite content. This may be part of the explanation as to why overall life satisfaction has little relationship with memory.

Table 3.7

Significant bivariate associations with self-rated memory

VARIABLE	SPEARMAN'S RHO (n = 32)	CONFIDENCE INTERVALS[#]	SIGNIFICANCE
Self-rated health	0.37	0.01–0.65	$p < 5\%$
Life satisfaction	0.19	–0.19–0.51	$p > 5\%$
Social relationships	0.39	0.04–0.64	$p < 5\%$
Self-ability to act	0.45	0.04–0.76	$p < 5\%$
Living to 100 is	0.56	0.31–0.76	$p < 5\%$

[#]Bootstrap $n = 5000$

CONCLUSION

This chapter has reported some findings on people who are living to very old ages and raised the issue that this group may well increase substantially in the future, redefining the term 'old age' to mean people in their 10th decade of life and beyond. In Laslett's (1989) taxonomy they are people who chronologically would fit into his fourth and final age of life. However, they appear to be living on, with some being reasonably content with their lot. They are not necessarily all in the frail and decrepit state Laslett imagined, with their status falling across a continuum of longer experiences of chronic ailments through to a compression of morbidity where illness is delayed to the end of life (Fries 2005). This emerging group may be showing us a more heterogeneous 'fifth age' where, through either evolutionary or engineered longevity, people can go on with a life that adapts to the gains and losses of ageing. Health professionals will need to be more cognisant of this heterogeneity and potential for life extension to ensure appropriate treatment is offered to all people.

In more detail, this exploratory research has investigated the important QoL concept in a small sample of highly selected centenarian respondents. As expected, the study found that overall self-rated health ranged from fair to good. Low scoring on ability to do things for oneself accords with the health problems most experience at this extreme age. Social relations were reported as being good and living to 100 years was generally seen as positive. However, memory was found to vary considerably among this group and seems to interact with most other dimensions of QoL. As predicted by the differential ageing perspective, it seems there are different subgroups among the centenarians whose health status and so on varies—good for some, not for others. The sample group as a whole appeared to score lower on most QoL domains than the general population. However, inconsistent with disengagement theory, the data suggest that for most centenarians whose memory is intact, QoL is fairly good. These people are, after all, remarkable survivors.

This demographic group is projected to increase rapidly in size in all industrialised societies and it is important that we have a better understanding of their health, sociodemographics and QoL at this age. Such an understanding will have important implications for developing appropriate health and social interventions at this and earlier ages, and can highlight valuable lessons about adding life to years rather than just years to life.

Reflective questions

1. What is the impact of living to 100-plus years on memory?
2. How do centenarians rate their quality of life? Why do you think this may be?
3. If you think about the probable age of their 'children', what impact may this have on community care?

Acknowledgment: The author specifically thanks and acknowledges the participants' and their significant others' informed consent and willing participation in this study. Also, Resthaven Retirement Homes in South Australia for their ongoing support and research assistance.

References

Administration on Aging, 1996. Estimates and projections of the older population 1990–2050. Online. Available: www.aoa.gov, 10 Sept 2003.

Andersen-Ranberg, K., Schrol, M., Jeune, B., 2001. Healthy centenarians do not exist, but autonomous centenarians do. Journal of the American Geriatrics Society 49 (7), 900–908.

Australian Bureau of Statistics, 1996. Census of population and housing Australia 1996, Cat No 2015.0. Commonwealth of Australia, Canberra.

Australian Bureau of Statistics, 2001. Year book Australia, Cat No 1301.0, various 1911–2001. Commonwealth of Australia, Canberra.

Australian Bureau of Statistics, 2002. Census of population and housing Australia 2001, Cat No 2015.0. Commonwealth of Australia, Canberra.

Australian Bureau of Statistics, 2003. Australian social trends, Cat No 4102.0. Commonwealth of Australia, Canberra.

Australian Bureau of Statistics, 2006. Census of population and housing Australia 2006, Cat No 2015.0. Commonwealth of Australia, Canberra.

Baltes, M., 1996. The many faces of dependency in old age. Cambridge University Press, Cambridge.

Baltes, P., Smith, J., 2003. New frontiers in the future of aging, Monograph. Max Planck Institute for Human Development, Germany.

Beard Belle, B., 1991. Centenarians: the new generation. Greenwood Press, Connecticut.

Birren, J., Bengston, V., 1988. Emergent theories of ageing. New York, Springer.

Booth, H., 2003. The future aged: new projections of Australia's elderly population. Australasian Journal on Ageing 22 (4), 196–202.

Booth, H., Tickle, L., 2004. Beyond three score years and ten. People and Place 12 (1), 15–26.

Cumming, E., Henry, W., 1961. Growing old: the process of disengagement. Basic Books, New York.

Fries, J., 2005. The compression of morbidity. The Milbank Quarterly 83 (4), 801–823.

Kannisto, V., 1994, Development of oldest-old mortality, 1950–1990, Monographs on Population Aging 1. Odense University Press, Odense.

Laslett, P., 1989. A fresh map of life. Cambridge University Press, London.

Maher, E., Cummins, R., 2001. Subjective quality of life, perceived control and dispositional optimism among older people. Australasian Journal on Ageing 20 (3), 139–146.

McCormack, J., 2000. Hitting a century: centenarians in Australia. Australasian Journal on Ageing 19 (2), 64–69.

McCormack, J., 2002. Acute hospitals and older people in Australia. Ageing and Society 21 (6), 23–27.

Medserve, 1998. Medical news. Online. Available: www.medserv.dk 18 Jan 2013

Ministry of Health, Labor and Welfare, 2003. Japan Times. Online. Available: www.japantimes.co.jp, 10 Sept 2003.

Moody, H., 1998. Aging: Concepts and controversies. Sage, California.

Neugarten, B., 1969. Continuities and discontinuities of psychological issues in adult life. Human Development 12, 121–130.

Perls, T., Bochenk, K., Freeman, M., et al., 1999. Validity of reported age and centenarian prevalence in New England. Age and Ageing 28 (2), 193–197.

Perls, T., Silver, M.H., 1999. Living to 100. Basic Books, New York.

Poon, L. (Ed.), 2006. The Georgia centenarian study. The International Journal of Aging and Human Development Special Issue 34, 1–17. Online. Available: http://www.publichealth.uga.edu/geron/research/centenarian-study, 31 Jan 2013.

Rowe, J., Kahn, R., 1987. Human aging: usual and successful. Science 237, 143–149.

Ruisdael, C., 2003. Centenarian Survey, Supercentenarian Interest Group. Online. Available: www.grg.org, 31 Jan 2013.

Sachdev, P., 2012. The Sydney centenarian study. Online. Available: http://www.med.unsw.edu.au/psychweb.nsf/page/brainage_centenarian, 18 Jan 2013.

Thatcher, D., 1999. The demography of centenarians in England and Wales. Office of National Statistics, UK.

United Nations, 2006. Population ageing UN publication, Sales No. E.06.X111.2

United Nations, 2010. World population ageing 1950–2050 UN publication. Online. Available: www.un.org, 31 Jan 2013.

Vaupel, J., Oeppen, J., 2002. Broken limits to life expectancy. Science 296, 1029–1031.

Wilkinson, T., Sainsbury, R.A., 1998. Census-based comparison of centenarians in New Zealand with those in the United States. Journal of the American Geriatric Society 46, 488–491.

CHAPTER 4

AGEING IN RURAL AREAS

Angela Greenway-Crombie, Peter Disler and
Guinever Threlkeld

Editors' comments

*Issues surrounding ageing in rural areas need to be urgently addressed. The authors
of this chapter suggest that the need to define what exactly is 'rural' would be a good
start. A change in healthcare planning is required so that equitable services to older
people living in areas that do not support specialist skills or have access to diagnostic
equipment can be provided. The added issue of culturally and linguistically diverse
people who live in rural areas contributes to the difficulty of providing services for
small groups. Preventive healthcare and monitoring the impact of chronic disease is
an issue mostly due to a lack of interdisciplinary teamwork and case management.
Attracting general practitioners and allied health professionals to rural areas has long
been a problem in Australia. There have been many programs that offer incentives
for these practitioners to work away from metropolitan areas, but these programs
do not seem to provide long-term commitment. The vignette provided highlights the
real problem of ageing in rural areas and the need for innovative ways to remain
independent at home.*

INTRODUCTION

Australia's population is ageing and this trend will continue into the foreseeable
future. Advances in medicine, living conditions and health literacy all
contribute to increased longevity, with the decreasing birthrate also impacting
on population ageing (Atterton 2008). The Australian population is projected
to increase by about 30% over the next 20 years; however, the number of
people aged 65 years or older is expected to rise by 90% and the number aged
85 years or older is anticipated to more than double in that time (Australian
Institute of Health and Welfare (AIHW) 2011). This population ageing has
significant implications for aged care service planning as 49% of Australians
aged 65–74 have five or more long-term health conditions, increasing to 70%
of those aged 85 and older (AIHW 2012a).

In Australia, like other developed countries, the population is growing older faster in rural areas than in metropolitan centres, with approximately 35% of Australians aged 65 and older living outside major cities (National Rural Health Alliance 2009). There remains an inequity in the health of rural populations compared with their metropolitan counterparts, with higher levels of disease risk factors and illness in people living in rural and remote areas than those in major cities (AIHW 2010, Humphreys & Gregory 2012). The ageing population presents a range of challenges for the health and aged care system, particularly in rural areas where workforce shortages, lack of access to specialist services and the sheer tyranny of distance are confounding factors.

Rural populations and service providers have a tradition of innovation in response to necessity, and indeed there are many initiatives currently underway that can add to our knowledge of how to best deliver care to older people in rural areas and to assist them to manage their ageing and their health in a positive way. Unfortunately many of these initiatives are not reported in the scholarly literature and healthcare professionals entering practice in the rural environment must brush up their investigative skills and learn to search the grey literature for reports and evaluations. Developing a network with colleagues in other rural settings is also a key to keeping abreast of innovation.

A recent article by Humphreys and Gregory (2012) provides a review of major rural health policies and programs in Australia and explores their progress in improving rural health outcomes over the past decade. The review suggests that positive progress has been achieved in acknowledging the need for interdisciplinary coordination of care to 'deal with the increased burden of chronic disease characterising an ageing rural population' (Humphreys & Gregory 2012 p 159). *The National Primary Health Care Strategy* and establishment of Medicare Locals, designed to create local networks of organisations to better coordinate the delivery of primary care services, hold promise. The review also indicates improvement in the provision of education and training to rural health professionals and in extended scope of practice initiatives; however, it identifies a number of barriers that continue to impede progress towards equitable health outcomes for all Australians. These ongoing barriers have key impacts on rural health resources, workforce and services and include: relationships between the Commonwealth and state governments; existing funding arrangements; siloed and metro-centric perceptions; and political expediency.

 Although some progress has been made to improve rural health over the past decade, we still have a long way to go to achieve equitable health outcomes for all Australians.

Providing interdisciplinary care for older people in rural areas has inherent difficulties. To start with, there is no internationally agreed definition of what exactly constitutes 'rural'! (Rygh & Hjortdahl 2007). This lack of universal definition reflects a wider debate about the characteristics that distinguish the rural context and which of these are most crucial in influencing outcomes for the rural population (Farmer et al 2012). The geographical approach seems to be the most commonly applied means of determining rurality and emphasises the relationship with major infrastructure and services, whereby a location is defined in relation to distance from major centres. The definition of a major centre, however, can also be debated when it comes to identifying the infrastructure essential to meet the needs of the surrounding population. There is also the sociological approach in determining rurality, which emphasises the differences between metropolitan and non-metropolitan contexts, underscoring the impact of socioeconomic, behavioural, attitudinal and perceptual characteristics of a defined area on access to services (University of Ballarat 2004).

In July 2011 Australia's official statistical geography classification changed. The Australian Bureau of Statistics (ABS) replaced the Australian Standard Geographical Classification (ASGC) with the Australian Statistical Geography Standard (ASGS). The ASGS reportedly defines more stable, consistent and meaningful areas than the ASGC and is now the essential reference for understanding and interpreting ABS spatial statistics. Old regions such as Census Collection Districts, Statistical Local Areas and Statistical Divisions have been replaced by the new Statistical Areas Levels 1 to 4 (SA1s–SA4s) and Greater Capital City Statistical Areas (ABS 2012).

There is no internationally agreed definition of what exactly constitutes 'rural'. In Australia the Australian Statistical Geography Standard is the official classification structure to determine rurality.

Official definitions take into account population density and distance to larger service centres; however, there is currently no classification of distance from the various health services that different population groups may require. We do know that the elderly population are not a homogenous cohort and that all people need a variety of services according to their specific and unique issues. It is not possible to describe every different need and initiative to address them, nor is it reasonable to make assumptions about what every older rural person will want access to in their community. This chapter therefore provides an overview and update of some of the main practice issues and innovations involved in delivering interdisciplinary healthcare to older people in rural Australia, using the term 'rural' to encompass all regional and remote settings.

RURAL DEMOGRAPHY

Approximately one-third of Australians live outside major cities and more than one-third of the rural population are aged 65 years and older. The proportion of the population who are Indigenous increases with remoteness, from 1% in major cities to 45% in very remote areas (AIHW 2012b). The ageing of the rural population is due to the national phenomenon of decreased fertility and additionally to the rural phenomena of the out-migration of youth and young adults and the in-migration of sea- and tree-changers. This pattern results in

20% of Australians living in communities with declining population (Larson 2011). Service development is especially challenging in the context of declining communities.

The care of older people entails much more than attention to health needs; however, health and health services are commonly of increasing significance in this period of life. The patterns of health and health services characteristic of rural Australia are different from those found in metropolitan areas and an understanding of these differences is important for those working with older people in rural communities and developing services to meet their needs. The further people live away from major cities, the less healthy they are likely to be with higher rates of morbidity and mortality.

The AIHW (2012c) cites coronary heart disease, other circulatory diseases, motor vehicle accidents and chronic obstructive pulmonary disease (such as emphysema) as the main contributors to higher death rates in regional and remote areas. There are clear differences in health service usage between rural and metropolitan areas, with lower rates of some hospital surgical procedures and general practitioner (GP) consultation, and generally higher rates of hospital admission in rural areas than in major cities. Health risk factors are also greater in rural areas, with rural people more likely than their major city counterparts to smoke and drink alcohol in harmful or hazardous quantities. The rural environment also plays a part in higher death rates, with more physically dangerous occupations and factors associated with driving (e.g. long distances, greater speed, isolation, animals on roads and so on) contributing to elevated accident rates and related injury death in country areas (AIHW 2012c).

The ageing of the Australian population is most pronounced in non-metropolitan areas, with this trend predicted to strengthen in coming years.

The older Indigenous population, like the older Australian population in general, has been growing at approximately 4% per year. The difference in life expectancy of Indigenous Australians compared with non-Indigenous Australians of course impacts on the definition of the term 'older'. Indigenous people aged 45 years and older are classified as the older population, whereas for the non-Indigenous population 'older' is over 75 years of age. This factor may contribute to the younger age profile of community aged care clients in remote and very remote communities (AIHW 2012d).

Recent initiatives focused on closing the gap between life expectancy of Indigenous and non-Indigenous Australians may see the rate of growth of the older Indigenous population increase further in future. Future planning of aged care services, particularly in remote and very remote areas, needs to take this increase into account as additional and culturally appropriate services will be required (AIHW 2011). Service planning will need to recognise the differing health profile of Indigenous Australians, such as higher rates of diabetes and younger age onset of chronic disease, and services will need to respond to this different pattern of health needs. A challenge will be to increase the numbers of

Indigenous people in the aged care workforce, including workers who are fluent in Indigenous languages (AIHW 2011).

Indigenous Australians are more likely to live in remote and very remote areas. The different pattern of health needs of the older Indigenous population will influence both the aged care services and workforce required in these areas to provide culturally appropriate care.

The population of rural communities is culturally and linguistically diverse (CALD). The concentration of post-war immigrants in major cities means that the representation of individual CALD groups in rural communities is often relatively small (Green 2001), posing the challenge of providing culturally appropriate services to small numbers. Patterns of settlement of some more recent immigrant groups have been more geographically dispersed (Hugo 2002), indicating that the cultural and linguistic diversity of those ageing in rural communities will increase.

Baby boomers are contributing to the sea/tree change and the ageing of our rural populations will be influenced by this movement (Ryan 2007). While the 'sea-change' and more recently the 'tree-change' movement of metropolitan dwellers has been motivated by a perception of more peaceful and fulfilling lifestyles in idyllic coastal and bush settings, the reality is that worldwide rural dwellers have poorer physical health status and tend to die younger than their urban counterparts (Allan et al 2008). Competing commitments to individualism and social activism have been observed as characteristic of this generation (Huber & Skidmore 2003, Olsberg & Winters 2005), although how these attitudes will shape expectations of health and aged care services as they move through the retirement decades is uncertain. Clearly this group will challenge existing assumptions about rural stoicism and become an influence for change in rural service planning and provision. The changing tone and role of the rural political voice and the widening of the rural political agenda were evident in 2010 during the formation of the Gillard minority government, and may be indicative of increasingly assertive advocacy from rural communities in future (Brett 2011).

Rural aged care services must be responsive to this demographic context, and to the differing needs characteristic of diverse rural communities. Older people in rural communities who are long-time residents of the country experience the cumulative effects of health disadvantage across the life course, which may intersect with other forms of rural, social and economic disadvantage (Beard et al 2009). Reliance on informal care, often provided by family members, has been shown to mask some of the care needs of older rural residents and to increase isolation from wider social networks (Winterton & Warburton 2011). And the care needs of those whose family live at a distance may be overlooked in communities where there is a strong expectation of informal care provided through family networks. International and local literature has identified the importance of place to older rural residents, both in maintaining identity (Winterton & Warburton 2012) and as a site of care (Bevan 2001, Castleden et al 2010). The desire to have control over end-of-life care and to die at home is a significant concern of older Australians (COTA 2012) and creates particular demands for the rural service system.

ACCESS TO HEALTH SERVICES

The rural/metropolitan differences in access to healthcare services are reflected in figures reported by Moates (2005) that show despite 30% of Australians living in 'the bush' they make up only 20% of Medicare rebates supplied by only 15% of the total medical workforce in Australia. This inequity is compounded by rural dwellers also having much lower private health insurance coverage than their urban counterparts, effectively directing more government funding to major cities rather than rural areas despite the greater need in the bush (Moates 2005).

A 2007 AIHW report (p 7) states:

> *Those who live away from Major Cities and for whom access to health services is restricted may be disadvantaged because of different access to:*
> * *preventive services such as immunisation and information allowing healthy life choices;*
> * *health management and monitoring;*
> * *specialist surgery and medical care;*
> * *emergency care, for example ambulance;*
> * *rehabilitation service after medical or surgical intervention;*
> * *aged care services.*

Older people living in rural areas need and deserve access to all of these services and limited access to any one of these can increase the need for others.

Access to palliative care and ancillary services such as transport, respite, aids and carer support is not only more limited in rural and regional areas but the actual scope of locally available services is often less comprehensive than those available in urban areas (Inder et al 2012, National Rural Health Alliance 2009).

Access to health and ancillary services is restricted in rural areas and the scope of services provided is less comprehensive than those in urban areas.

A range of factors can have a negative impact on service access in rural areas and these will vary for different groups and individuals within different communities (Davis & Bartlett 2008). Some of these factors are explored below.

Tyranny of distance and cost

Sheer distance can be a large barrier to accessing services in rural Australia, whether this is for an older person travelling hours for general and specialist healthcare or for a personal care attendant travelling out to a rural property three times a week to assist with showering and personal care tasks. Providing both general and specialist medical services, and indeed most community and aged care services in rural areas, is hampered by distance and lack of a population base with a critical mass to justify local service provision. Tyranny of distance is compounded by the financial burden of both travel and the cost of accessing services. Add to these costs the emotional and physical burden often placed on older people and their carers and you start to calculate the enormity of the issue for rural older people.

Transport issues

There is minimal public transport infrastructure in most rural areas of Australia. Where public transport is available it may not actually help rural older people to access services due to timetabling, routes and expense (National Rural Health Alliance 2005). Davis and Bartlett (2008) point out that public transport arrangements in many rural areas are often ad hoc and community and volunteer transport services are not well coordinated, 'often failing to meet the real needs of older people' (p 58).

Economic forces

Local and global economic forces affect both the experiences of older people and the availability of services in rural Australia. Many small rural towns have suffered from drought and the impacts of economic slowdown, losing much of their community infrastructure such as post offices, pharmacies and banks (Davis & Bartlett 2008; Horton et al 2010). Climate change and the pattern of increasing frequency of major weather events have an economic impact and bring new health issues for older people and challenge service requirements, including in the area of emergency management of older people in rural communities. These rural towns also continue to lose both aged and community care services because of increased costs of goods and services (mainly due to transport costs) and no critical population mass to benefit from economies of scale. The increased cost of operating an aged care facility in rural areas and the smaller number of people who require the service makes them commercially unviable (National Rural Health Alliance 2009).

Rural stoicism

Country people have a reputation as being tough and resilient. Studies have shown that rural dwellers tend to have different health beliefs and values with high levels of stoicism and fatalism often leading to delayed presentation and diagnosis and resulting in poorer prognosis and survival (Howatt et al 2006). Rural older people tend to use health services less often and delay seeking healthcare, which may be due to stoicism and hardiness; however, this may also be through necessity because the services aren't readily accessible (Davis & Bartlett 2008). There is some evidence this stoicism is changing, at least at the political level, and rural older people may not be so accepting of service inequalities in future.

> **A range of factors impact on access to services by older people in rural Australia, including local and global economic forces.**

ACCESS ISSUES IN REMOTE AUSTRALIA

While the population profile and demography of remote areas varies between communities, remote areas generally have slower population growth, more children but fewer young adults and fewer older people than in metropolitan areas. Access to resources tends to decrease with remoteness and the affordability and availability of commodities such as food and petrol is often significantly less in remote Australia. In particular, remote areas are less likely to have access to basic food items such as fruit and vegetables (Services for Australian Rural and Remote Allied Health (SARRAH) 2013a).

Australians living in rural and remote communities have less access to health services and to health and allied health professionals (AHPs) than those living in metropolitan areas. For example, access to GPs in remote areas is 45–67% of the level of access enjoyed by those in metropolitan areas (Health Workforce Australia (HWA) 2013). Remote communities are characterised by limited local healthcare services, limited private health services and an absence of specialist services. Workforce shortages and high staff turnover negatively impact on service access. Remote populations are also widely dispersed; significant travelling distances and limited and costly transport options further compound access to services (SARRAH 2013b).

Initiatives such as outreach services, primary healthcare and telehealth are seeking to address some of the challenges in accessing health services in remote communities, particularly for older people.

PROFESSIONAL PRACTICE IN THE RURAL CONTEXT

A study examining pharmacist and social worker perceptions of their 'fit' within rural communities highlighted 'access to care, local context and individual, personal and professional issues as factors that impinge on healthcare service provision' (Allan et al 2008 p 7).

Aptly entitled *You have to face your mistakes in the street: the contextual keys that shape health service access and health workers' experiences in rural areas*, the study (Allan et al 2008) reminds us that the traditional disease model of healthcare service provision fails to include the variety of social, individual, subgroup and population group factors that affect the health environment and subsequent status of the whole of Australia.

Rural health professionals face their patients in the street on a regular basis. Rural communities pride themselves on community cohesiveness and engagement. Imagine providing often distressing diagnoses and knowing the most intimate of details about a person, being responsible for the management of these, and running into them at the supermarket, post office, a sporting event or other public forum! Worse still, imagine running into their sons, daughters, spouse or other significant person in their life who want you to bring them 'up to date with what's happening' with their loved one while you're in the middle of aisle 5 at the local supermarket or during interval at the school play!

Establishing relationships and gaining the trust of rural older people is the first challenge for rural health professionals; maintaining it in a community where everyone already seems to know what is happening with everyone else before it even happens is almost impossible. Even when that relationship is clearly established with individuals, it is difficult to maintain the professional–personal balance.

A sense of belonging is essential to emotional wellbeing. Being on call 24/7 to address the health and care needs of a community may evoke feelings of worth and belonging but the ability to sustain this lifestyle is restricted. Many rural health professionals never really 'knock off'. Personal experience and discussion with other regional and rural health professionals identifies that if you live in or near a town small enough for people to know who you are and that you are a health professional, you will be contacted in times of need—no matter what day or time that need occurs.

A sense of belonging is essential to emotional wellbeing.

Enmeshed in the rural community, health and aged care practitioners easily become isolated from their professional communities. It can be a struggle to build or maintain supportive professional relationships; few systems are in place to ensure access to supervision and professional development, and higher education is frequently beyond reach or too difficult to accommodate with workload (Blue 2002, Department of Health and Ageing 2008, Green & Lonne 2005).

In this context, it is not surprising to find that family relationships may become strained (Lonne & Cheers 2001), with evidence of the significant impact of partners' and children's experiences on decisions to leave rural and remote practice (Chenay et al 2003, Veitch & Crossland 2005).

Opportunities for specialisation are limited and the expectations on generalist practitioners are substantial. The scarcity of various professions involved in health and aged care across regional and remote settings creates opportunities for interdisciplinary and multidisciplinary care. If high-quality care is to be provided in this setting respect between professions is crucial, with little room for excessive vigilance in boundary maintenance between the professions, and the sharing of skills and knowledge across the professions essential. Interpersonal and inter-organisational skills must be exemplary if the thin spread of services and personnel across large distances is to effectively meet the needs of those ageing in our rural communities (Lonne & Darracott 2006, Munn 2003).

RURAL HEALTH WORKFORCE SHORTAGES IMPACTING ON INTERDISCIPLINARY CARE OF OLDER PEOPLE

A substantial challenge in providing equitable access to people living in regional and remote areas is that, unlike major cities, non-metropolitan populations are dispersed and clustered. Towns exactly the right size to support one, two or three doctors, nurses and allied health workers are very rare—more usually they would support a fraction of a health worker or, for example, more than one but less than two. In these situations, a single worker may practise in one town and also service one or more others. Either way, someone has to travel, with routine and emergency access potentially compromised and/ or the health worker spending substantial amounts of time travelling rather than consulting with patients.

(AIHW 2003 p 4)

Anyone working in health or aged care in rural settings will attest to the shortage of key health professionals and to the difficulty in recruiting and retaining staff, yet reliable data about the rural workforce is scarce. The *Report on the Audit of Health Workforce in Rural and Regional Australia* (Department of Health and Ageing 2008) provides the most comprehensive view to date of workforce shortages impacting on health and aged care beyond our cities. Current shortages and issues of maldistribution are anticipated to compound in the coming decade as the rural health workforce (on average nine years older than the all-industry average) ages, reduces work hours and retires (Community Services and Health Industry Skills Council submission to Productivity Commission 2005). Calls to extend the working lives of baby boomers may be significant for addressing rural workforce shortages (CEDA 2009). An emerging pattern of fly-in fly-out health workers for rural and remote communities addresses some problems of workforce shortages but may create others. Both these strategies to address rural workforce issues are currently the subject of research. The geographic distribution of public and private services also has a negative impact on the rural health workforce. Private services dwindle with increasing distance from major cities, and as private services become more scarce so do the many professions whose members have a preference for private practice.

NURSING

Representing approximately half the total health workforce nationally, and more often employed in the public sector than any other group in that workforce (Department of Health and Ageing 2008 p 17), nurses form the backbone of the rural health and aged care services. The distribution of nurses is a little more even than that of GPs; however, state comparisons undertaken for the recent workforce audit highlight significantly lower numbers in inner regional areas of Western Australia and South Australia, remote areas of Queensland, and outer regional and remote Tasmania (Department of Health and Ageing 2008). Nurses specialising in aged care are in short supply.

Shortfalls in the nursing workforce are forecast to continue and will have a disproportionate impact on regional, rural and remote areas that currently rely on the nurse, who may be the sole health professional in the community, to provide a broad range of services (HWA 2012a).

MEDICAL

The rural medical workforce is key to maintaining the health and wellbeing of older people living in rural areas and driving their input into interdisciplinary care is critical. While the optimal ratio of GPs to population has yet to be established, there is widespread agreement that there is a rural medical workforce shortage in Australia (Department of Health and Ageing 2008, May et al 2007). Aided by effective campaigning from the medical profession, this area of workforce shortage has received great public and government attention. In 1998 the shortage was so critical that the rural workforce agencies (RWAs) were established in all states and the Northern Territory (White et al 2007). The initial purpose of the RWAs was to 'promote and facilitate the supply, recruitment, retention, education, support and better distribution of GPs in rural and remote areas' (White et al 2007 p 2). We are yet to see evidence of any impact on the health of the rural older population.

In March 2012 HWA released the *Health Workforce 2025* report, which provides an analysis of the future supply of the Australian health workforce in a range of scenarios. The report predicts that the current distribution of GPs will remain inequitable between rural and urban populations and notes that poor distribution doesn't necessarily mean poor supply. The report states that 'there is little purpose in having an adequate aggregate workforce supply unless it is distributed beyond metropolitan Australia' (HWA 2012a p 157).

Shifting the medical workforce away from cities is indeed challenging. One of very few studies that focus on GP perceptions of initiatives to improve recruitment and retention of the rural medical workforce is a study by Jones et al (2004). They reported increased Medicare remuneration and better access to after-hours and on-call arrangements as essential to recruiting and retaining GPs outside cities (Jones et al 2004 p 5). More recently recruitment and retention of rural GPs has been linked to: poor infrastructure, resources and supervision; increasing work pressures; limited clinical training capacity; and the trend towards sub-specialisation (Department of Health and Ageing 2008 p 38). Medical specialists report that rural recruitment and retention is adversely affected by limited training places, professional isolation, and a population too dispersed to support specialist service infrastructure (Department of Health and Ageing 2008 p 39).

  Better remuneration for Medicare consultations and improved access to after-hours and on-call arrangements were ranked as the most important interventions for both attracting and retaining rural GPs.

ALLIED HEALTH

Data about the allied health workforce is difficult to isolate, in part because definitions of this group vary widely. According to the AIHW (2012a), AHPs form approximately 17% of Australia's health workforce with availability of these services decreasing in line with distance from major metropolitan centres. The underrepresentation of AHPs in rural areas is seen even in professions that have an adequate supply of qualified workers, such as pharmacy, with the Pharmaceutical Society of Australia reporting that 72% of pharmacists are located in major cities (Senate Community Affairs Committee 2012). The Australian Psychological Society estimates that approximately 79.5% of psychologists work in metropolitan and major regional centres and the Australian Dental Association has identified that the number of dentists is over three times higher for major cities compared with remote areas (Senate Community Affairs Committee 2012). Salary differences between geographical areas and between the public and private sector deter dentists from non-metropolitan practice and this discrepancy in remuneration may also affect other professions (Department of Health and Ageing 2008).

There is also some evidence of high rates of allied health staff turnover in regional and remote settings. For instance, research with social workers has identified workers in rural settings experience higher levels of stress and lower levels of job satisfaction than their metropolitan peers. Scant preparation for rural practice in undergraduate courses and poor employer support in adjusting to rural practice often provide the backdrop to such an experience of stress (Lonne & Cheers 2004a, 2004b).

 There is evidence of high rates of allied health staff turnover in regional and remote settings.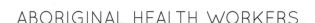

ABORIGINAL HEALTH WORKERS

Census 2006 data indicates that the one area where numbers don't actually decrease with increased remoteness is Aboriginal health workers, with it reporting that 'the number of Aboriginal and Torres Strait Islander health workers increases from 1 per 100,000 in the major cities, to 50 per 100,000 in remote areas and 190 per 100,000 in very remote areas of Australia' (Senate Community Affairs Committee 2012 p 14). Despite these numbers there remains an issue of undersupply in remote areas as the majority of Indigenous people, particularly older Indigenous people, live in remote locations.

Aboriginal health workers have usually lived in the community in which they work and have developed lasting relationships with the community and with the various government agencies (Mitchell & Hussey 2006). They are usually based in Aboriginal community-controlled health services and offer a broad range of primary healthcare services including immunisations, screening, referrals, community health education and patient transport. Aboriginal health workers who have completed the Certificate Level III in Aboriginal and Torres Strait Islander health are eligible to provide services under the Medicare CDM items (Allied Health Professions Australia (AHPA) 2013). Increasing access to Aboriginal health workers in remote communities would be of great benefit to older Indigenous Australians.

EDUCATING THE RURAL HEALTH WORKFORCE

To help address some of the rural health workforce shortage issues a range of strategies have been introduced focusing on attracting rural students to the study of medicine, nursing and allied health, and providing undergraduate experience in rural settings. These include locating university courses in regional settings (Chater 2008).

Rural clinical schools have been established for a number of disciplines such as medicine, nursing and physiotherapy, with particularly significant investment in this strategy for addressing medical shortages in rural areas. The premise behind these clinical schools is that students who are trained in rural and regional areas are more likely to practise in rural and regional areas. Referred to as the 'rural pipeline' strategy (Murray & Wronski 2006), the pipeline consists of recruiting students from rural backgrounds, providing education in rural settings, emphasising rural issues in curriculum, providing rural clinical experience and articulating rural postgraduate training pathways. The success of these approaches in increasing the representation of non-metropolitan students in undergraduate courses is clear (Chater 2008 p 315), but there is not yet evidence of the ultimate success of this strategy in attracting medical graduates to settle in rural areas. Recent research shows evidence that the combination of a student selection policy that favours students from rural areas and high-quality rural clinical experience is strongly linked to undergraduate medical students' intention to practise rurally (Walker et al 2012). We will wait to see if this intention translates into action. The increasing collocation of health undergraduates in rural clinical schools will enhance shared allocation and distribution of a range of multidisciplinary training facilities and resources, and will increase a shared understanding of each discipline and provide the environment in which effective models of interdisciplinary healthcare to the rural elderly can be developed.

Rural clinical schools have been established for a number of disciplines such as medicine, nursing and physiotherapy.

Clinical placement shortages confront education providers in all the health and allied health disciplines. Through the *National Partnership Agreement on Hospital and Health Workforce Reform 2008*, government initiatives such as the HWA Clinical Training Funding (CTF) program have been introduced to help address the identified health workforce issues. In 2010, HWA pledged $425 million to support more than 1.7 million additional clinical placement training days for medicine, nursing and AHPs over a three-year period.

Increasing the number of students undertaking clinical training placements in rural areas, and providing them with a positive learning experience while undertaking their clinical training, is essential to the future recruitment and retention of a skilled workforce in rural and regional health and aged care services. The quality of this experience is pivotal, as poor rural clinical placement experience has been found to be a deterrent to entry to rural practice (Walker et al 2012).

Rural organisations experience a number of barriers and challenges in providing clinical training placements. Individually, these organisations do not have the critical mass of staffing or students of their urban counterparts, and subsequently they have limited resources to support growth in student numbers and placement days. Three of the main barriers to clinical training placement growth in the majority of rural organisations include: lack of student accommodation; lack of clinical training learning space (e.g. tutorial rooms); and lack of appropriately skilled and qualified clinical training supervisors, teachers and tutors. HWA CTF funds are being used to support clinical supervision, student accommodation, fitting out of training spaces and purchasing essential training equipment, addressing the main barriers faced by rural organisations (HWA 2011a).

Other HWA initiatives aimed at increasing the capacity and skills of the health workforce, and that are particularly relevant in rural areas, include the Clinical Supervision and Support Program, which aims to expand clinical supervision capacity and competency (HWA 2011b) and the Simulated Learning Environments Program, which is increasing access to simulated learning techniques for students in regional, rural and remote settings (HWA 2011c). The use of simulated learning allows the rural health workforce to experience the full range of healthcare encounters across the spectrum, from healthy ageing in the community, to care of deteriorating older patients in an acute setting.

The Rural Health Education Foundation (RHEF), established in 1992, is a non-profit organisation 'dedicated to delivering free health education to healthcare teams in remote and rural Australia and their communities' (RHEF 2012). RHEF provides its programs through a range of formats considered most appropriate for access by rural health professionals, including digital satellite technology, the internet (with live webcasting), DVDs and other television services. The programs feature interactive presentations from medical, nursing and AHPs who are leaders in their field and the panels usually include at least one rural health professional. RHEF estimates that its satellite network reaches more than 90% of rural doctors and other health professionals.

For rural health professionals, reducing the travel and time impost in accessing contemporary continuing professional development opportunities is most welcome. Videoconferencing is becoming increasingly popular as a vehicle for rural health education, with university and other education providers now using videoconferencing as part of their curriculum for rural students, and specialist services and/or organisations utilising videoconferencing to provide education sessions aimed at upskilling rural GPs and health professionals.

The advantages for rural health professionals in accessing education through online or e-learning are also now being realised. Rural health professionals can undertake e-learning opportunities at a time that suits them, with a program that suits them and in a place that suits them. Many e-learning modules are also free. The flexibility of e-learning is also attractive from a provider perspective both in reaching the maximum target audience and reducing costs of providing traditional modes of education in rural areas. The changing expectations of learners in a modern internet-connected society is a key driver for e-learning and advances in technology have increased interactivity through multimedia production, making e-learning modules more appealing to both verbal and visual learners.

INITIATIVES SUPPORTING INTERDISCIPLINARY CARE FOR OLDER PEOPLE IN RURAL AREAS

TELEHEALTH AND TELEMEDICINE

Advances in information communications technology (ICT) are making inroads into the provision of health services to people living in rural and remote Australia. Telemedicine is defined as 'the use of information and communications technology to provide healthcare services to individuals who are some distance from the healthcare provider. Telehealth is defined more broadly and includes administration and training in addition to clinical services' (Moffatt & Eley 2010 p 276). Although not a new concept, with nurses and other health workers in remote areas having relied on radio and telephone support since the early 1900s, improvements in telecommunication networks across rural Australia over the past decade has certainly enhanced its uptake (Ellis 2004).

From 1 July 2011 Medicare Benefit Schedule (MBS) items were introduced to enable online video consultation with a specialist including:
- medical practitioners (including GPs, specialists or consultant physicians)
- midwives
- nurse practitioners
- practice nurses and Aboriginal health workers on behalf of a medical practitioner and under the clinical supervision of the medical practitioner.

These MBS incentives have seen 19,698 telehealth services provided to 10,301 patients by more than 3098 practitioners as at the end of May 2012. Approximately 23% of these services were provided in major cities, with the majority provided in regional Australia (approximately 69%) and around 8% in remote Australia. GPs/nurse practitioners/midwives provided the most services (7138) followed by consultant physicians (6660) (Department of Health and Ageing 2012a).

From 1 November 2012 the MBS telehealth items were amended to require the patient and specialist to be at least 15 km apart, except residents in aged care facilities or patients of an Aboriginal medical service. This change was announced in the 2012–13 federal budget to ensure that 'funding is targeted at patients for whom distance is a genuine barrier to accessing specialist care' (Department of Health and Ageing 2012b).

Videoconferencing is probably the most common and simple form of telehealth and has a multitude of uses from a metropolitan psychiatrist 'seeing' a patient with mental health issues in a remote location and being able to monitor their body language, mood and other signs that complement diagnosis, to case conferencing with multiple care providers in a variety of rural, metropolitan and international locations, to 'providing psychosocial support and training to groups of isolated carers' (Van Ast & Larson 2007 p 1).

Reported benefits of telehealth and telemedicine for rural patients include reduced travel and cost burden, improved access to locally provided specialist service, and improved quality of existing clinical services (Moffat & Eley 2010). Moffat and Eley (2010) also identified direct benefits to rural health professionals including local access to continuing professional development activities, ability to provide an enhanced local service and indirect benefits through experiential learning from close contact with specialists and a perception of reduced isolation.

Telehealth has led to innovations in the way that many clinical services can now be offered to rural communities.

Remote monitoring is another innovative means of harnessing telehealth technologies to capture and transmit important health information to relevant health professionals. Devices and sensors that monitor vital signs 'combined with either the internet or other broadband carrier systems have enabled physiological parameters such as blood pressure and ECG to be monitored and transmitted automatically to hospitals' (Meade & Dunbar 2004 p 2). This technology is becoming increasingly accurate, simple, unobtrusive and cost-effective, making it an attractive option in under-resourced rural and remote areas. Recording and sending clinical information from a patient living in a rural town to a health professional in a regional or metropolitan centre allows them to assess and manage that person's health status without the patient or professional needing to travel long distances, given the associated travel, accommodation and time costs involved. However, caution is needed to ensure the gains in access that can be offered through telehealth do not jeopardise the appropriateness of services by neglecting the context of remotely situated service recipients (Lonne & Durracott 2006).

Improvements in telecommunications infrastructure, ICT support and training, combined with its cost-effectiveness and variety of ways it can be utilised, makes telehealth an effective vehicle to provide interdisciplinary care to older people in rural and remote areas. The full potential of telehealth is still under exploration. However, it is essential that initiatives be examined at a national level to ensure those rural and remote populations living near state and territory borders are not disadvantaged by incompatible systems and regulations that currently influence models of cross-border healthcare (Webber 2005). The current embryonic stage of telehealth in Australia means that the legal issues involved in its use across states and jurisdictions have not been fully tested (Australian Nursing and Midwifery Council (ANMC) 2007).

NATIONAL REGISTRATION AND ACCREDITATION FOR HEALTH PROFESSIONALS

The National Registration and Accreditation Scheme (NRAS) for health practitioners commenced on 1 July 2010. The NRAS was established by state and territory governments through the introduction of consistent legislation in all jurisdictions. The Australian Health Practitioner Regulation Agency (AHPRA) administers the NRAS and professions currently regulated under the NRAS include:
- Aboriginal and Torres Strait Islander health practice
- Chinese medicine
- chiropractic
- dental practice
- medical radiation practice
- medicine
- nursing and midwifery
- occupational therapy
- optometry
- osteopathy
- pharmacy
- physiotherapy
- podiatry
- psychology.

There is potential for national telehealth and other interdisciplinary care initiatives in rural areas to be enhanced through this national system. Many cross-border issues in providing interdisciplinary care to older adults can be addressed if the government also reflects this national recognition in allowing not only professionals but also services to work across geographic borders.

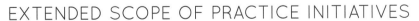

National registration and accreditation for health professionals may address some of the cross-border issues in providing interdisciplinary care to older adults.

EXTENDED SCOPE OF PRACTICE INITIATIVES

Face-to-face access to the full spectrum of health professionals in rural areas is decreasing in reality and in community expectations. The ageing of the Australian population is reflected in the ageing of our health workforce. According to a study by Kilpatrick et al (2007) 38% of health and community services workers in Australia are aged 45 years or older. The high percentage of the health workforce close to retirement age and the ageing of the general population has provoked an array of initiatives aimed at up-skilling 'paraprofessionals', with rural and remote areas in particular becoming 'home to a set of innovative service delivery models such as up-skilling therapy assistants to work across several areas, as well as a range of community-based solutions' (Kilpatrick et al 2007 p 3).

The rural health workforce shortage has seen the development of a range of advanced practice roles to help combat the overall lack of traditionally trained health professionals. Workforce redesign initiatives that increase the efficiency and effectiveness of the available workforce and improve workforce distribution, particularly in under-resourced rural areas, are critical to a sustainable health service system.

Although relatively new in Australia, nurse practitioners (NPs) have been providing healthcare in other countries such as the United States since the 1960s. In Australia the first two NPs were endorsed in rural New South Wales in 2000 (Australian College of Nurse Practitioners 2012). Although uptake of the NP role in Australia has been relatively slow, attributed in part to the lack of access by NPs to the Pharmaceutical Benefits Scheme (PBS) and the MBS until 2009 (Driscoll et al 2012), as of September 2011 there were 595 authorised NPs nationally, and many more working towards endorsement, although the exact number is not known (Department of Health 2011). The potential value of the NP role in rural settings is recognised, however, barriers do exist. Some of the barriers in developing and implementing NP roles in rural areas include access to tertiary education, creating a sustainable number of NP positions and financial cooperation from community and acute providers (Haines & Critchley 2009).

The potential value of the NP role in rural settings is recognised; however, barriers exist and include access to tertiary education, creating a sustainable number of NP positions and financial cooperation from community and acute providers.

NPs are performing a range of activities historically in the sole domain of medical practitioners such as prescribing medications and ordering a range of diagnostic testing within established guidelines including achieving academic and clinical competency. Other nurses, particularly those in rural and remote areas, may work at an advanced practice level that is often not recognised. Unlike registered nurses or NPs 'advanced practice nursing has no national recognition or agreed role definition' (Cant et al 2011 p 180). CRANA*plus*, founded by remote area nurses from across Australia, describes remote health professionals as specialist practitioners who undertake appropriate educational preparation for their practice, which is to provide and/or coordinate a diverse range of healthcare services for remote communities (CRANA*plus* 2012). There is, however, no specific national registration through AHPRA for remote area nursing.

Workforce redesign initiatives that increase the efficiency and effectiveness of the available workforce and improve workforce distribution, particularly in under-resourced rural areas, are critical to a sustainable health service system.

The responsibilities of enrolled nurses (ENs) have also expanded with the introduction of medication-endorsed ENs. Undertaking appropriate study enables ENs to administer a range of medications by most routes (including intravenous). This extended scope of practice is particularly relevant to rural aged care where staffing a residential aged care facility with the appropriate skill mix can be a substantial challenge.

Introducing extended scope of practice or advanced practice roles often evokes concern from health professionals who may be affected by the changes. Some of these concerns are valid, whereas other concerns seem to be based more on the human tendency to resist change. Adopting the expanded role of ENs has not been uniform across all health services and indeed there is evidence that individual wards and units within individual health services differ in the extent to which they allow their ENs to practise within their legal scope (Eagar et al 2010).

Eagar et al (2010) also purport that the introduction of unregulated and unqualified care workers such as assistants in nursing (AIN) and patient care attendants (PCAs) further complicates the nursing scope of practice issue in Australia. Some employers view unregulated workers as a more cost-effective option to registered nurses and this may have impacts on quality of care, particularly in rural aged care, which already struggles with the high costs of service provision associated with rurality.

AHPs are also in short supply, particularly in rural areas of Australia. This shortage of AHPs has led to developing an allied health assistant (AHA) workforce (Moore 2011). AHAs undertake Allied Health Assistant Certificate IV training and can focus on various skill sets such as occupational therapy, physiotherapy and community rehabilitation. Of course, supervision and ongoing assessment of competency can be challenging in rural areas where AHPs are not available to provide appropriate supervision. Initiatives such as remote supervision models are being investigated as a way to support the rural AHA workforce.

Research into developments in the paramedic role hold promise for rural communities. A rural expanded scope of practice model has been proposed based on research into existing innovation in rural paramedic practice (Mulholland et al 2009, O'Meara et al 2012). Critical elements of this model include: enhanced rural community engagement; emergency response; situated practice in either institutional or out-of hospital settings; and recognition of involvement in primary care as a first point of contact when people have a health problem. Such a model expands paramedic involvement across the cycle of care and extends sites of practice to include the community and the hospital.

The potential role of physician assistants (PAs) is also being considered to augment and extend services traditionally provided by GPs and physicians. In the American health system, PAs are an established provider of medical services, with the role developed more than 50 years ago. The Netherlands, South Africa and some Canadian provinces have recently introduced the PA role as a licensed profession and other countries including England, Scotland, New Zealand and Australia have trialled US-trained PAs in a range of health services (HWA 2012b).

The Australian College of Rural and Remote Medicine (ACRRM) supports the introduction of the PA role in Australia and suggests that the introduction of PAs would assist rural GPs to continue to provide medical leadership and support in a flexible way within their traditional team-based healthcare approach. 'The National Rural Health Alliance (NRHA) and ACRRM believe there is an urgent need for PAs in rural and remote Australia to support the GP primary care and GP proceduralist workforce' (HWA 2012c p 12).

Traditional health professional roles are changing to meet the changing demands of our population. 'An ageing of our population and a reduced socioeconomic base have altered healthcare needs in rural areas. Rural communities now require health services involving a more diverse range of promotive, preventive, chronic and social care' (Mahnken 2001 p 1).

The growth of telehealth initiatives in interdisciplinary models of care for older people in rural areas suggests the future rural health workforce will be required to have an advanced level of telecommunications skills in their advanced practice repertoire!

LIVING LONGER AND LIVING BETTER IN THE BUSH

In 2012 the Australian Government released its Living Longer Living Better aged care reform package. The package provides $3.7 billion over five years allocated to:

- helping people stay at home
- helping carers access respite and support
- delivering better residential aged care
- strengthening the aged care workforce
- supporting consumers and research
- ensuring better health connections
- tackling the nation's dementia epidemic
- supporting older Australians from diverse backgrounds
- building a system for the future.

The reforms acknowledge that, in general, it is more expensive to deliver aged care services in regional, rural and remote Australia than in urban areas. In response the government provides a viability supplement to eligible providers on top of other funding. In January 2010 the government increased the viability supplement by over 40% in recognition of the higher costs faced by rural aged care providers. 'As a result of the aged care reform package, the government is projected to provide more than $280 million in viability supplements to aged care providers over the next five years' (Commonwealth of Australia 2012 p 12).

The package also recognises that aged care facilities in regional, rural and remote areas also face higher building costs than those in urban areas. The government will combine its current aged care capital grants programs into a single 'Rural, Regional and Other Special Needs Building Fund', with around $51 million available for the fund each year (Commonwealth of Australia 2012).

In total, the aged care reform package component aimed at ensuring the sustainability of aged care services in regional, rural and remote areas of Australia totals approximately $108 million. Reflecting on the multitude of complex issues facing rural older people, we can only hope that the government reforms really will enable older Australians to live longer and to live better in the bush.

Vignette

Innovations in interdisciplinary models are 'driving' the care of rural older people

A major issue in rural areas is driving. Fifty-five percent of deaths on Victorian roads in 2012 were in country areas and there is a growing trend in the number of older drivers losing their lives on Victorian roads (Transport Accident Commission 2013). Moreover, mortality data only partly reflect the situation as the disabling effects of non-fatal injury may have profound effects on the injured person; on a global level the World Health Organization estimates that 1.2 million people die annually as a result of road accidents and a further 50 million people are disabled thereby (Ameratunga et al 2006).

Much has been written about the effect that cognitive impairment has on the ability to drive safely, and it has been suggested that a driving assessment should be carried out for all people in whom dementia is diagnosed, and repeated at least twice annually (Lovell & Russell 2005). Australian research has suggested that although GPs are concerned about this problem, their knowledge about how to proceed is variable, and their approach inconsistent (Snellgrove & Hecker 2002).

To many older people, being told they have to stop driving is a highly significant event and perceived as the end of independence. In rural areas the effects may be even more profound, as public transport is poor or non-existent, and driving into town may be the only way that supplies are obtained and social or community relationships maintained. Moreover, outside metropolitan areas, there is a serious lack of skilled driving assessors (usually occupational therapists with specific training). Anecdotal experience suggests that the risk of losing their licence may dissuade many rural elderly people from seeking medical help for dementia or memory problems at all, and this is compounded by the lack of funding to subsidise driving assessments. Traditional models of driving assessment and subsequent management needs review, particularly in rural areas.

Take the case of 'Harriet'. Harriet led a full life. She retired from her profession as a well-known and respected lawyer in a small rural community some years ago. Though her partner of many years died 10 years ago, she has continued to live alone on her 25-acre block on the river, which is 15 minutes out of town, with her horses and dogs. In her retirement she has been an active member of the community, exercising her love of animals as a committed volunteer for the RSPCA and involving herself in social pastimes like playing Scrabble and Bridge.

Harriet visited her GP expressing concern at her developing inability to make words playing Scrabble, which she has always excelled at. This was followed by a series of minor, but potentially dangerous, incidents involving lapses of memory. She also fell and fractured her hip. The GP assessed Harriet as unfit to drive.

The loss of her licence had far-reaching implications for Harriet and her way of life. Harriet was adamant that she didn't want to leave her small farm or lose her animals for whom she continued to care for competently. Without her own transport *and* without any public transport, however, she became isolated and unable to continue with her usual functional activities. In fact it really became impossible for her to sustain her life, practical and social, in the country. 'Losing my licence was the beginning of the end for me,' Harriet said later. Small matters like getting bread and milk or hay for the horses became large obstacles. It was not feasible to depend on friends and neighbours to ferry her about constantly, and if anything urgent arose, she was trapped by her situation. Harriet moved into a low-level aged care home, which she perceived as her only option.

Harriet's is a common story for older people living in rural areas. If we as health professionals are committed to maintaining quality of life as well as quantity of life then new models that support people to maintain their lifestyles across their life span are essential.

Increased access to preventive healthcare measures, such as increasing GP uptake of the MBS items that include the 75+ health assessments, case conferencing, care planning and chronic disease management items and providing access to specialist services such as geriatricians and cognitive, dementia and memory services (CDAMS) clinics through new technologies such as telehealth initiatives, will help to prevent the impact of ageing on lifestyle. Early referral to Aged Care Assessment Teams (ACATs) that can perform comprehensive assessments of older people's needs and refer them to appropriate multidisciplinary professionals, such as occupational therapists who can investigate home safety requirements and physiotherapists who can provide strength training exercises, along with referral to relevant Home and Community Care (HACC) services such as personal or home care services to assist with shopping, and voluntary organisations to provide transport to social outings and assistance to feed animals etc., could have produced very different outcomes for Harriet and for many others like her.

If, as government policy suggests, we are truly committed to maintaining independence of older people and supporting them in their own homes then the traditional models of healthcare for older people in rural areas need to change. Despite the challenges that the ageing population brings, and despite the rural workforce shortages affecting all health professions, the sheer distance to travel with its associated costs and the professional practice issues inherent in rural healthcare, there are current and future innovations in the provision of interdisciplinary healthcare that are reflective of policy and that improve the quality of life for older people in rural areas of Australia. We just need to make them the 'norm'.

CONCLUSION

The ageing of our population has far-reaching impacts that will stretch the finite resources and the creativity of government, health professionals and local communities to provide the most appropriate models of care to older people. There is no greater challenge than that of meeting the diverse needs of the significantly expanding cohort of the rural elderly. Despite the problems inherent in distance and in rural lifestyle, improving interdisciplinary service provision and 'putting our money where our mouth is' in maintaining the independence of older people to live in their own homes will reap great rewards with benefit for the quality of life for both rural older people and for the often under-resourced but ingenious and dedicated health professionals who support them.

Reflective questions

1. Think of ways aged care services could be delivered to rural populations that would increase access to specialist care. How would you cost this?

2. What are some advantages of living in a rural area that would entice a healthcare professional to practise there?

3. The use of technology is improving education and clinical services for rural areas. Telehealth services are increasing, but what are the pitfalls of such technology for older people?

4. The need for flexibility in funding services is very apparent. How could a rural health program for older people be more effective if funding could be restructured?

Acknowledgment: Thank you to Sally Disler for contributing the vignette.

References

Allied Health Professions Australia (AHPA), 2013. Aboriginal health workers. Online. Available: http://www.cdm.ahpa.com.au/HealthcareProfessionals/AlliedHealthProfessionals/AboriginalHealthWorkers/tabid/148/Default.aspx, 22 Feb 2013.

Allan, J., Ball, P., Alston, M., 2008. You have to face your mistakes in the street: the contextual keys that shape health service access and health worker's experiences in rural areas. Rural and Remote Health 8, 835. Online. Available: www.rrh.org.au, 21 Mar 2008.

Ameratunga, S., Hijar, M., Norton, R., 2006. Road traffic injuries: confronting disparities to address a global health problem. The Lancet 367, 1533–1540.

Atterton, J., 2008. Demographics of the ageing rural population. Working with Older People 12 (3), 19–22.

Australian Bureau of Statistics, 2012. Population estimates and Australia's new statistical geography: the new Australian statistical geography standard. Online. Available: http://www.abs.gov.au/ausstats/abs@.nsf/Products/3218.0~2011~Main+Features~Population+estimates+and+Australia's+new+statistical+geography?OpenDocument, 15 Aug 2012.

Australian College of Nurse Practitioners, 2012. What is a nurse practitioner. Online. Available: http://www.acnp.org.au/content/what-is-a-nurse-practitioner.html, 14 Aug 2012.

Australian Institute of Health and Welfare, 2003. Rural, regional and remote health: a study on mortality. Cat. No. PHE 45. AIHW, Canberra. Online. Available: http://www.aihw.gov.au/publications/phe/rrrh-sm/rrrh-sm.pdf, 18 Mar 2008.

Australian Institute of Health and Welfare, 2007. Rural, regional and remote health: a study on mortality (2nd edition). Rural health series no.8 PHE 95. AIHW, Canberra. Online. Available: www.aihw.gov.au, 18 Mar 2008.

Australian Institute of Health and Welfare, 2010. Australia's health 2010. Australia's health series no. 12. Cat. no. AUS 122. AIHW, Canberra. Online. Available: http://www.aihw.gov.au/publication-detail/?id=6442468376&tab=2, 14 Aug 2012.

Australian Institute of Health and Welfare, 2011. Australia's welfare 2011. Australia's welfare series no. 10. Cat. no. AUS 142. AIHW, Canberra.

Australian Institute of Health and Welfare, 2012a. Australia's health 2012. Australia's health series no.13. Cat. no. AUS 156. AIHW, Canberra.

Australian Institute of Health and Welfare, 2012b. Rural health demography. Online. Available: http://www.aihw.gov.au/rural-health-demography/, 15 Aug 2012.

Australian Institute of Health and Welfare, 2012c. Impact of rurality on health status. Online. Available: http://www.aihw.gov.au/rural-health-impact-of-rurality/, 15 Aug 2012.

Australian Institute of Health and Welfare, 2012d. Aged care packages in the community 2010–11: a statistical overview. Aged care statistics series no. 37. Cat. No. AGE 69. AIHW, Canberra.

Australian Nursing and Midwifery Council, 2007. Guidelines for nurses and midwives on telehealth practice. Online. Available: http://www.anmc.org.au/docs/guidelines_and_position_statements/Guidelines%20on%20Telehealth%20Practice.pdf, May 2008.

Beard, J.R., Tomaska, N., Earnest, A., et al., 2009. Influences of socioeconomic and cultural factors on rural health. Australian Journal of Rural Health 17 (1), 10–15.

Bevan, C., 2001. An ageing society; issues and challenges. Australasian Journal on Ageing 20, 15–22.

Blue, I., 2002. Characteristics of Australian rural health care professional practice. In: Wilkinson, D., Blue, I. (Eds.), The new rural health. Oxford University Press, South Melbourne.

Brett, J., 2011. Fair share country and city in Australia. Quarterly Essay 1–67.

Cant, R., Birks, M., Porter, J., et al., 2011. Developing advanced rural nursing practice: A whole new scope of responsibility. Collegian 8 (4), 177–182.

Castleden, H., Crooks, V.A., Schurman, N., et al., 2010. It's not necessarily the distance on the map …' using place as an analytic tool to elucidate geographic issues central to rural palliative care. Health and Place 16 (2), 284–290.

CEDA, 2009. Silver lining: Keeping baby boomers at work to counter Australia's demographic deficit. Online. Available: http://ceda.com.au 24 Sep 2012.

Chater, A.B., 2008. Looking after health care in the bush. Australian Health Review 32 (2), 313–318.

Chenay, H., Campbell, S., Wilson, E., 2003. The 21st century GP: recruitment and retention: Discussion Paper, Institute for Sustainable Futures, Rural Faculty RACGP.

Commonwealth of Australia, 2012. Living Longer. Living Better. Online. Available: http://www.health.gov.au/internet/publications/publishing.nsf/Content/CA2578620005D57ACA2579E2007B9DFC/$File/D0769%20Living%20Longer%20Living%20Better%20SCREEN%20070512.pdf, 14 Aug 2012.

COTA, 2012. Summary report on the conversations on ageing. Available: https://www.cotamembership.org.au/australia/Achieving/cma.aspx, 18 Aug 2012.

CRANA*plus*, 2012. About us. Online. Available: http://www.crana.org.au/2-about-us.html, 15 Aug 2012.

Davis, S., Bartlett, H., 2008. Healthy ageing in rural Australia: issues and challenges. Australasian Journal on Ageing 27 (2), 56–60.

Department of Health, 2011. Nursing in Victoria: nurse practitioner frequently asked questions, State Government of Victoria. Online. Available http://www.health.vic.gov.au/nursing/furthering/practitioner/nurse-practitioner-frequently-asked-questions, 14 Aug 2012.

Department of Health and Ageing, 2008. Report on the audit of health workforce in rural and regional Australia, April 2008. Commonwealth of Australia, Canberra.

Department of Health and Ageing, 2012a. Telehealth statistics. Online. Available: http://www.mbsonline.gov.au/internet/mbsonline/publishing.nsf/Content/connectinghealthservices-factsheet-stats, 15 Aug 2012.

Department of Health and Ageing, 2012b. 2012–2013 Budget: changes to telehealth. Online. Available: http://www.health.gov.au/internet/mbsonline/publishing.nsf/Content/connectinghealthservices-2012-13BudgetFactsheet.htm, 15 Aug 2012.

Driscoll, A., Harvey, C., Green, A., et al., 2012. National nursing registration in Australia: a way forward for nurse practitioner endorsement. Journal of the American Academy of Nurse Practitioners 24, 143–148.

Eagar, S.C., Cowin, L.S., Gregory, L., et al., 2010. Scope of practice conflict in nursing: a new war or just the same battle? Contemporary Nurse 36 (1–2), 86–95.

Ellis, I., 2004. Is telehealth the right tool for remote communities? Improving health status in rural Australia. Contemporary Nurse 16, 3. Online. Available: http://www.contemporarynurse.com/archives/vol/16/issue/3/article/2051/is-telehealth-the-right-tool-for-remote, 18 May 2008.

Farmer, J., Munoz, S., Threlkeld, G., 2012. Theory in rural health. Australian Journal of Rural Health 20, 185–189.

Green, A., 2001. Bush politics. In: Lockie, S., Bourke, L. (Eds.), Rurality bites: the social and environmental transformation of rural Australia. Pluto Press, Sydney.

Green, R., Lonne, B., 2005. Great lifestyle, pity about the job stress: occupational stress in rural human service practice. Rural Society (doi: 10.5172/rsj.351.15.3.253.

Haines, H., Critchley, J., 2009. Developing the nurse practitioner role in a rural Australian hospital: A Delphi Study of Practice Opportunities, Barriers and Enablers. Australian Journal of Advanced Nursing 27 (1), Sept/Nov 30–36.

Health Workforce Australia (HWA), 2011a. Annual report 2010–2011. Online. Available: https://www.hwa.gov.au/sites/uploads/health-workforce-australia-annual-report-2010-2011.pdf, 15 Aug 2012.

Health Workforce Australia (HWA), 2011b. Clinical supervision and support program—Directions Paper April 2011. Online. Available: http://www.hwa.gov.au/sites/uploads/clinical-supervision-support-program-directions-paper-april-2011.pdf, 15 Aug 2012.

Health Workforce Australia (HWA), 2011c. Simulated Learning Environments Program update December 2011. Online. Available: https://www.hwa.gov.au/sites/uploads/20120215_final_update_aussett_v1.pdf, 15 Aug 2012.

Health Workforce Australia (HWA), 2012a. Health workforce 2025—doctors, nurses and midwives—Volume 1. Online. Available: https://www.hwa.gov.au/sites/uploads/health-workforce-2025-volume-1.pdf, 14 Aug 2012.

Health Workforce Australia (HWA), 2012b. The potential role of physician assistants in the Australian context Volume 2—Literature Review. Online. Available: https://www.hwa.gov.au/sites/uploads/hwa-physician-assistant-report-volume2-literature-review-20120816.pdf, 20 Aug 2012.

Health Workforce Australia (HWA), 2012c. The potential role of Physician Assistants in the Australian context—final report. Online. Available: https://www.hwa.gov.au/sites/uploads/hwa-physician-assistant-report-20120816.pdf, 20 Aug 2012.

Health Workforce Australia (HWA), 2013. Rural and remote health workforce innovation and reform strategy. Online. Available: http://www.hwa.gov.au/work-programs/workforce-innovation-and-reform/rural-and-remote-health-workforce, 22 Feb 2013.

Horton, G., Hanna, L., Kelly, B., 2010. Drought, drying and climate change: Emerging health issues for ageing Australians in rural areas. Australasian Journal on Ageing 29 (1), 2–7.

Howatt, A., Veitch, C., Cairns, W., 2006. A descriptive study comparing health attitudes of urban and rural oncology patients. Rural and Remote Health 6, 563. Online. Available: www.rrh.org.au, 14 Aug 2012.

Humphreys, J., Gregory, G., 2012. Celebrating another decade of progress in rural health: What is the current state of play? Australian Journal of Rural Health 20, 156–163.

Huber, J., Skidmore, P., 2003. The new old: why baby boomers won't be pensioned off. Demos, London. Online. Available: http://www.demos.co.uk/files/thenewold.pdf, 2 Jul 2008.

Hugo, G., 2002. Australia's changing non-metropolitan population. In: Wilkinson, D., Blue, I. (Eds.), The new rural health. Oxford University Press, South Melbourne.

Inder, K.J., Lewin, T.J., Kelly, B.J., 2012. Factors impacting on the well-being of older residents in rural communities. Perspectives in Public Health 132 (4), 182–191.

Jones, J.A., Humphreys, J.S., Adena, M.A., 2004. Rural GPs' ratings of initiatives designed to improve rural medical workforce recruitment and retention. Rural and Remote Health 4, 314. Online. Available: www.rrh.org.au 9 Mar 2008.

Kilpatrick, S.I., Johns, S.S., Millar, P., et al., 2007. Skill shortages in health: innovative solutions using vocational education and training. Rural and Remote Health 7, 623. Online. Available: www.rrh.org.au 9 Mar 2008.

Larson, A., 2011. Doing more for fewer: health care for declining rural communities' Ch 13. In: Luck, G.W. et al. (Eds.), Demographic change in Australia's rural landscapes, 307 Landscape Series 12, doi10.1007/978-90-481-9654-8_13.

Lonne, B., Cheers, B., 2001. Adjusting to rural practice: a national study. Paper presented to Australian Association of Social Workers National Conference. Melbourne, Victoria, 23–26 September.

Lonne, B., Cheers, B., 2004a. Practitioners speak: a balanced account of rural practice, recruitment and retention. Rural Social Work 9, 244–254.

Lonne, B., Cheers, B., 2004b. Retaining rural workers: an Australian study. Rural Society 14 (2), 163–177.

Lonne, B., Darracott, R., 2006. Rual and remote communities. In: Chui, W.H., Wilson, J. (Eds.), Social work and human services best practice. The Federation Press, Sydney.

Lovell, R.K., Russell, K.L., 2005. Developing referral and reassessment criteria for drivers with dementia. Australian Occupational Therapy Journal 52, 26–33.

Mahnken, J.E., 2001. Rural nursing and health care reforms: building a social model of health. Rural and Remote Health Online. Available: http://www.rrh.org.au/publishedarticles/article_print_104.pdf, 21 Mar 2008.

May, J., Jones, P.D., Cooper, R.J., et al., 2007. GP perceptions of workforce shortages in a rural setting. Rural and Remote Health 7, 720. Online. Available: www.rrh.org.au, 21 Mar 2008.

Meade, B.J., Dunbar, J.A., 2004. A virtual clinic: telemetric assessment and monitoring for rural and remote areas. Rural and Remote Health 4, 296. Online. Available: www.rrh.org.au, 21 Mar 2008.

Mitchell, M., Hussey, L., 2006. The Aboriginal health worker. Medical Journal of Australia 184 (10), 529–530.

Moates, A., 2005. The rural urban health divide. Chisholm Health Ethics Bulletin 11 (1), 4–7. Online. Available: http://search.informit.com.au/search;action=doSearch, 18 May 2008.

Moffat, J.J., Eley, D.S., 2010. The reported benefits of telehealth for rural Australians. Australian Health Review 34, 276–281.

Moore, S., 2011. Allied Health Assistants: A new wave of health workers. Australian Polity 2, 1. Online. Available http://australianpolity.com/australian-polity/allied-health-assistants-a-new-wave-of-health-workers, 15 Aug 2012.

Mulholland, P., O'Meara, P., Walker, J., et al., 2009. Multidisciplinary practice in action: the rural paramedic—it's not only lights and sirens. Journal of Emergency Primary Health Care 7 (2), Article 6.

Munn, P., 2003. Factors affecting service coordination in rural South Australia. Australian Social Work 56 (4), 305–317.

Murray, R.B., Wronski, I., 2006. When the tide goes out: health workforce in rural, remote and Indigenous communities. Medical Journal of Australia 185 (1), 37–38.

National Rural Health Alliance, 2005. Older people and aged care in rural, regional and remote Australia: national policy position. Online. Available: http://www.agedcare.org.au/what-we-do/policies-and-position/policies-pdfs/Rural_remote_policy05.pdf, 14 Aug 2012.

National Rural Health Alliance, 2009. Ageing in rural, regional and remote Australia. Fact Sheet 3. Online. Available http://nrha.ruralhealth.org.au/cms/uploads/factsheets/fact-sheet-03-ageing.pdf, 14 Aug 2012.

Olsberg, D., Winters, M., 2005. Ageing in place: intergenerational and intrafamilial housing transfers and shifts in later life: Australian Housing and Urban Research Institute. Online. Available:http://www.ahuri.edu.au/publications/p70223/, 2 Jul 2008.

O'Meara, P.F., Tourle, V., Stirling, C., et al., 2012. Extending the paramedic role in rural Australia: a story of flexibility and innovation. Rural and Remote Health 12, 1978. Online. Available: http://www.rrh.org.au, 20 Sep 2012.

Productivity Commission, 2005. Australia's health workforce. Position paper. Productivity Commission, Canberra.

Rural Health Education Foundation, 2012. About us. Online. Available: http://www.rhef.com.au/about-us/, 14 Aug 2012.

Ryan, K., 2007. Palliative care for an ageing population: a rural based model? Or 'For whom the bell tolls'. PhD Thesis. Online. Available: http://wallaby.vu.edu.au/adt-VVUT/uploads/approved/adt-VVUT20070517.162333/public/01front.pdf, 29 Apr 2008.

Rygh, E.M., Hjortdahl, P., 2007. Continuous and integrated health care services in rural areas. A literature study. Rural and Remote Health 7, 766. Online. Available: www.rrh.org.au, 18 Mar 2008.

Services for Australian Rural and Remote Allied Health (SARRAH), 2013a. Demography and population. Online. Available: http://www.sarrahtraining.com.au/site/index.cfm?display=143626, 22 Feb 2013.

Services for Australian Rural and Remote Allied Health (SARRAH), 2013b. Online. Available: http://www.sarrahtraining.com.au/site/index.cfm?display=143624, 22 Feb 2013.

Senate Community Affairs Committee, 2012. The factors affecting the supply of health services and medical professionals in rural areas. August 2012. Commonwealth of Australia. Online. Available: http://www.aph.gov.au/Parliamentary_Business/Committees/Senate_Committees?url=clac_ctte/rur_hlth/report/index.htm, 15 Aug 2012.

Snellgrove, C.A., Hecker, J.R., 2002. Driving and dementia: general practitioner attitudes, knowledge and self-reported clinical practices in South Australia. Australasian Journal On Ageing 4, 210–212.

Transport Accident Commission, 2013. Police announce final 2012 road toll. Online. Available: http://www.tac.vic.gov.au/media-room/media-releases/media-release-items/police-announce-final-2012-road-toll2, 1 May 2013.

University of Ballarat, 2004. Defining the focus on 'rural' and 'regional' research. Position Paper No.1. Regional Research Framework. Online. Available: http://www.ballarat.edu.au/ard/research/irrr/docs/1DefinitionsofRuralandRegional.doc, May 2008.

Van Ast, P., Larson, A., 2007. Supporting rural carers through telehealth. Rural and Remote Health 7, 623. Online. Available: www.rrh.org.au, 18 Mar 2008.

Veitch, C., Crossland, L.J., 2005. Medical family support needs and experiences in rural Queensland. The International Electronic Journal of Rural and Remote Health 5 (4), 467.

Walker, J.H., DeWitt, D.E., Pallant, J.F., et al., 2012. Rural origin plus a rural clinical school placement is a significant predictor of medical students' intentions to practice rurally: a multi-university study. Rural and Remote Health 12, 1908. Online. Available: http://www.rrh.org.au, 4 Sep 2012.

Webber, K.M., 2005. General practice hospital integration in rural and remote Australia: summary of findings. Australian Rural Health Education Network. Online. Available: http://www.arhen.org.au/docs/gphi-irra-summary.pdf, 21 May 2008.

White, C.D., Willett, K., Mitchell, C., et al., 2007. Making a difference: education and training retains and supports rural and remote doctors in Queensland. Rural and Remote Health 7, 700. Online. Available: www.rrh.org.au, 21 May 2008.

Winterton, R., Warburton, J., 2011. Models of care for socially isolated older rural carers: barriers and implications. Rural and Remote Health 11, 1678. Online. Available: http://www.rrh.org.au, 4 Sep 2012.

Winterton, R., Warburton, J., 2012. Ageing in the bush: The role of rural places in maintaining identity for long term rural residents and retirement migrants in north-east Victoria, Australia. Journal of Rural Studies 28 (4), 329–337.

CHAPTER 5

YOUNGER PEOPLE IN RESIDENTIAL AGED CARE FACILITIES

Sally Garratt and Anne Kelly

Editors' comments

This chapter examines the issues surrounding the admission of younger people to residential aged care facilities. The number of younger people with a disability is growing, largely due to accidents and illnesses that have now got improved medication and treatments to prolong life, and improved care systems in the community. Accommodation services are not keeping up with service provision needs and specialist housing is limited (Kirby 2012). Aged care facilities are often the only place to obtain 24-hour care with some nursing skill base to manage clinical issues. The lifestyle that younger people wish to continue becomes difficult as lack of staff time and poor environments impact on achieving satisfactory outcomes. People who have younger onset dementia form a different cohort to younger people with physical disabilities. A mix of generations with complex care needs can work if there is commitment to address person-centred care and the resources made available to provide it.

Sally can be seen and heard in Session 2 of Evolve.

INTRODUCTION

Traditionally, residential aged care facilities (RACFs) in Australia cater for the over 65-year age group and entry into a service is governed by the Aged Care Assessment Service (ACAS) (2012). The number of people who are surviving longer with chronic illnesses such as multiple sclerosis or motor neuron disease (MND) is increasing, as is the number with an acquired brain injury (ABI) from accidents that leave younger people with lifelong disability (Kirby 2012). Younger people with an ABI are often kept in hospital or rehabilitation units longer than optimal because they have no other options for assisted living.

They are admitted to an RACF as a default option because there is no other place that can provide the complex care they need.

The problems that arise over mixing generations in such care facilities are complex and often require more skill than the current staff mix of an RACF can provide. Skilled nursing care and rehabilitation programs are difficult to organise on RACF budgets and environments are often not conducive to the lifestyle of a younger person.[1]

THE CURRENT SITUATION

The Young People in Nursing Homes National Alliance (www.ypinh.org.au) was formed to lobby for more age-appropriate care for young people with a disability. The statistics they produce are updated each year and for 30 June 2010 are outlined in Table 5.1.

The number of beds occupied by younger people with a disability in RACFs was 6456 in 2010. This number is likely to increase unless more appropriate housing is developed (Young People in Nursing Homes National Alliance 2012). (Note: The Young People in Nursing Homes Alliance is now Young People In Residential Aged Care or YPIRAC.)

The Commonwealth Government Senate Community Affairs Committee in 2005 enquired into quality and equity in aged care (Senate Community Affairs Committee 2005). They established that there was a need to improve the capacity of the current system to meet the needs of younger people with a disability. In February 2006 the Council of Australian Governments (COAG) agreed on an initiative—the Younger People with disability in Residential Aged Care (YPIRAC)—which had three main objectives (AIHW 2012):

- to move younger people with a disability living in an RACF into appropriate supported disability accommodation where it can be made available, and if that is the person's choice
- to divert younger people with a disability who are at risk of admission to an RACF into more appropriate forms of accommodation
- to enhance the delivery of specialist disability services to those younger people with a disability who choose to remain in an RACF or for whom an RACF remains the only available and suitable supported accommodation option.

The YPIRAC program has assisted by moving younger people to more appropriate accommodation and providing enhanced services (such as targeted community support and access) within RACFs. The funding for this program ended on 30 June 2011. Victoria has continued the initiative in developing the My Future My Choice program. This program is for people under 50 years of age and is targeting the same objectives as the YPIRAC program. Evaluation of this project by the Summer Foundation and Monash University found the project had made significant differences in the lives of younger people with a disability (Summer Foundation 2011). Although the project reduced or

....
[1]This chapter does not discuss the particular issues of people with an intellectual disability.

Table 5.1

Number of young people in nursing homes, by state

STATE/AGE	0–9	10–19	20–29	30–39	40–49	50–59	60–64	UNDER 65
NSW	0	0	16	49	239	959	1100	2363
Vic.	0	0	12	21	112	634	749	1528
Qld	0	0	X	26	102	509	628	1285
SA	0	0	X	9	42	201	221	473
WA	0	0	X	X	47	201	283	531
Tas.	0	0	0	X	13	54	94	161
NT	0	0	0	X	6	15	29	50
ACT	0	0	0	X	X	28	37	65
Australia	**0**	**0**	**28**	**105**	**561**	**2601**	**3161**	**6456**

X denotes cells that contain small cell numbers (1–5), which makes individuals potentially identifiable. The figures do not separate younger onset dementia as this is considered to be aged care.

Source: Young People in Nursing Homes National Alliance 2012

changed admission to RACFs there is still a need for changes to community housing options and service provision. If this does not occur there will still be an estimated 200 people under aged 50 admitted to RACFs each year in Australia (Winkler 2007).

 The YPIRAC program has assisted by moving younger people to more appropriate accommodation and providing enhanced services.

At the time of writing the Commonwealth Government is advising state governments to put funding into a disability insurance scheme that will provide extra funding for care of people who have a disability (www.nds.org.au). There is disagreement over the level of contribution from the states and territories to establish this scheme; however, levels of funding from each state and territory government and the Commonwealth by way of an additional 0.5% levy on Medicare payments from the community seemed to have been agreed upon and the National Disability Insurance Scheme Bill received Royal Assent on 28 March 2013. It has now become law. Finalisation of the details and costings may not be completed until 2015.

The need for accommodation for those who have a disability has been recognised by governments at both the state and the federal levels, but understanding the complexity of care and the costs of providing the skill base required for quality outcomes is yet to be made evident.

Examples of ill-health states/diseases that cause disability in younger people include:

- ABI from accidents
- brain injury from neurological surgery to remove tumours
- genetic problems (e.g. Down syndrome) that parents have previously managed but now cannot as life expectancy of these people has increased and parents are ageing
- multiple sclerosis (MS) and MND
- severe forms of arthritis or lupus
- younger onset vascular accidents (stroke)
- younger onset dementia.

While all of the above create special needs the most common is rehabilitation to reduce the impact of the injury or disease and lessen or at least slow the physical and mental deterioration.

ADMISSION TO AN RACF

All admissions to residential aged care services come through aged care assessment services/teams (ACAS/Ts). Cross-program collaboration is necessary between the ACAS and the Victorian government's Disability Services program. The *Disability Services Aged Care Assessment Program Operational Guidelines* (Department of Human Services 2009 p 4) state that:

> *In assessing whether younger people with disabilities should enter aged care residential facilities … delegates should be aware of the Commonwealth's view that residential*

aged care facilities focusing on the needs of aged people rarely, if ever, enhance the quality of life or offer the least restrictive accommodation option for younger people with disabilities. Entry to the type of care should have been approved only after all other care alternatives have been demonstrably exhausted.

The *Disability Act 2006* (Part 1) defines disability and the target group for disability services as:

(a) A sensory, physical or neurological impairment, or an acquired brain injury, or any combination thereof that:
  (i) is, or is likely to be, permanent; and
  (ii) causes a substantially reduced capacity in at least one of the areas of self-care, self-management, mobility or communication; and
  (iii) requires significant ongoing or long-term episodic support; and
  (iv) is not related to ageing; or
(b) an intellectual disability; or
(c) a developmental delay ...

This definition excludes people with a primary psychiatric disability. However, where a person with a disability has a co-existing, but not primary, psychiatric disability and may require care in an RACF, Disability Services and ACAS will invoke the principles and processes of this protocol (ACAS 2009 p 5).

Because disability services mainly target those people younger than 50 years of age and dementia is associated widely with old age, younger people with dementia often fall through the gap (Alzheimer's Australia 2012). There are major differences between younger people with motor disability or an ABI and a person who has younger onset dementia. Dementia is considered to be an aged care problem and those people who are younger than 50 and require residential care have no option but to enter RACFs.

Because disability services mainly target those people younger than 50 years of age and dementia is associated widely with old age, younger people with dementia often fall through the gap.

FUNDING

Lack of choice in living arrangements means the options for a younger person's lifestyle to continue as they wish are considerably reduced. There are limited supported residential houses or facilities and family care at home often requires more support than is available. RACFs operate on budgets established by government assessment procedures essentially focused on caring for older people through the Aged Care Funding Instrument (ACFI). The amount of funding assumed for each resident does not cater for managing complicated rehabilitation programs and the extra resources that a young person is likely to require.

REHABILITATION

Extensive physiotherapy is required to move limbs and reduce contractures in younger people who have strokes, MND, multiple sclerosis or other diseases that impede mobility. A person who has an ABI has special needs to relearn speech, swallowing and communication and staff need to be able to understand specific disability-related behaviours. Activities designed for older people may not suit the level of mental and/or physical action that rehabilitation of younger people requires. Deterioration of muscle function, compromised/lack of bladder and bowel control and immobility, development of pressure sores and contractures are important for any age group, but younger people usually have a longer life span with their disability and associated problems resulting from inadequate or inappropriate care.

Initially rehabilitation after an ABI, for example, is focused on returning cognitive, sensory-perceptual and motor skills with strategies implemented as soon as possible after the injury. Passive therapy may be commenced even if the person is unconscious. Once a program of rehabilitation has begun it must be continued for as long as the person requires it. This means staff of RACFs need to know the reason for a special program, how to do it, how to assess issues that may arise and outcomes that occur (Carr & Shepherd 2002).

Assessment becomes the key indicator of the progress or otherwise of the therapy being given. Continuing assessment by physiotherapists should be instigated and staff taught the correct techniques to follow on a daily basis. The ongoing cost of therapists is built into the funding for RACFs for older people but does not account for the special and extensive needs of younger people with a disability.

Without an approach that focuses on rehabilitation and independence increased disability is easily achieved. Of great concern, however, is increased disability that can develop very quickly after admission into residential care. It arises when staff perform tasks for a person that they are able to do themselves. Independence can very quickly turn to dependence. Continuing assessment should identify failing skills and enable development of strategies to maintain independence as long as possible. Meaningful activities need to be seen as clinical interventions for health, self-esteem, a sense of worth and value (Hoeman 2002).

Of great concern, however, is increased disability that can develop very quickly after admission into residential care. It arises when staff perform tasks for a person that they are able to do themselves.

BUILDING DESIGN

Most RACFs have single bedrooms and appropriate bathrooms that will accommodate wheelchairs. The space required for larger or motorised wheelchairs or scooters is not always readily available, nor is the ability to recharge batteries from power sources easily accommodated. Motorised wheelchairs and scooters require undercover housing, with power supply points within easy access of the person using them. Only newer, purpose-built facilities have considered building this requirement into their homes.

Having motorised wheelchairs or scooters also presents problems when there are frail older people walking through corridors or in lounge/recreational spaces that are not designed to accommodate such vehicles. Parking motorised vehicles or large extended wheelchairs in corridors also presents an occupational health and safety issue for both residents and staff. The authors have had experience with these issues and they are not easily resolved within current RACFs.

Designing dementia-friendly environments is discussed in Chapter 21 so will not be covered here.

FREEDOM OF CHOICE

The ability to choose lifestyle patterns such as mealtimes, bathing schedules, outings, inviting friends for coffee, music and the use of technology can be difficult for any resident of an aged care facility. Routinised daily activity that suits the facility's staffing patterns and work schedules constrain the choices available. For example, the choice of bathing in the morning or at night may simply not be an option because of a limited number of staff rostered for that shift. While meals can be heated in microwaves for later dining in some facilities this does affect the flavour. Excluding care staff from the kitchen, or family providing food for occupational health and safety reasons, further reduces flexibility and choice. There have been instances reported where food brought into a facility could not be stored in the kitchen refrigerator in case it was 'tainted'. Alcohol may not be permitted in some facilities or is monitored closely through 'happy hours' usually conducted weekly. The ability to manage self-directed medication as required may also cause concern for younger people who, prior to admission, have been able to administer their own pain relief or other drugs as needed. Lack of control over one's life, whatever the age, can lead to unhappiness and is a precursor for depression (beyondblue 2012).

> **Lack of control over one's life, whatever the age, can lead to unhappiness and is a precursor for depression.**

RISK TAKING

For younger people who still wish to maintain outside interests that might contain an element of risk, residential aged care service providers need to accept freedom of choice that may entail some risk taking and encourage any activity that brings pleasure. Decisions about maintaining outside activities remains the domain of the person and their family based on their ability to cope. It is not the role or the right of organisations to make such decisions unless there is a demonstrable threat to a duty of care.

More flexible approaches, guidelines and protocols are required if residential aged care services are to deliver the creative, innovative and responsive care that younger people need. It is a challenge to an industry that is focused on the care and support of older people.

LEISURE AND LIFESTYLE

Younger people have a need for interaction with other people of their own age group who share the same or similar interests. Generally this means going outside the facility for communal socialisation. Arrangements to attend concerts, restaurants, sporting events or to experience community participation in support groups are usually undertaken by other organisations or family members and, for younger people without good family support, the difficulty in accessing community events is even more pronounced. Often younger people have no contact with external events at all (Summer Foundation 2007).

> **Younger people have a need for interaction with other people of their own age group who share the same or similar interests.**

UNDERSTANDING BEHAVIOUR

The conditions that result in younger people living in RACFs may also leave a person with a compromised immune system and increased incidents of infection. This can mean a level of hospitalisation unusual for the age cohort. In addition, when younger people live in aged care facilities for a period of time they are likely to encounter more frailty and death because of the age of other residents than is 'normal' experience for their age. This can become an issue when relationships are formed with an older person and then the older person dies. This disenfranchised grief (Doka 2002) is often not recognised or supported. While death is part of the life trajectory in aged care it is more common.

Depression is a common symptom following loss of abilities, and life plans are drastically changed. For younger people in RACFs this is profound and the incidence of major depression higher. Major or clinical depression is when the symptoms are affecting how the person copes and these symptoms are not changed by any non-pharmacological interventions such as attempts to alter the environment or counselling. Such depression needs formal psychiatric assessment and treatment (Fann et al. 2009).

Frustration and anger are understandable and emotional liability is often present. The swings in mood are difficult for staff to understand and endeavouring to 'cheer the person up' does not help. Often anger is directed at the closest family member or a staff member.

The behavioural changes that occur in people who have dementia can be hard for a younger person with an ABI, MS or MND who is also living in the RACF to understand. Wandering into another's personal space, being unable to communicate verbally, taking objects belonging to another and demonstrating a lack of concern over another's abilities can profoundly and adversely affect another resident's quality of life.

Verbal abuse should not be tolerated from any resident without some intervention. Screaming and inappropriate language can be deterred by careful assessment of any unmet need and interventions to address these gaps or behaviour management techniques such as leaving the room, making it clear that such behaviour will not be listened to, setting clear rules of tolerance and using strategies such as time out in a space by themselves. Because of a lack of insight by the person with the disability into the cause of their behaviour it may be difficult to change and/or for the person to realise it intimidates older residents in an RACF. Neuropsychological assessment and advice or referral to a primary care assessment and treatment team (PCAT) will assist staff to understand the causes of various behaviours and develop an evidence-based care plan.

Neuropsychological assessment and advice or referral to a primary care assessment and treatment team will assist staff to understand the causes of various behaviours and develop an evidence-based care plan.

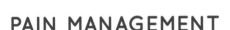

PAIN MANAGEMENT

Muscular degeneration and nerve involvement, spasticity, cognitive diseases and motor diseases (e.g. arthritis) can cause considerable pain on moving a limb or trying to communicate (Shumway-Cook & Woollacott 2001). Assessing pain usually relies on the ability of the person to verbalise discomfort and, for people who cannot verbally self-report, staff need to be able to astutely observe the person (see Ch 15). Any noticeable change in behaviour, facial grimacing, screaming, moaning, refusal to move or cooperate may indicate pain. Where a person cannot self-report, pain relief may be trialled to see if the behaviour changes and the person settles. Proxy assessments will demonstrate whether the behaviour is pain related so appropriate measures can be implemented.

INTIMACY AND SEXUAL EXPRESSION

For younger people living in residential aged care the opportunity for intimate visits from family and friends is crucial and should be encouraged by providing for overnight visits and a welcoming environment built on an ethos of tolerance and respect for all. Disability, whether physical or cognitive, does result in many losses for a person, but the ability and need to express sexuality and sensuality can remain for the duration of one's life. For many younger people entering care, their admission can result in the abrupt end to any such expression. This is often driven by staff attitudes and the environments created for people in care (see Ch 16).

YOUNGER ONSET DEMENTIA DIAGNOSIS AND CARE

There has been much discussion in recent years about issues specific to people living with younger onset dementia. People with younger onset dementia are those diagnosed with a type of dementia occurring before the age of 65 years. It is estimated that 16,000 people in Australia have younger onset dementia. This represents 0.6% of all people with dementia; however, the true prevalence is uncertain due to issues regarding early diagnosis (Access Economics 2009).

Alzheimer's disease is the most common form of dementia in the under-65 age group, currently at 30% (Alzheimer's Australia 2012). Frontotemporal dementia is the second most common form of dementia and has different pathways that depend on which part of the brain is most affected. If the initial disease affects the frontal lobe then the main changes are in behaviour and personality. In the temporal lobe loss of language skills predominate (progressive aphasia). The pathology of dementia is different and with current scan techniques the changes can be detected (Alzheimer's Australia 2009).

A person with younger onset dementia often needs extra consideration for support at home because the dementia may appear when they are in full-time employment, actively raising a family, financially responsible for a family and physically strong and healthy (Deloitte Access Economics 2011).

Younger people tend to face more barriers in the diagnosis of dementia, especially in the early stages, because dementia is regarded as a disease of old age, and signs in younger people may be thought to relate to other health issues. For younger people with a frontotemporal dementia the first sign may be a change in personality or behaviour. This compounds the problems of early diagnosis and they can often be first diagnosed with depression, stress, anxiety and even menopause. Depression is misdiagnosed in 30–50% of people with younger onset dementia, the final diagnosis often taking 12–18 months. (Alzheimer's Australia 2009).

Younger people tend to face more barriers in the diagnosis of dementia, especially in the early stages, because dementia is regarded as a disease of old age.

People who develop dementia at a young age may have recently had to leave employment, may have financial obligations such as mortgages, young families and undoubtedly dreams for the future. They are often physically strong and healthy and therefore can behave in ways that other people find challenging. They also may have more awareness of their disease trajectory and difficulty with accepting losses. Carers of people with younger onset dementia are often themselves in full-time employment and have the added responsibility of children. Diagnosis affects people beyond the immediate family including parents, friends and workmates. The needs specific to younger people with dementia have been publicly discussed through forums and consumer groups. The recent aged care reforms handed down by the Commonwealth

Government, specifically the Living Longer Living Better package, promises $268.4 million dollars over the next five years to address the issue of dementia, including a number of plans specifically addressing the requirements of people with younger onset dementia. A total of $23.6 million will be provided to enable younger people with dementia to access improved coordinated care and support, assisted by what the announcement calls 'dementia key workers' (Department of Health and Ageing 2013). This funding will also help younger people with dementia continue to actively participate in the community through the development and dissemination of information about dementia for community groups (Alzheimer's Australia 2012). Under the Living Longer Living Better program, funding for dementia key workers is available to organisations offering dementia-specific programs. The Alzheimer's Australia, Tasmania group have been granted funds for a specific worker to assist younger onset dementia clients.

DEVELOPING A THERAPEUTIC APPROACH TO CARE

There have been many models of care produced and programs implemented to improve the lives of younger people with disability. However, very little research has been done to evaluate outcomes of these programs. As the disability/disease progresses approaches to care may need to change and other ways to provide a meaningful life found. People with younger onset dementia usually do not present for admission to an aged care facility until they are advanced in the illness trajectory. The family or close friends recognise that they finally cannot cope with the behavioural changes and physical deterioration. Being admitted because of a loss of cognitive ability that will continue to deteriorate when you are 40–55 years of age makes any adjustment to the new environment difficult.

There are many models for caring for people in RACFs that may also improve the quality of life of younger people with a disability, be it from dementia, an ABI or other causes, and these include the following four.

 There are many models for caring for people in RACFs, which may also improve the quality of life of younger people with disability.

THE EDEN ALTERNATIVE

Dr Bill Thomas created the Eden Alternative way of living for aged care facilities in 1990 when working as a geriatrician in a large care facility. He identified that helplessness, boredom and loneliness were the three needs of the human spirit and that these were not being addressed in a meaningful way. To create an environment that promoted meaning and uplifted the spirit he saw that animals, plants, children, staff and family members should all be involved in creating a home with many connections to the outside community. The model stresses the need to change the environment and move from a medical model and institutional care to one of relaxation and harmony. To ensure these changes occur and everyone is familiar with the approach takes commitment from management and a shift in allocation of resources (Mackenzie 2003). Evaluation is still being undertaken with scarce publication of results.

PROGRESSIVELY LOWERED STRESS THRESHOLD (PLST)

This model was developed by Hall and Buckwalter (1987) and is based on the premise that as dementia progresses the capability of the person to cope with stressors decreases. The key to maintaining a less stressful environment is to reduce stimuli such as noise levels, limiting choice or options, and activity that is outside the competency of the person. Limiting choice ensures the person is not overwhelmed in decision making and options such as meals served one course at a time limits the problem of not knowing how to commence eating. Careful cueing of the surrounding spaces is an essential factor. There has been limited research published on this model (Hall & Buckwalter 1987).

ENHANCED LIFESTYLE THROUGH OPTIMAL STIMULUS (ELTOS)

ELTOS was developed through adapting the PLST model when action research into this model made the authors aware that people react to different levels of stimuli and that reducing the whole environment to a lower level was not a solution. Cultural differences must be considered and certain activities that were noisy and enjoyable no matter what the level of dementia present were found to be effective (Garratt & Hamilton-Smith 1985). An example of this was the Greek community's love of loud music and dancing that may not be shared by others in a facility. Adaptation to create an environment that allows for optimal levels of stimuli is challenging but can be achieved. The need to 'know the person' is essential to provide an environment that is not overwhelming but provides sufficient stimulation to maintain a meaningful lifestyle.

MONTESSORI METHODS

Montessori methods for dementia are 'based on a set of clearly articulated principles primarily developed from the original theories and principles developed by Maria Montessori' (Elliot 2012). The theory originated from the work done by Dr Montessori for developmentally delayed children and the belief that a controlled environment and purposeful activity based on the needs, capacity, skills and interests would assist learning. Montessori's philosophy (vision) makes a perfect mission statement for dementia care: *To enable individuals to be as independent as possible, to have a meaningful place in their community,* to have *high self-esteem,* and to have the chance to make *choices* and *meaningful contributions* to their community. In adapting this approach for dementia care the environment must be supportive for the cognitive loss occurring. There is a strong rehabilitative focus on activity that creates meaningful and purposeful responses related to daily roles and routines (Elliot 2012).

Person-centred care (see Ch 7) is common to all approaches and if embraced will improve the lives of residents, families and staff.

Vignette 1

A 90-bed RACF admitted a man aged 46 who had suffered a haemorrhage in his brain with a resulting haematoma near the basal ganglia. This resulted in an inability to care for himself and, because his wife worked, there was no choice but to admit him because of the severity of his poor motor control and his unstable behaviour. On admission he was depressed and did not want to take part in any social events in the facility. Eventually funds were donated so he could have a motorised wheelchair and the occupational therapist provided training in how to drive it.

He became much more stable and began to socialise now he had some independence. The family stopped trying to take him home but would take him outside for longer periods and walk with him. Unfortunately he had another small event similar to a transient ischaemic attack (TIA) that caused more loss of motor control.

This interfered with his ability to feed himself but he persevered, making mealtimes an ordeal for both him and the staff. Frustration and anger resulted in food being thrown and often refused. Staff made him milkshakes and anything they could get him to eat because he was losing weight.

The next major difficulty became handling his wheelchair. The only way he was able to stop it moving was to drive it into the nearest wall or object in front of him. This resulted in four broken glass doors and damage to furniture, a dishwasher and dented walls. To remove the chair was the last link of independence he had, but he was becoming a danger to others, many of who were aged over 80 and frail. A family conference was called and much anger expressed by all parties as costs of repairs were mounting and the family had no finances to assist. They considered that the RACF was responsible for damages and the management was more concerned about the other residents' safety.

Finally it was agreed that the occupational therapist would reassess his ability to manage his chair and his use of it would be restricted to certain times of the day. The staff would not assist him into his chair until after lunch and he could only go up one corridor and the external courtyards until teatime. The occupational therapist was compromising because she knew it would be taking his independence away to remove the chair altogether.

He was not happy about any of this and was verbally abusing staff who ignored most of the temper displays. There were complaints about his behaviour from other residents and visitors and management obtained a referral and visit from the psychiatric team to help.

Medication assisted but it was very difficult to obtain satisfactory results. If too much was given he slept all day, and too little did nothing to ameliorate his behaviour. He was totally intolerant of people who had dementia and would call them wandering idiots and shout at them to get out of his way. This was distressing for all concerned.

Eventually he had a major stroke resulting in hospitalisation, where he remained until he died.

The family considered he did not get the care they thought he needed but were unable to support him socially or handle his psychological problems. Staffing levels were not able to be adjusted to give him the personal company he desired.

Vignette 2

Mrs X was admitted to an RACF because, at aged 49, she had early-onset dementia and had reached a stage where her husband could not continue to care for her and keep working. His work as a lawyer was busy and they needed to keep his income at the present level to maintain two children studying at university. The grief and loss this family sustained when their mother and wife began to behave in an uninhibited way was profound. Mrs X would remove her clothes, swear at staff, proposition visitors and generally behaved in a way very much out of her usual character.

Finally she couldn't remember her children's names or want any connection with her husband. She was still physically active but some motor control was a problem because she couldn't remember how to feed herself and her movements were becoming slower.

Reflective questions—vignette 1

1. How can the needs of various age groups with different levels of disability be met in RACFs?

2. Are there differences in needs for various disabilities? Discuss this and consider how these needs could increase clinical care.

3. How would a facility prepare care staff to provide appropriate care for complex care needs?

4. Identify the care issues in the case study and plan a strategy to improve care.

Reflective questions—vignette 2

1. How would you assist this family to cope with their loss and grief?

2. As younger onset dementia usually affects the frontal lobes explain the change in behaviour of this 49-year-old woman.

3. How would you deal with the overt sexual behaviour?

CONCLUSION

This chapter has raised issues surrounding the admission of younger people who have a disability, either physical or cognitive, to an RACF. The rehabilitative strategies to reduce further decline are an important feature of care and require a consistent application for positive outcomes. Emotional, psychological and social inclusiveness must also be assessed and considered in providing care. The current funding of RACFs make it difficult for management to increase allied health support such as physiotherapy, personal activities in the community and engagement of a younger cohort to visit in the facility. The use of community agencies for additional support and family involvement in the lifestyle of younger people in RACFs needs to be facilitated and encouraged. Every person is unique and has the right to receive care that is sensitive to their own situation—care that respects relationships with both significant others and the community and where the individual is honoured and included in all aspects of decision making. A person's right to have the opportunity to be involved in meaningful activity and to continue with current roles does not disappear because of residential care admission. Where a rehabilitative approach forms the basis of care it will enable each person to function to their highest possible level.

A person's identity is at risk when there is a necessity to move into residential care. All of a sudden the disability/dementia is seen rather than the person; it can be as if a mask is slid over their face when they enter through the facility door. Previous roles of father, mother, husband, wife, lover, worker, bill-payer, gardener, cook and friend must be encouraged to continue, perhaps in a different way, but still continued. This is essential if the person is to experience a sense of self and their place in their community. An RACF cannot do anything about a person's diagnosis with a deteriorating disease but they are able to support a person's goals, choices and dignity, self-esteem and sense of worth.

References

Access Economics, 2009. Keeping dementia front of mind: incidence and prevalence 2009–2050. Canberra.

Aged Care Assessment Service, 2012. How can Aged Care Assessment Teams (ACATs) help you (updated paper). Online. Available: www.agedcareaustralia. gov.au, 1 May 2013.

Alzheimer's Australia, 2009. Quality dementia care. Canberra.

Alzheimer's Australia, 2012. HOPE Newsletter. Issue 11, July: 1–5. Canberra.

Australian Institute Health and Welfare, 2012. Younger people with disability in residential aged care 2010–2011. Online. Available: http://www.aihw.gov.au/ WorkArea/DownloadAsset.aspx?id=10737421563, 31 Jan 2013.

Beyondblue, 2012. Information papers. Online. Available: www.beyondblue.org.au/ dep, 15 Jan 2012.

Carr, J., Shepherd, R., 2002. Neurological rehabilitation: optimizing motor performance. Butterworth Heinemann, Oxford.

Commonwealth Government Senate Community Affairs Committee, 2005. Quality and equity in aged care. Chapter 5. Commonwealth Government, Canberra.

Deloitte Access Economics, 2011. Dementia across Australia 2011-2050. Deloitte Access Economics, Melbourne.

Department of Health and Ageing, 2013. Living Longer Living Better website. Australian Government. Online. Available: www.livinglongerlivingbetter.gov.au, 31 Jan 2013.

Department of Human Services, 2009. Disability Services Aged Care Assessment Program Operational Guidelines. State Government of Victoria, Melbourne.

Doka, K., 2002. Disenfranchised grief: new directions, challenges, and strategies for practice. Research Press, Ill.

Elliot, G., 2012. Montessori methods for dementia: focusing on the person and the prepared environment. Franklin Press Moonah, Tasmania.

Fann, J.R., Hart, T., Schomer, K.G., 2009. Treatment for depression after traumatic brain injury: a systematic review. Journal of Neurotrauma 26 (12), 2383–2402.

Garratt, S., Hamilton-Smith, E., 1985. Rethinking dementia: an Australian approach. Ausmed, Melbourne.

Hall, G., Buckwalter, K.C., 1987. Progressively lowered stress threshold: a conceptual model for care of adults with Alzheimer's disease. Archives of Psychiatric Nursing 1 (6), 399–406.

Hoeman, S.P., 2002. Rehabilitation: process, application and outcomes, third ed. Mosby, St Louis.

Kirby, T., 2012. Hope for young disabled in elderly care homes. The Lancet 378 (9789), 387–388.

Mackenzie, D., 2003. The Eden alternative. In: Hudson, R. (Ed.), Dementia nursing: a guide to practice. Ausmed, Melbourne.

Shumway-Cook, A., Woollacott, M., 2001. Motor control: theory and practical applications, second ed. Lippincott Williams & Wilkins, Philadelphia.

Summer Foundation, 2007. Younger people in residential aged care: support needs, preferences and future directions. Department of Human Services, Melbourne.

Summer Foundation, 2011. Quality of life evaluation report 2011. Summer Foundation, Melbourne.

Winkler, D., 2007. Summer Foundation report: younger people in residential aged care. Melbourne.

Young People in Nursing Homes National Alliance, 2012. 2009 statistics. Online. Available: www.ypinh.org.au/Statistics, 8 Aug 2012.

CHAPTER 6

COMMUNITY SUPPORT FOR OLDER AUSTRALIANS: ISSUES AND FUTURE DIRECTIONS

Yvonne Wells and Bridget Regan

Editors' comments

Older people say they prefer to 'stay at home' if possible until they die. This requires care and support to be delivered in the community. While we would all agree this sounds great it does have consequences and relies very heavily on families, friends and communities. This chapter provides an overview of the current situation, a vision for community cares and explores some of the barriers that need careful consideration and planning.

Yvonne Wells features in Session 1 of Evolve.

INTRODUCTION

Our focus in this chapter will be on government funded programs that provide assessment and community services to older people living in the community. We will be looking at emerging issues and new directions in the provision of community care to older people.

In Australia, the system of care and supports for older people is broadly divided in two streams—residential care, which is provided in hostels and nursing homes, and community care, which is provided in people's homes and community settings. However, older people also use a range of other services and supports. They are high users of health and hospital services; people over the age of 65 account for approximately half of all patient days in public hospitals (Australian Institute of Health and Welfare (AIHW) 2012). They use public and private housing services; about 5% live in retirement villages (Retirement Villages Association 2010). Finally, transport and other community services are vitally important to older people (World Health Organization (WHO) 2007).

Australian and state governments currently fund a range of community care programs. Generally, these are of four broad types: assessment and information; the Home and Community Care (HACC) program; a range of packaged care programs, which provide case management as well as direct assistance; and services that are directed to specific subgroups of older people.

It is important to understand the context in which these services are provided. Most significantly, the community care system for older Australians may be about to undergo radical change as a result of the recent Productivity Commission inquiry (Productivity Commission 2011) and the Australian Government's policy response, Living Longer Living Better (Department of Health and Ageing 2012a).

THE AUSTRALIAN COMMUNITY SERVICE SYSTEM

The Australian aged care system is characterised by a mix of types of provision and a high degree of collaboration between all levels of government, service providers and the community (AIHW 2007). The Australian Government has the major role of funding both residential and community aged care services. It establishes the policy directions in consultation with state and territory governments and the aged care industry and consumers, and provides the bulk of administrative support.

In Australia, community services are provided by local government, not-for-profit, and for-profit organisations. Not-for-profits (NFPs) are defined as agencies that do not distribute profits or surpluses to personal owners or shareholders. They provide a substantial proportion of community care in Australia. Most (about 84%) of community care packages are delivered by charitable and other not-for-profit community-based providers. The remaining 16% are provided by commercial organisations, and state, territory and local governments (Department of Health and Ageing 2010). NFPs are critically important in providing aged care tailored to particular culturally and linguistically diverse (CALD) communities (Productivity Commission 2011).

Although residential care continues to receive most of the funding (about 66% of the 11 billion Australian dollars spent in 2009–10 on aged and community care (Productivity Commission 2011), a shift in funding towards community care has occurred and is likely to continue in the future. The following sections describe the major service types available in Australia.

AGED CARE ASSESSMENT PROGRAM

Since it was established in 1984, the Aged Care Assessment Program (ACAP) has been an important and integral part of Australia's aged care system. The core objective of the ACAP is to assess the needs of frail older people comprehensively and to facilitate access to available care services appropriate to their needs. Aged care assessments also determine eligibility for Australian Government-subsidised residential aged care and packaged care services.

The ACAP has been a gatekeeper for access to intensive levels of care in both residential and community settings and has enabled the Australian

Government to implement planning targets for subsidised care. However, state and territory governments are responsible for the day-to-day operation and administration of the ACAP.

In 2009–10 the ACAP completed nearly 170,000 assessments of people in their target group, which is defined as people aged 70 and older or Indigenous people aged 50 or older; about 7.5% of all people in the target group received an assessment. Nearly half of the assessments (41%) were of people aged 85 years or older. More than 114,000 people were given approvals to enter residential care, and 69,000 were approved to use packaged care (Productivity Commission 2012).

The ACAP has developed differently in different places, and the scope and role of the ACAP varies to some degree between the various states and territories. However, reforms adopted since 2006 are addressing inconsistency by setting key performance indicators, implementing a set of validated assessment tools, and providing national training resources for ACAP staff. All Australian jurisdictions are actively involved in redeveloping assessment processes to better meet the existing and emerging needs of older Australians and to reduce the burden of assessment to provider and client.

HOME AND COMMUNITY CARE

The HACC program is the main provider of home-based care services in Australia. It provides a range of services to both frail older people and younger people with disability as well as their carers. The program was created in 1984 (via the *Home and Community Care Act 1985*) and brought together into one system a range of separately funded programs.

The HACC program provides maintenance and support services for people in the community whose independence is at risk. The program aims to prevent premature or inappropriate admission to residential care (Productivity Commission 2012). A wide range of services is provided under HACC, including assessment, domestic assistance and home maintenance, personal care, food services, respite care, transport, allied healthcare and community nursing. Services provided under HACC are not rationed by the Australian Government, and provision varies between states and territories. In 2009–10 more than 930,000 people received support from HACC and almost 13 million hours of services were provided. In addition, HACC provided over four million meals, nearly two million transport trips, and over six million dollars' worth of home modifications. While two-thirds of HACC clients are aged 70 years or older (69%), HACC also supports younger people in the community with disabilities, and almost 11% of people who use HACC are aged under 50 years (Productivity Commission 2012).

In the past, HACC has been funded jointly by the Australian Government and state and territory governments. The state and territory governments were responsible for managing the program while the Australian Government maintained a broad strategic role. However, from July 2012, the Australian Government took full funding, policy and operational responsibility for HACC services for older people in all states and territories (except Victoria and Western Australia, where basic community care services will continue to be delivered under a program funded by both the Australian Government and the state government). The state and territory governments will continue to fund and administer HACC services for people under the age of 65 or under 50 for Aboriginal and Torres Strait Islander people.

Since 2006 the nature of services provided under the HACC program has been changing, particularly in Victoria and Western Australia, in response to a range of pressures, including changing philosophies of care (described in more detail below) and a recognition by state governments that the service system needed to be re-designed. These shifts in HACC have been towards wellness and re-ablement approaches. In Western Australia, the Home Independence Program (HIP) targets older home care clients when first referred for assistance, while the Personal Enablement Program (PEP) is designed to meet the needs of clients who are exiting an acute episode of care in hospital. These programs are targeted at clients with no dementia. In Victoria, the approach has been developed as the Active Service Model (ASM).

PACKAGED CARE

In addition to the HACC system, the Australian Government supports aged care packages in the community and residential care places. The costs of packaged care are borne by the Australian Government, with some co-contributions from clients. Packaged care provides case management as well as direct care services, and eligibility is determined through an ACAP assessment. Packaged care, like residential care, is rationed. The Australian Government has set targets of 113 places per 1000 people aged 70 or older: 44 in high level residential care, 44 in low level residential care, and 25 in packaged community care. Over three-quarters of approved providers of packaged care are private, not-for-profit agencies (AIHW 2012).

A key feature of community packaged care is that care services are provided to approved care recipients on a planned and managed basis. Community Aged Care Packages (CACPs) are intended to provide community-based 'low level' care to people who would otherwise require a low care (hostel) residential place. The CACP program was established in 1992, and has grown rapidly; in 2009–10, nearly 60,000 people received a CACP (AIHW 2012).

A key feature of community packaged care is that care services are provided to approved care recipients on a planned and managed basis.

In 1998 the Extended Aged Care at Home (EACH) program was introduced as a pilot program for frail older people with complex needs who require a high level of in-home care. The program was supplemented in 2004–05 by the EACH-D program, which provides care packages for people with dementia who experience behaviours of concern and psychological symptoms that impact on their ability to live in the community. In 2009–10 more than 10,000 people received an EACH package and 4800 people received an EACH-D package (AIHW 2012).

Table 6.1 provides rates of operational aged care places per 1000 in the population aged 70 or older for the 12 years from 1999 to 2011. Operational

Table 6.1

Provision of residential care and aged care packages per 1000 aged 70+

	HIGH-CARE RESIDENTIAL	LOW-CARE RESIDENTIAL	CACPS	EACH	EACH-D	TRANSITION CARE	TOTAL
1999	45.7	40.5	8.5				94.7
2000	44.2	40.3	10.9				95.4
2001	43.6	39.4	14.3				97.3
2002	42.4	40.5	15.0				97.9
2003	42.2	42.0	15.5				99.7
2004	41.6	42.4	15.6	0.5			100.1
2005	41.8	43.4	16.3	0.9			102.4
2006	41.8	43.8	18.2	1.3	0.3	0.3	105.7
2007	41.6	44.0	19.0	1.7	0.6	0.8	107.7
2008	42.8	44.5	20.1	2.1	1.0	1.0	111.5
2009	42.6	44.2	19.9	2.2	1.0	1.1	111.0
2010	42.8	44.0	20.6	2.7	1.2	1.3	112.5
2011	42.5	43.3	21.3	3.8	1.9	1.5	114.3

Data from various Productivity Commission Reports on Government Services, Operational care places per 1000 people aged 70 years or older, available at <www.pc.gov.au/gsp/rogs>.

care places do not include places or beds that have been approved but are not yet filled, and the number of operational care places is a measure of access. As can be seen from the total column in this table, the provision of aged care places per population aged 70 and over has been growing steadily. However, the number of places in residential care has been levelling off or even decreasing, while the number of funded packages has been increasing. This recognises increasing demand for community care in preference to residential care.

RESPITE

The aim of the National Respite for Carers Program (NRCP) is to contribute to the support and maintenance of caring relationships between carers and care recipients by facilitating access to information, respite care and other support appropriate to the carer's individual needs and circumstances, and those of the care recipient (Department of Health and Ageing 2012b). The NRCP assists carers with information, respite care and support. More than 650 respite services and 54 Commonwealth Respite and Carelink Centres across Australia are funded under the program.

For the purposes of this program, respite care is defined as a care arrangement whose primary purpose is giving the carer a short-term break from their usual caring role or assistance with the performance of their caring role on a short-term basis (Department of Health and Ageing 2012b). Respite services are delivered to carers and the people they care for in a variety of settings, including homes, day centres, host families and residential overnight cottages. In 2010–11 the NRCP assisted nearly 130,500 people (Productivity Commission 2012).

The vital role of carers was recognised in the government's National Carer Strategy, which was designed following a community consultation process and launched in 2011. The strategy is intended to improve the current provision of assistance for carers and complements reforms which are currently occurring across the aged care system and in related healthcare systems.

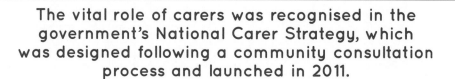

The vital role of carers was recognised in the government's National Carer Strategy, which was designed following a community consultation process and launched in 2011.

OTHER COMMUNITY CARE SERVICES

The Australian Government supports a range of other relatively small programs to provide community care for older people. Services similar to those funded under the HACC and packaged care programs are provided to by the Department of Veterans' Affairs (DVA) under the Veterans' Home Care and Community Nursing programs. In 2009–10 there were about 77,000 clients of the Veterans' Home Care program, making it second only to the HACC program in terms of the numbers of older people it assists (AIHW 2012).

The Transition Care Program was established relatively recently, in 2004–05, as a jointly funded initiative between the Commonwealth and states and territories. The Transition Care Program is for older people who would otherwise be eligible for residential aged care. To enter the program, clients must be assessed by an Aged Care Assessment Team (ACAT) while they are still a hospital inpatient. A TCP provides goal-oriented, time-limited, therapy-focused care to help older people at the conclusion of a hospital stay. It may include low-intensity therapy (such as physiotherapy, occupational therapy and social work) and nursing support or personal care. It is intended to help older people complete their restorative process and optimise their functional capacity, while assisting them and their family or carer to make long-term care arrangements. Transition care can be provided either in a home-like residential setting or in the community. The average duration of care is seven weeks, with a maximum duration of 12 weeks that may in some circumstances be extended by a further six weeks.

Finally, a range of services is provided in mixed delivery settings that are designed to provide flexible care or specific support. For example, multipurpose services (MPSs) support the integration and provision of health and aged care services for small rural and remote communities where standard programs may not be viable if provided separately: day therapy centres deliver services such as physiotherapy, occupational therapy, podiatry and speech therapy to individuals or groups of clients to assist them to maintain or recover their independence; the National Aboriginal and Torres Strait Islander Flexible Aged Care Program aims to provide flexible, culturally appropriate aged care to older indigenous people close to their homes and communities; the Long Stay Older Patients initiative funds acute care services to support older people to maintain function while waiting for an appropriate residential care place to become available; and the Innovative Pool supports programs where mainstream aged care services might not meet the needs of specific locations or target groups and trials of new programs prior to them being rolled out as part of mainstream service provision. For example, the Consumer Directed Care (CDC) program is currently supported by Innovative Pool funding.

CARERS AND THE INTERFACE BETWEEN FORMAL AND INFORMAL CARE

Formal, publicly funded services represent only a small proportion of total assistance provided to frail older people. Extended family and partners are the largest source of emotional, practical and financial support for older people: about 76% of people aged 60 and over living in the community in 2009 who required help with any task received assistance from informal care networks of family, friends and neighbours (compared with 56% who received help from formal services: ABS 2009). Many people receive assistance from both formal aged care services and informal sources. In Australia, the essential role of informal carers in assisting older people to remain in the community is recognised through the provision of HACC services to carers and services such as the National Respite for Carers Program (NRCP).

Formal, publicly funded services represent only a small proportion of total assistance provided to frail older people.

The literature on long-term care for the older population has focused on trade-offs among different types of personal care in order to address the 'woodwork effect'; the concern that public coverage for home care could cause a reduction in informal care (Agree et al 2005). However, studies have generally found that formal home care does not substitute for, or crowd out, informal care, and, in many cases, supplements informal care (Tennstedt et al 1996). Cohen et al (2000), in a North American study of informal carers, found that whether or not formal care substitutes for informal care is related to the characteristics of the caregiver. For adult children formal care sometimes substitutes for informal care, but this is not generally the case for spouses. Where the informal caregiver provides eight hours per week or less of help with activities of daily living (ADLs), paid help also tends to be low, but where the informal caregiver is providing large amounts of ADL help, paid help is also used for large blocks of time.

Informal carers actually facilitate formal care provision. Few older clients, either in the United Kingdom or the United States, receive formal care alone (Davey & Patsios 1999). Similarly, our analysis of the ACAP minimum dataset (Howe et al 2006) shows that clients with no carer are *less* likely to be using services than clients with a carer, and clients with co-resident carers are the group most likely to be using HACC and CACPs.

Little attention has been paid to where the cultures of the formal and informal sectors clash. A gulf may develop between the ways in which families perceive the task of care provision for someone who is sick or disabled and the way in which professional carers approach the task (Levine & Murray 2004). This gulf can lead to mutual incomprehension, disagreements, and even conflict. At worst, professionals ignore families' perceptions and preferences, while families fail to comply with healthcare directions; professional carers perceive well-meaning family carers as interfering, while family carers see professionals as uncaring and unsympathetic; and each views the other as incompetent. This is particularly a risk where formal care is highly medicalised and removed from everyday experience.

TENSIONS AND PRESSURES IN THE AGED CARE SYSTEM

The combined effects of population trends, fiscal pressures and developments in service delivery models have increased pressure to ensure that resources available to the community aged care services are used in the most effective manner. This section of the chapter introduces some of these pressures and the next section describes some key concepts and solutions suggested to address them.

POPULATION

As with many western nations, our dramatically ageing population poses significant challenges for governments (WHO 2002). The large baby boom generation is ageing and the number of older people is projected to increase rapidly. As the youngest of the surviving baby boomers reaches 65 years of age in 2031, the population aged 65 years and older is projected to reach 5.4 million in Australia (more than double the number in 1999) and will represent 22% of the total population (compared with 12% in 1999). As the youngest baby boomers reach 85 years of age in 2051, importantly, the population aged 85 years and older is projected to reach 1.3 million (more than five times the number in 1999) and to represent 5% of the total population (Trewin 2001).

In spite of steady growth in funding, all providers report that demand for services exceeds their capacity to supply them. Factors such as an increase in the number of clients remaining at home with complex care needs; difficulties accessing residential care; shorter hospital stays; more outpatient and day treatments; lack of post-acute home care provision from private hospitals; and higher community awareness and expectations about the benefits of the HACC program have all contributed to rising demand (Wittenberg et al 2004).

In spite of steady growth in funding, all providers report that demand for services exceeds their capacity to supply them.

In some countries, this increasing demand has resulted in longer waiting lists for clients assessed as having low level care needs. This is cause for concern, as research has suggested that risk may be imposed on clients if delivery of small amounts of critical services—targeted at clients at the time need is expressed—is delayed, or if services are not available at all (Elkan et al 2001, LaPlante et al 2004). If people with lower level needs are neglected, the opportunity to provide restorative services, at a time when clients are likely to retain sufficient capacity to maximally benefit, may be lost. It should be noted that a person's need for services is related not just to their level of functional dependence, but also to their circumstances, especially the extent to which they have support from their family and community.

The steadily rising demand for services also continues to place pressure on many traditional community care providers to maintain services, sometimes over many years—for example, the provision of domestic services or meals-on-wheels—to all eligible clients in the community (Howe et al 2006, Parker 2001, Pilkington 2006). In some countries, this has resulted in longer waiting lists or cessation of service for those clients assessed as having low-level care needs.

In the absence of any further improvements in the effectiveness of our health and community care systems, it is unlikely there will be any deceleration in the growing demand for home care services. Rather, systemic issues are likely to have an increasing impact, including ongoing difficulties recruiting and retaining community care staff and the projected decline in family care with an increase in women entering or remaining in the workforce.

FUTURE AVAILABILITY OF CARERS

In the 1990s considerable concern was expressed about the future availability of carers for frail older people. Reasons for anticipating a potential decline in informal care include: declines in family size (Clarke 1995) and the proportion of older people who live with their children (Grundy 2000); rises in divorce rates, childlessness and employment rates among married women (Clarke 1995, Hancock 2002, Rowland 2007); and shifts in the nature of kinship obligations, especially in relation to filial responsibilities (Gans & Silverstein 2006).

In response to this concern, Carers Australia commissioned the National Centre for Social and Economic Modelling (NATSEM) to examine demographic and carer data from the Australian Bureau of Statistics (NATSEM 2004). The study projected a significant increase in the numbers of older people likely to need informal care in Australia between 2001 and 2031 along with a smaller increase in the numbers likely to be carers. At the same time, shifts in the composition of the disabled and carers' populations were also projected, and both were predicted to include higher proportions of older people. Hence, there may well be increasing pressures on informal carers in the future. This, however, is not necessarily a cause for panic. Other OECD countries have already met the demands of the changing population structure that Australia is expected to encounter in the next few years.

COMMUNITY EXPECTATIONS

Both the community and governments have been aware for many years that the provision of community care services results in an overall improvement in the quality of life and maintenance of a basic standard of living for many frail older adults in the community *and* may reduce or delay high intensity, high cost services such as residential care or hospital admission (Elkan et al 2001). The majority of services were previously provided in a largely standardised way to all eligible clients, and often acted to substitute for activities previously undertaken by the individual prior to them experiencing difficulties with looking after themselves.

A growing number of critics suggested that community care programs in Australia were not as successful as they could have been because they relied on an outdated 'dependency' model of service provision rather than a newer focus on activity, independence and successful ageing (Baker 2006, Glendinning et al 2008, Hallberg & Kristensson 2004, Lewin et al 2006, O'Connell 2006). Services have often lacked an emphasis on the promotion of healthy lifestyles and daily routines, social support, exercise, and autonomy and control, despite strong evidence that these are strongly linked to the maintenance of health and independence in older adults (Peel et al 2004, Seeman & Crimmins 2001).

Many approaches to community care provision still give insufficient attention to an individual's rehabilitative potential, and, via well-meaning attempts to assist, may actually prevent people from participating in important physical and social activities (e.g. shopping and cooking). Older people may become entrenched in a 'sick role', characterised by an absence of self-motivation, and the view that because they are aged or unwell they must remain dependent upon continuous professional management of care (O'Connell 2006). The funding mechanisms that underpin many services also limit the capacity for services to provide restorative care. Many services are funded for short, task-focused events, which makes it difficult to use a flexible, goal-oriented approach to underpin a more restorative program (Ware 2002). Some staff may also believe that bed rest is beneficial for a frail or sick older individual, despite considerable evidence to the contrary (Baker 2006). Staff may exacerbate this situation by emphasising task completion and doing as much as they can for the client, rather than to trying to assist the client to do things for themselves.

> **The funding mechanisms that underpin many services also limit the capacity for services to provide restorative care.**

Such practices within community care services for frail older adults contrast sharply with the highly progressive movements that have occurred with other groups in developed countries over the previous 50 years. Older adults have not been entitled to the same empowerment-oriented and independence-focused approaches as other groups with disabilities: for example, the concepts of normalisation and social role valorisation, which transformed approaches to the management of intellectual disability (Wolfensberger 1972), the large-scale deinstitutionalisation of people with psychiatric and intellectual disabilities, the emergence of more flexible community management models (Mansell 2006), and, more recently, the chronic disease self-management movement from the US (e.g. Chodosh et al 2005). As the highly educated and proactive baby boomer generation enters retirement age, criticism of outmoded approaches is likely to intensify (Someya & Wells 2008).

KEY CONCEPTS IN COMMUNITY AGED CARE

Changes in community expectations have been mirrored in gerontology and the development of new models of community aged care. The discussion below outlines some of these concepts.

SUCCESSFUL AGEING

A key concept that has emerged in attempting to rethink how to address the needs and maximise the health and wellbeing of our ageing population is that of 'successful ageing' (Browning & Kendig 2003, 2004). Impetus for a conceptual shift towards more active, restorative models of care is mirrored by conceptual developments that have occurred within gerontology about what constitutes successful ageing.

Many traditional approaches to aged care emphasised rest, comfort, assistance and support. It has been suggested that this dependency model shares some features with the outdated 'disengagement theory' (Cumming & Henry 1961), popular in gerontological research in the 1960s. This theory proposed that in the normal course of ageing, people gradually withdraw or disengage from social roles as a natural response to lessened capabilities and diminished interest, and disincentives from the broader society to participate. Older people are viewed as happy to retire from work or family life, in order to make room for younger individuals. While winding down and preparing for death, they are then free to pursue other solitary, passive activities.

Recent theories of successful ageing have undergone a major shift in emphasis. The focus is now much more on the promotion of activity and active participation in society in order to maximise the physical and mental wellbeing of people as they age, rather than any suggestion that older adults should disengage from activities or society (Buys & Miller 2006).

Over the previous 15 years, broad-based theoretical frameworks have been developed to articulate the components of healthy ageing and relevant outcome measures (Buys & Miller 2006). A variety of terms have been used to describe these frameworks, including 'healthy ageing', 'productive ageing' and 'successful ageing'. WHO published an 'Active Ageing' framework (WHO 2002), designed to overcome key criticisms and incorporate all the most important aspects of previous frameworks. The term 'active ageing' was chosen to emphasise the valuable contribution older people make to their families, communities and society. It is defined as: 'the process of optimising opportunities for physical, social and mental wellbeing throughout the life course, in order to extend healthy life expectancy, productivity and quality of life in older age' (WHO 2002 p 12). The framework emphasises the value of continued involvement across six life domains: social, economic, civic, cultural, spiritual, and physical. The phrase 'engaged in life' captures its underlying philosophy.

Conceptually, WHO's definition of active ageing comprises three key pillars:
- participation: lifelong learning, paid and unpaid work
- health: achieving and maintaining good physical and mental health in later life
- safety: ensuring the protection, safety and dignity of older people by addressing the social, financial and physical security rights and needs of people as they age.

While the quality of the ageing experience will be determined by all three key pillars, there is some ongoing dispute about their relative importance. The West Australian Active Ageing Taskforce has suggested that participation, not health, should be the central pillar of the model. They also suggested that engagement in social and family connections should be placed under the participation pillar rather than the health pillar (Government of Western Australia 2003). Australian survey findings on older people's perceptions of what constitutes successful ageing are consistent with the Western Australian perspective; that participation, including participation in social activities, is central to older adults' views of what constitutes successful ageing (Buys & Miller 2006).

RESTORATIVE CARE AND PROMOTION OF WELLNESS

The concept of 'wellness' has been used for at least 30 years, but over the previous decade it has become a key concept in approaches to community care for older adults. Wellness refers to a state of optimal physical and mental health, especially when maintained by a healthy diet, exercise, and other habits. From an ecological viewpoint, wellness depends on the dynamic relationship between people and the quality of their physical and social environment (McMurray 2007). The term wellness has been used to emphasise a substantially broader definition of health than the more traditional one narrowly focused on the presence or absence of symptoms of illness (Crowther et al 2002).

The concept of 'wellness' has been used for at least 30 years, but over the previous decade it has become a key concept in approaches to community care for older adults.

The focus within health services has shifted over the previous 50-year period from treatment to prevention. Only half a century ago, community services were scarce and people typically went to their local hospitals for one-off treatment for an acute event or illness. Medications and technologies to prolong the lives of people who were frail or elderly were largely ineffectual. Improvements in medicine have resulted in individuals living much longer and chronic conditions (e.g. diabetes, arthritis, obesity and depression) are now more common. These conditions often require ongoing treatment in the community, and choices about lifestyle, such as exercise, diet and social connectedness, contribute to their emergence. Thus governments have focused on *primary prevention* of disease directed at all age groups (e.g. exercise promotion or quit smoking campaigns). *Secondary prevention* involves the early identification of disease or illness in order to teach individuals self-management strategies to avoid further exacerbation or decline. *Tertiary prevention*, in which efforts are made to rehabilitate remaining function wherever possible, is also effective in many cases (Godfrey 2001).

Evidence suggests that adopting wellness strategies is advantageous in all age groups, including the oldest (McWilliam et al 2000, Ryburn et al 2009). Strategies to enhance wellness include physical activity (e.g. through shopping, cooking and gardening), utilising aides and equipment, improving nutrition, developing new coping strategies to deal with episodes of depressed mood or stress, and increasing supportive social networks to avoid social isolation.

Restorative approaches to home care have been proposed as a way of reducing dependency in home care provision and to improve our capacity to cope with growing demand for care, via more timely and preventative services. An emerging body of evidence suggests that such programs are effective, including health promotion, occupational therapy and assistive technologies, physical therapy and social rehabilitation (McWilliam et al 2000, Ryburn et al 2009).

Governments in Australia have become interested in restorative programs following the success of re-enablement teams within the UK, where in 2010

88% of councils had a scheme in place or were establishing one (Pilkington 2010). Re-enablement typically refers to intensive and time-limited multidisciplinary home care service interventions developed for people with poor physical or mental health, to help them learn or re-learn the skills necessary to manage their illness and to participate maximally in everyday activities. The majority of programs are relatively unselective and target clients at the beginning of their home care career, while others are targeted to specific clients post-discharge from hospital. Programs vary widely in their structure, staff skill mix, and nature of interventions, although they share general principles, such as a focus on helping people 'to do' rather than 'doing to or for', a specific outcome focus, and defined maximum duration. Each service provides comprehensive assessments and time-limited (up to two months) programs of rehabilitation in the client's own home. Teams usually comprise occupational therapists, social workers, and home care agency staff; some teams also include physical therapists. Usually, these services are available to the range of frail older adults and younger people with disability who would be eligible for home care services in the UK. Some councils have made participation in such a program compulsory prior to commencement of home care services as usual.

Evaluations of the approach have supported it as having benefits for both service providers and older people. The City of Edinburgh Council Home Care Re-ablement Service, introduced in 2008, had been shown to reduce the number of hours of support required by clients at the end of their six-week period of re-ablement—by some 41%. Clients liked the service because it allowed them to regain their independence quickly and gave them the confidence to undertake tasks for themselves (McLeod & Mair 2009).

A prospective longitudinal study of home care re-ablement services examined the immediate and longer term impacts of home care re-ablement, the cost-effectiveness of the service, and the content and organisation of re-ablement services. People who received home care re-ablement were compared with a group receiving conventional home care services, and both groups were followed for up to one year (Glendinning et al 2010). Re-ablement was associated with a significant decrease in subsequent service use. However, these lower costs were almost entirely offset by the higher cost of the re-ablement intervention itself. Equally important, re-ablement also resulted in improvements in users' health-related quality of life and quality of life up to ten months after re-ablement, in comparison with users of conventional home care services.

In Australia several pilot studies involving time-limited multi-component restorative home care programs have been trialled. These include the development and evaluation of the Home Independence Program (HIP) by the private home care provider Silver Chain in Western Australia (Lewin et al 2006, Silver Chain 2007), the Supported Independent Living Collaborative in Queensland, and the implementation of pilot programs across the state of Victoria. The West Australian state government has also funded the rollout of a broad-based training package within a range of existing home care providers outlining the principles of restorative care. The Wellness Approach to Community Homecare, or WATCH (O'Connell 2006) has now been formally recognised as a key priority for its home care system.

Lewin and Vandermeulen (2010) evaluated the HIP model by following up 200 clients both at the end of the re-ablement service and three and 12 months later. While this evaluation showed promising results, a later randomised controlled trial in which 750 community dwelling older people received either HIP or usual HACC home care services was more convincing. This trial showed that at three months, 78% of those who received restorative care no longer required a support service, compared with 31% of the control group, and at 12 months 86% of the intervention group no longer required a service, compared with 57% of the control group. Furthermore, over two years, the HIP group was less likely than the control group to use hospital emergency services (Lewin 2010).

The Victorian Department of Health (formerly the Department of Human Services) has developed a new service delivery model, the Active Service Model (ASM) (Department of Human Services 2008), in response to the perceived limitations of current approaches to service provision and increasing demands on the home and community care system. The model aims to incorporate conceptual developments in service delivery which have emerged from disability care provision in other sectors, an understanding of factors known to promote successful ageing, and theoretical developments in gerontology.

The Department of Health funded eight pilot projects in HACC from 2006 to 2008. These projects included a range of HACC activities, such as home help and garden maintenance, nutrition and physical exercise, and continence management. A series of evaluations concluded successful programs require both a shared vision and understanding about the aims and objects of the project from as early as possible in the planning and strong, ongoing leadership. Interventions were well-received by clients and were most successful when they forged strong relationships between staff and clients. Improved assessment processes and access to allied health expertise was highlighted as fundamental to success. Finally, workforce development and resources were seen as necessary for further development of the program (see Department of Health 2012a). Several programs to train staff in the ASM approach have since been instituted.

In Victoria all HACC-funded agencies developed an ASM initial implementation plan for 2010–11. The plan was to focus on identifying a summary of strengths, challenges and opportunities the organisation could see in moving to an ASM approach. In 2011–12 agencies were asked to review these plans and build on their experiences to develop new plans.

The adoption of an active service model involves a paradigm shift in the organisation of care, with substantial changes in service culture and challenges to the perception of ageing. The key features of the new active service model include:

- an emphasis on capacity building or restorative care to maintain or promote a client's capacity to live as independently as possible (the overall aim is to improve functional independence, quality of life and social participation)
- an emphasis on a holistic, person-centred approach to care, which promotes client wellness and active participation in decisions about care
- an attempt to provide more timely, flexible and targeted services capable of maximising the client's independence.

Implementing the ASM with a client may refer to very specific work involving just a single component (e.g. assisting a client to regain capacity for personal care following an acute episode such as a stroke), but it could also involve a broader range of services targeted at someone whose independence has slowly diminished, because of frailty or a chronic condition, with the aim of helping them to regain a degree of functional autonomy, self-confidence and connectedness with the outside world. In any case, an active service model implies a coming together of a range of strategies and services to promote wellness and independence within the limitations imposed by disease or disability for each individual.

Vignettes

The following vignettes have been adapted from the ASM pilot projects that have operated throughout Victoria. They are intended to highlight how some of the Active Service Model core components can be operationalised.

Mrs Andelucci

After a stroke left her with limited use of her left arm and poor mobility, Mrs Andelucci experienced depression and short-term memory loss. She was heavily reliant on social support and home help. She was rarely cooking for herself or taking care of even basic housekeeping tasks.

During the activity and nutritional program offered at the planned activity group that she regularly attended, Mrs Andelucci identified four goals:

* to improve her stamina and flexibility (a physiotherapist developed a strength training program and her home care worker encouraged her to carry it through)
* to learn to dance
* to do more cooking (she asked the home care worker to support her to buy ingredients and prepare basic meals in advance)
* to get involved in her community as a volunteer.

Mrs Andelucci quickly reaped the benefits of this focus on her own wellbeing. Within three months she felt she had turned a corner, happily observing her new 'get up and go'. Mrs Andelucci had become more motivated about doing some of her housework, and was thoroughly enjoying cooking with the support staff and having food in the freezer. She felt physically more confident and was enjoying seeing new friends at the dance classes she had started attending.

ASM components

Health promoting

Capacity building

Access to skilled staff

Holistic

Social inclusion

Flexible and responsive

The planned activity group staff utilised goal setting and care planning to identify the tasks Mrs Andelucci valued. Access to the most appropriate support was coordinated to provide services that were flexible and tailored to her needs; providing opportunities for health promotion, capacity building and social inclusion.

Mr and Mrs Cooper

Mr and Mrs Cooper were referred to their local council by their general practitioner for a home care service. The assessor found that Mr Cooper used to do most of the house cleaning tasks prior to his recent hospital admission for a fall and other complicated medical issues. Mr Cooper had reduced mobility and was not able to vacuum or wash the floor. Mrs Cooper was on 24-hour oxygen and experienced shortness of breath after minimal exertion during cleaning tasks.

Following assessment, a plan was put in place to increase both their physical capacity as well as strategies to facilitate their ability to resume cleaning tasks. Mr Cooper was referred to physiotherapy for an ongoing exercise group to increase his mobility following hospitalisation and Mrs Cooper was engaged in home care tasks with alternative techniques and equipment.

On review, Mrs Cooper had purchased her own motorised carpet sweeper and was cleaning a few rooms at a time. She had purchased a microlite mop and was managing to wash the floors well. The local council instituted a reduced ongoing service of 0.5 hours per month to vacuum the corners. Mrs Cooper commented: 'There's a big difference. The gadgets you've recommended have made cleaning a lot easier. Now I can last longer.'

Mrs Cooper received a timely and coordinated service to respond to a need that was only evident to the home care staff. The home staff member had been provided with training and support structures to assist him to connect Mrs Cooper to an appropriate service. This had a significant impact on her quality of life and confidence to reconnect to her community and family.

ASM components

Detailed assessment

Capacity building

Skilled staff

Functional exercise

Flexible and responsive

Without a detailed assessment, it is likely that Mr and Mrs Cooper would have received an ongoing fortnightly home care service that would have completed tasks for them. They were motivated to do as many of these tasks themselves and were assisted to simplify the tasks and build their capacity.

The council also provided a monthly service to address their unmet need.

Source: Department of Human Services 2008

Restorative approaches have also been implemented in New Zealand. Research here on the perceptions of paid caregivers showed that the restorative home care intervention has a substantial positive impact on paid caregiver job satisfaction. This appeared to be due to improved training, increased support and supervision, and improved flexibility. The intervention also resulted in substantially reduced staff turnover (King et al 2012).

PERSON-CENTRED CARE

The notion of 'person-centred care' has been adopted in several developed countries (Dowling et al 2006). Described in more detail elsewhere in this book (see Ch 7), it refers to a range of approaches that share a common goal: the prioritisation of the holistic range of care needs of the person receiving care and their carers (Department of Human Services 2003). Such approaches can be contrasted with services that are more oriented towards the priorities of an organisation or its staff (i.e. routines, time and tasks) or towards the provision of expert treatment for a specific illness or body part. Such services often provide a relatively mass produced or wholesale type of service, and take a very traditional view that service users are passive recipients of expert care, who do not need to be involved or take an active part in decision making or the development of services.

The concept of person-centred care aims to re-orient service delivery in two main ways. First, it counters the emergence of organisation or illness-centric systems that may be detrimental to the quality of holistic client care (Mansell & Beadle-Brown 2004). Second, it is a set of techniques that enable people to take a lead in planning all aspects of how the service they receive is delivered (Mead & Bower 2000).

Within the UK, person-centred care has been adopted as a central pillar of public policy for the development of health and community support for people, and has been clearly articulated within key policy documents since the late 1980s (Dowling et al. 2006), including the recent white paper, *Our health, our care, our say: A new direction for community services*, which placed emphasis on a person-centred approach (Department of Health 2006). Within Australia there has also been an emphasis on the concept of person-centred care in the release of the policy *Improving health care for older persons: A policy for health services* (Department of Human Services 2003). The development of the active service model for home care provision also falls within this framework, as it aims to increase the effectiveness of the HACC sector in improving health and quality of life outcomes, via the adoption of a more person-centred approach to care delivery.

A review of the literature on person-centred care concluded that evidence in the literature on the approach was limited but largely supports its effectiveness (NARI 2006). An Australian comparison of person-centred care, dementia care mapping (an approach that attempts to identify experiences from the resident's point of view) and usual care for people with dementia in residential care concluded that both interventions were successful in reducing agitation (Chenoweth et al 2009).

CONSUMER-DIRECTED CARE

Consumer-directed care (CDC) is a practical extension of a person-centred care model, with its emphasis on client and carer choice, empowerment and self-management. Under this approach participants choose the services they receive and have a say in the choice of staff and timing of services. Participants may in some cases be able to manage an individual budget for services. In some models, participants have been allowed to hire friends or family to provide care. In the past few years, consumer-directed care has come to denote particular services in which consumers are allowed to hire, train, supervise and pay their own workers, and, if necessary, to fire them.

 Consumer-directed care is a practical extension of a person-centred care model, with its emphasis on client and carer choice, empowerment and self-management.

Innovative programs have been developed in Europe and the US, and various types of programs have been tested internationally. In a review, Tilly and Rees (2007) argued that the evidence suggests that consumer-directed care may, in some cases, result in better care and greater satisfaction for participants and their families than for those who receive services from home care agencies. Quality of care has been found to be at least as good as it is in traditional programs, and there has been no systematic evidence of abuse or neglect of participants in CDC programs.

In 2004 the American National Council on Disability (NCD) conducted a literature review on consumer-directed care. It found the best studied examples of consumer direction have been in the area of long-term care, where consumer control of resources and direction of caregivers has been tested as an alternative to agency-directed community care. The review indicated that while virtually all consumers express a preference for community-based care, interest in consumer-directed or consumer-oriented healthcare models varies. Younger individuals seem to be more interested in consumer direction than older individuals. Nevertheless, interest in consumer direction is evident across a range of disabilities and ages. The conclusion of the review is that most studies of consumer-directed care demonstrate positive outcomes in terms of consumer satisfaction, quality of life, and perceived empowerment. There is no evidence that consumer direction compromises safety. Individuals who have participated in consumer-directed systems express strong preference for consumer direction and satisfaction with their care. However, there is conflicting evidence on the issue of cost effectiveness, perhaps due to variations in study design (NCD 2004).

Consumer-directed care has now been trialled in Australia. An early qualitative evaluation (Ottman et al 2009) indicated that CDC had the potential to empower people with disabilities and their carers. In 2010–11 and 2011–12 the Innovative Pool Program funded 1,000 consumer-directed care (CDC) packages and 400 consumer-directed respite care (CDRC) packages. The evaluation of this initiative (KPMG 2012) set out to assess the effectiveness of consumer-directed care approaches in the Australian community aged care context by examining the implementation, operation, impact and cost of the initiative. The predominant model implemented here offered participants 'enhanced choice' (KPMG 2012) of supports with providers maintaining responsibility for coordinating and managing packages. Other models incorporated different levels of participant control and self-management. As participant control increased and participants moved towards managing their package themselves, the level of support, coordination and management undertaken by providers decreased. The evaluation found that most participants were able to manage their package to some degree. However, few took on a substantial self-management role. Even after a short period of operation, CDC appeared to have a positive impact on participants' level of satisfaction with various aspects of their life, such as their ability to participate in social and community activities, and their health and wellbeing. The packages provided considerable benefits for carers from being able to plan supports and from being simply involved—sometimes for the first time—in the planning process. However, providers incurred some set-up and ongoing costs.

TARGETING

Targeting is one possible response to financial constraints. It can be defined as the principles and practices which providers adopt in making decisions about the allocation of services to individual clients and between clients among the client population they serve. Given that the resources available to HACC are limited, targeting necessarily requires consideration of the outcomes that can be achieved for different clients, taking into account their relative needs (NARI & BECC 1999).

The focus of discussion on targeting is usually at the individual client level. However, some decisions about resource allocation are also made at other levels as funds move from government to provider organisations in different regions, and from organisations to services (NARI & BECC 1999). These levels of decision-making shape the level and mix of services that can ultimately be allocated to clients and carers. Decisions made by providers about allocating resources in smaller or larger amounts to one or another individual client cannot be considered in isolation from the other levels of decision-making. Even at the individual client level, resource allocation decisions are not one-off, but repeated as the client moves along the pathway from initial eligibility for service, to assessment and care planning, to possible review and re-assessment, and to eventual discharge when the service is no longer needed or because of a change in care arrangements or move to residential care (NARI & BECC 1999).

The debate about targeting of community care services in the US began in the 1980s when extensive demonstration projects that aimed to establish whether community care could reduce the use of nursing home care were initiated under the umbrella of the National Long-Term Care Channelling Demonstration. By the early 1990s, a large body of literature reporting evaluations of these projects was available. The results of most of these evaluations—based largely on aggregate accounts of outcomes for total client populations—were, at best, ambiguous. The failure to produce more conclusive results was frequently attributed to poor targeting. Calls for 'better' targeting in turn opened up discussion as to what this might mean and how it could be achieved (Howe et al 2006).

More convincing evidence of the effectiveness of community care began to emerge from a modelling exercise using data from the Channelling

Demonstration (Greene et al 1995). The authors argued that much of the failure to find convincing evidence for the efficacy of community care was due to design shortcomings in most of the earlier evaluations, particularly the failure to disaggregate the effects of particular kinds of services for particular groups of clients. Greene et al (1995) went on to develop a transition probability model and used data from the Channelling projects to show more effective outcomes could have been achieved with different distribution of the same resources.

The most recent formulation of the targeting debate in the US was set out by Weissert et al (2003), who analysed home and community care in the US over more than three decades, discussed several longstanding shortcomings in existing targeting policy, and proposed an alternative called 'titrating'. This model suggests that simple 'in or out' targeting should be replaced with an approach that takes account of the effectiveness (E) of home care services in mitigating the risks, the risk (R) of adverse outcomes and the value (V) of the outcomes achieved relative to those avoided. The ERV model calls for titrating care rather than targeting clients. The proposed titrating model would be generous in eligibility—that is, access to services would be relatively easy—but the number of resources actually allocated to each client would be carefully calibrated. The ERV model does not deny any services to low dependency clients, but allocates more services to high dependency clients only when the additional inputs will achieve a cost effective reduction in risk of an adverse outcome.

Robust evidence from diverse studies shows that small amounts of service, provided early, are worthwhile. Provision of small amounts of service is effective in restoring functional decline in particular, and also protects against a range of adverse outcomes. Elkan et al (2001) provided an excellent systematic review and meta-analysis of the impact of home-based support on older people. They reviewed 15 studies of home visiting, of which 13 were randomised controlled trials and two were quasi-experimental designs. The home visit could comprise of surveillance, support, health promotion, and the prevention of ill health, but excluded specialist visits such as district nursing or community psychiatric nursing. The study demonstrated a positive impact of home visits on reducing mortality and admission to residential care. The effectiveness of an intervention did not depend on whether it was targeted at at-risk older people or more widely.

The evidence of the benefits to clients of using only limited services is particularly strong in comparison to those using no services and reporting unmet need for assistance. In Australia and elsewhere, many of those receiving no formal assistance are at high levels of dependency and so face considerable risks of adverse outcomes.

Specific allied health interventions are among those for which there is strong evidence of positive outcomes. For example, Lin et al (2004) demonstrated the effect of low intensity home-based physical therapy (only once a week for 10 weeks) on activities of daily living and physical motor function in clients who had suffered a stroke. A Cochrane collaboration meta-analysis showed that individual exercise programs, as well as group programs and tai chi, are effective in reducing falls and the risk of falling in older people living in the community (Gillespie et al 2009). These and similar studies support the development of more active interventions within the HACC system to support client independence. The evidence to support the benefits of aids and equipment is also strong, particularly to support walking among the population aged 80 years and over (Freedman et al 2006).

The evidence for case management is more mixed. However, some studies have shown that provision of case-managed services can delay admission to residential care for people with dementia. In the UK, for example, Challis et al (2002) showed that fewer people in an intervention group that received intensive case management were admitted to residential care during a two-year period than people in a control group. In the US, Gaugler et al (2005) analysed data on more than 4700 carers and 5300 care recipients. They showed that early use of community services is likely to be of more benefit both for carers and care recipients than if service use is delayed. For carers in the earlier stages of their role, use of in-home services such as personal care or help with chores predicts a delay in admission to residential care. The authors suggested that earlier results which had shown equivocal relationships between use of community services and admission to residential care may be attributed to the studies' lack of consideration of the timing of service provision.

In Australia Doyle et al (2005) reviewed the literature on the use of case management for people with dementia living in the community. They concluded that although earlier studies indicated that case management could precipitate admission to residential care, more recent studies have generally found that case management delays admission. Importantly, some evidence indicates that the earlier community services are provided, the longer the delay in admitting a person with dementia to residential care.

The evidence is mixed in relation to the outcomes of additional levels of services, including case management. An underlying reason for limited success is that higher levels of service provision are generally associated with higher levels of dependency, making it increasingly difficult for additional services to moderate the effects of multiple dependencies. A second reason is the lack of consistency in allocation of services to clients; variations in provision are often unrelated to client dependency or other relevant characteristics.

The evidence suggests that a combination of strategies that maintain the current broad-based eligibility and access to the basic tier of services, and a refinement of comprehensive assessment and access to progressively higher levels of care, could achieve more consistency in access and improved effectiveness of service delivery at different levels of care.

THE ROLE OF ASSESSMENT

A shift towards restorative models of service provision has demanded a change in assessment practices. However, by itself, assessment of older people requiring care is a valued service that may lead to positive outcomes. Randomised controlled trials have shown that comprehensive assessment of older people has demonstrated benefits in terms of functional status and quality of life (Kuo et al 2004). Among well-functioning older people, comprehensive assessment can delay the onset of disability (Büla et al 1999) and reduce re-admission to acute care. For example, Caplan et al (2004) reported a randomised controlled trial of elderly patients at Prince of Wales Hospital, Sydney, who, on discharge, either received a comprehensive geriatric assessment and interventions or the usual care. Patients who received a comprehensive geriatric assessment as well as a multidisciplinary intervention maintained physical and mental function better than those who did not. The authors recommended that all patients aged over 75 presenting to an emergency department should be referred for comprehensive assessment.

A shift towards restorative models of service provision has demanded a change in assessment practices.

While the major provider of assessment services in Australia, the ACAP is not the only provider. The complexity and potential duplication of assessment processes for older adults within the community sector was analysed by Eagar et al (2005), who identified at least eight types of assessment ranging from collection of basic demographic and personal information to determine eligibility for specific services to wide-ranging in-depth assessment across physical, social, and psychological and cognitive function. Multiple assessment systems and tools are employed in the community aged care sector with wide variation in the use of standardised assessment procedures. For example, the screening tools that are widely used in HACC, the ACAP assessment and CACP assessment differ substantially from one another (AIHW 2004). Foreman et al (2004) reported a similar high level of variation between regions and providers in comprehensive assessment processes, tools, point of entry and balance between breadth and depth.

As noted previously, a move to more standardised and integrated approaches to assessment has been a theme of the reform agenda, along with what is being assessed and how the assessment is conducted. Assessment, no matter how streamlined and standardised, is only useful to the extent that it can inform effective service provision. The challenge for the current assessment reform agenda is not only to improve assessment processes in terms of reducing duplication of assessment, introducing more standard, valid and reliable processes, and facilitating transfer of assessment information between care settings and care episodes, but also to deliver assessment outcomes that can contribute to the new models of care emerging in the sector. This means moving away from reliance on a deficit-focused assessment and towards an approach that encompasses client strengths and assets and informs goal-setting that is client-centred and restorative in nature. In addition, assessment processes should recognise that, for a frail older person, as care needs change with time so assessment processes need to be both progressive (more information will be required over time as the older person's support needs increase), and recursive (the person's status in relation to service requirement should be reviewed on a regular basis).

In an attempt to move assessment away from a deficit model, Victoria has introduced the Living at Home Assessment (LAHA) as part of the HACC program. This person-centred assessment of the person and their family or carer's needs leads to a care plan and individualised service responses (Department of Health 2012b). The first step in implementation of the HACC Assessment Framework was to designate 100 HACC-funded organisations as

HACC Assessment Services. A mix of local councils, health and community health services, nursing services, Aboriginal community controlled organisations and community service organisations were so designated early in 2008.

THE PRODUCTIVITY COMMISSION REVIEW AND AUSTRALIAN GOVERNMENT RESPONSE

The National Health and Hospitals Reform Commission, in its report *A Healthier Future for All Australians* (2009), indicated that the aged care system needed significant reform to meet the challenges of an older and increasingly diverse population. In response, the Australian Government commissioned the Productivity Commission to develop detailed options for redesigning Australia's aged care system to ensure that it could meet the challenges it will face in coming decades. In 2010–11 the Productivity Commission conducted an extensive public inquiry into the future of aged care in Australia. In the course of this inquiry, the commission consulted widely with older Australians, their carers, aged care providers, government agencies and other interested parties. The PC released a final report in August 2011 (Productivity Commission 2011). This report highlighted a significant number of challenges in the aged care system. It described the system as difficult to navigate, and services and consumer choice as limited. The quality of services is variable, with inconsistencies and inequities in coverage of needs, pricing, subsidies and user co-contributions. Workforce shortages are exacerbated by low wages, and some workers in the system have insufficient skills to meet the tasks they are required to perform.

The Productivity Commission's report included a series of recommendations in 10 key areas, which included: funding mechanisms; the nature and quality of care and housing services; an emphasis on diversity; support for carers and volunteers; the need for better policy research and evaluation; and a possible implementation timetable. Importantly, the PC recommended that there be a single gateway for accessing services, a single system of integrated and flexible care packages, and a focus on re-ablement. The Productivity Commission also recommended that the basis for provision of aged care services shift from a rationed system to an entitlement-based one in which people would be funded to receive care and support according to their assessed needs.

The Australian Government responded to the Productivity Commission's report firstly with a series of community consultations by Minister Butler and COTA (Council on the Ageing 2012) and secondly with a policy initiative: Living Longer Living Better. This aged care reform package is intended to 'build a responsive, integrated, consumer-centred and sustainable aged care system, designed to meet the challenges of population ageing and ensure ongoing innovation and improvement (Department of Health and Ageing 2012a p 16).

Other key government directions include a range of proposals to assist people to remain living at home, to support carers, to change the funding of residential care, to up-skill the workforce, and to promote research and evaluation. Special areas of attention include better healthcare, including primary care, tele-health and palliative care, and attention to dementia and diversity. The government has proposed new ways to access the system, including a national call centre and a My Aged Care website. Finally, the government has endorsed a positive ageing agenda.

The government has recognised that limited data and evidence are available in aged care. This means that both providers and users of aged care are not as well informed as they could be in making decisions about care and support needs. More research is needed to evaluate current services and to provide an evidence base for future directions.

The reforms will be implemented in three phases from 2013–14 to 2021–22 and include funds to support the development of more residential aged care facilities in areas of greatest need (including rural and remote areas) and to expand home care services. Two new types of home care packages will be introduced from July 2013 to allow a seamless continuum of care at home. The new packages will support people with basic and intermediate care needs and will complement the existing CACP and EACH packages. A new dementia supplement will also be introduced from July 2013 to support people with dementia receiving care at home and in residential care settings (AIHW 2012).

There has been broad agreement with the government on the general direction set in the new policy. In mid-2012, Kendig commented:

> The reforms outlined in the Living Longer Living Better report align with important values about what older people (and their carers) want—to stay in their own homes for as long as possible. There's an emphasis on a fairer, more accountable, and more sustainable financial system. Inconsistencies in existing funding arrangements will be addressed and consumer protections strengthened. And the proposed Gateway and My Aged Care website service have potential to improve transparency and access to services.

(Kendig 2012)

However, since then, aspects of the implementation of the policy, including the redirection of funds away from residential care to workforce training, have become highly contested. In addition, it is not clear to what degree the current Opposition would implement Living Longer Living Better if elected. Without bi-partisan political support, it is difficult to know what the future of the policy reforms might be.

CONCLUSION

Community care is an essential and growing component of aged care services in Australia. Demand for community services is likely to grow in response to population ageing and this growth in demand is likely to be accelerated if existing social and demographic trends result in decreased availability of informal carers, as has been predicted. Moreover, future users of community care services are likely to have more complex and diverse needs as the current trends in dependency levels among community-dwelling older Australians and differential ageing rates among different migrant groups in Australia carry forward into the future as expected. Increased demand on community aged care service will continue to direct attention to the need to develop effective strategies that ensure the best use of funds and to the related but more general question of what we should be trying to achieve through the provision of such services.

The challenge for the community care sector in this context is to ensure the projected expansion of community care occurs in parallel with movement towards more coordinated, responsive effective care that enhances the autonomy and dignity of older Australians. Emerging models of care which are more closely aligned with broader conceptualisation of positive ageing and client-centred and consumer-directed care provide examples of what may be possible in terms of service delivery and point the way for development of the sector. It is to be hoped that the broad directions pointed out by the Productivity Commission's review will guide change and reform in community aged care in coming years.

Reflective questions

1. The three key pillars of active ageing (WHO 2002) will impact on the ways in which services are delivered in Australia. How can local communities act to facilitate these positive changes?

2. If participation is the most important way to improve a sense of wellbeing and improve social inclusion, then a funding shift will need to occur. What impact will this have on services?

3. Promoting wellness and independence through a restorative approach to care is an exciting approach and is already affecting service delivery in Australia. What barriers might prevent this approach reaching its full potential?

4. In Australia, an entitlement approach may well replace rationing in community aged care. What are the costs and benefits of this approach for older individuals and service providers?

References

Agree, E.M., Freedman, V.A., Cornman, J.C., et al., 2005. Reconsidering substitution in long-term care: when does assistive technology take the place of personal care? The Journals of Gerontology Series B: Psychological Sciences and Social Sciences 60, S272–S280.

Australian Bureau of Statistics, 2009. Disability, ageing and carers, Australia: summary of findings, 2003, Cat. No. 4430.0. Online. Available: http://www.abs.gov.au/AUSSTATS/abs@.nsf/DetailsPage/4430.02009?OpenDocument, 24 Apr 2013.

Australian Institute of Health and Welfare, 2004. The comparability of dependency information across three aged and community care programs. AIHW Cat, No. AGE 36. Canberra.

Australian Institute of Health and Welfare, 2007. Older Australia at a glance. AIHW Cat, No. AGE 52. Canberra.

Australian Institute of Health and Welfare, 2012. Aged care packages in the community 2010–11: a statistical overview. Aged care statistics series no. 37. Cat. no. AGE 69. AIHW, Canberra.

Baker, D., 2006. The science of improving function: implications for home healthcare. Journal for Healthcare Quality 28 (1), 21–28.

Browning, C., Kendig, H., 2003. Healthy ageing: a new focus on older people's health and well-being. In: Liamputtong, P., Gardner, H. (Eds.), Health care reform and the community. Oxford University Press, Sydney, pp. 182–205.

Browning, C., Kendig, H., 2004. Maximising health and well-being in older people, in hands on health promotion. In: Moodie, R., Hulme, A. (Eds.), Hands on health promotion. IP Communications, Melbourne, pp. 374–388.

Büla, C.J., Bérod, A.C., Stuck, A.E., et al., 1999. Effectiveness of preventive in-home geriatric assessment in well-functioning community-dwelling older people: secondary analysis of a randomized trial. Journal of the American Geriatrics Society 47 (4), 389–395.

Buys, L., Miller, E., 2006. The meaning of 'active ageing' to older Australians: exploring the relative importance of health, participation and security. Refereed proceedings of the 39th Australian Association of Gerontology Conference, Sydney, Australia.

Caplan, G.A., Williams, A., Daly, B., et al., 2004. A randomised controlled trial of comprehensive geriatric assessment and follow up after discharge of elderly from the Emergency Department—The DEED II study. Journal of the American Geriatrics Society 52 (9), 1417–1423.

Challis, D., von Abendorff, R., Brown, P., et al., 2002. Care management, dementia care and specialist mental health services: an evaluation. International Journal of Geriatric Psychiatry 17 (4), 315–325.

Chenoweth, L., King, M.T., Jeon, Y.-H., et al., 2009. Caring for Aged Dementia Care Resident Study (CADRES) of person-centred care, dementia-care mapping, and usual care in dementia: A cluster-randomised trial. Lancet Neurology 8, 317–325.

Chodosh, J., Morton, S., Morjica, W., et al., 2005. Meta analysis: chronic disease self-management programs for older adults. Annuals of Internal Medicine 143, 427–438.

Clarke, L., 1995. Family care and changing family structure: bad news for the elderly? In: Allen, I., Perkins, E. (Eds.), The future of family care for older people. HMSO, London, pp. 19–49.

Cohen, M.A., Weinrobe, M., Miller, J., 2000. Informal caregivers of disabled elders with long-term care insurance. U.S. Department of Health and Human Services, Office of Disability, Aging and Long-Term Care Policy, and LifePlans, Office of Disability, Aging and Long- Term Care Policy Report: Washington, D.C.

Council on the Ageing, 2012. Summary report on the conversations on ageing. Online. Available: http://www.cota.org.au/lib/pdf/COTA_Australia/public_policy/conversations_final_report.pdf, 24 Apr 2013.

Crowther, M.R., Parker, M.W., Achenbaum, W.A., et al., 2002. Rowe and Kahn's model of successful ageing revisited: positive spirituality—the forgotten factor. The Gerontologist 42 (5), 613–620.

Cumming, E., Henry, W., 1961. Growing old. Basic Books, New York.

Davey, A., Patsios, D., 1999. Formal and informal community care to older adults: comparative analysis of the United States and Great Britain. Journal of Family and Economic Issues 20 (3), 271–299.

Department of Health and Ageing, 2010. 2009–2010 Aged care approvals round results. Australian Government, Canberra. Online. Available: www.health.gov.au/acar2009–10.

Department of Health and Ageing, 2012a. Living Longer Living Better. Australian Government, Canberra. Online. Available: http://www.health.gov.au/internet/

publications/publishing.nsf/Content/ageing-aged-care-reform-measures-toc, 24 Apr 2013.

Department of Health and Ageing, 2012b. Respite service providers' program manual. Australian Government, Canberra. Online. Available: http://www.health.gov.au/internet/main/publishing.nsf/Content/ageing-carers-nrcp.htm, 24 Apr 2013.

Department of Health, 2006. Our health, our care, our say: a new direction for community services. Department of Health, London. Online. Available: http://www.dh.gov.uk/en/Publicationsandstatistics/Publications/PublicationsPolicyAndGuidance/DH_4127453.

Department of Health, 2012a. Active service model policy context. Online. Available: http://www.health.vic.gov.au/hacc/projects/asm_policy.htm#hacc, 24 Apr 2013.

Department of Health, 2012b. Assessment in the HACC program. Online. Available: http://www.health.vic.gov.au/hacc/assessment.htm, 24 Apr 2013.

Department of Human Services, 2003. Improving care for older people: a policy for health services. State Government of Victoria, Melbourne.

Department of Human Services, 2008. Victorian HACC active service model discussion paper. State Government of Victoria, Melbourne. Online. Available: http://www.health.vic.gov.au/hacc/projects/asm_project.htm#disc, 24 Apr 2013.

Dowling, S., Manthorpe, J., Cowley, S., et al., 2006. Person-centred planning in social care: a scoping review. University of London, Joseph Rowntree Foundation, York.

Doyle, C., Ward, S., Rees, G., 2005. EACH Dementia Development Research Project: Review of Best Practice in Dementia Care. Unpublished report to Australian Department of Health and Ageing, Canberra.

Eagar, K., Owen, A., Marosszeky, N., et al., 2005. National intake assessment project: progress report on the development of the Australian Community Care Needs Assessment instrument. Centre for Health Service Development, University of Wollongong.

Elkan, R., Kendrick, D., Dewey, M., et al., 2001. Effectiveness of home-based support for older people: systematic review and meta-analysis. British Medical Journal 323 (7315), 1–8.

Foreman, P., Thomas, S., Gardner, I., 2004. The review and identification of an existing, validated, comprehensive assessment tool. Report prepared for Aged Care Branch, Victorian Department of Human Services. La Trobe University, Australian Institute for Primary Care.

Freedman, V.A., Agree, E.M., Martin, L., et al., 2006. Trends in use of assistive technology and personal care for late-life disability 1992–2001. The Gerontologist 46 (1), 124–127.

Gans, D., Silverstein, M., 2006. Norms of filial responsibility for aging parents across time and generations. Journal of Marriage and Family 68, 961–976.

Gaugler, J.E., Kane, R.L., Kane, R.A., et al., 2005. Early community-based service utilization and its effects on institutionalization in dementia caregiving. The Gerontologist 45 (2), 177–185.

Gillespie, L.D., Robertson, M.C., Gillespie, W.J., et al., 2009. Interventions for preventing falls in older people living in the community. Cochrane Database of Systematic Reviews Issue 2. Art. No.: CD007146. DOI:10.1002/14651858.CD007146.pub2.

Glendinning, C., Clarke, S., Hare, P., et al., 2008. Progress and problems in developing outcomes-focused social care services for older people in England. Health and Social Care in the Community 16, 54–63.

Glendinning, C., Jones, K., Baxter, K., et al., 2010. Home care re-ablement services: investigating the longer-term impacts (prospective longitudinal study). Working paper No. DHR 2438. Social Policy Research Unit, University of York, York UK.

Godfrey, M., 2001. Prevention: developing a framework for conceptualizing and evaluating outcomes of preventive services for older people. Health and Social Care in the Community 9 (2), 89–99.

Government of Western Australia, 2003. Active Ageing Taskforce. Report and Recommendations. Minister for Community Development, Perth.

Greene, V.L., Lovely, M.E., Miller, M., et al., 1995. Reducing nursing home use through community long-term care: an optimization analysis. Journal of Gerontology 50B (4), S259–S268.

Grundy, E., 2000. Co-residence of mid-life children with their elderly parents in England and Wales: Changes between 1981 and 1991. Population Studies 54, 193–206.

Hallberg, I.R., Kristensson, J., 2004. Preventive home care of frail older people: a review of recent case management studies. Journal of Clinical Nursing 13 (6B), 112–120.

Hancock, L., 2002. The care crunch: Changing work, families and welfare in Australia. Critical Social Policy 22, 119–140.

Home and Community Care Act 1985. Online. Available: http://www.austlii.edu.au/au/legis/cth/consol_act/hacca1985221/sch1.html, 24 Apr 2013.

Howe, A., Doyle, C., Wells, Y., 2006. Targeting in community care. Australian Department of Health and Ageing. Online. Available: http://www.health.gov.au/internet/publications/publishing.nsf/Content/ageing-twf-targeting-report.htm, 24 Apr 2013.

Kendig, H., 2012. Moving in the right direction for better aged care. Online. Available: http://theconversation.edu.au/moving-in-the-right-direction-for-better-aged-care-6582, 24 Apr 2013.

King, A.I.I., Parsons, M., Robinson, E., 2012. A restorative home care intervention in New Zealand: perceptions of paid caregivers. Health & Social Care in the Community 20, 70–79.

KPMG, 2012. Evaluation of the Consumer Directed Care Initiative. Online. Available: http://www.health.gov.au/internet/main/publishing.nsf/Content/ageing-cdc-evaluation.htm, 24 Apr 2013.

Kuo, H., Scandrett, K., Dave, J., et al., 2004. The influence of outpatient comprehensive geriatric assessment on survival: a meta-analysis. Archives of Gerontology and Geriatrics 39 (3), 245–254.

LaPlante, M.P., Kaye, S.H., Kang, T., et al., 2004. Unmet need for personal assistance services: estimating the shortfall in hours of help and adverse consequences. Journal of Gerontology 59B (2), S98–108.

Levine, C., Murray, T.H. (Eds.), 2004. The cultures of caregiving: conflict and common ground among families. JHU Press, USA.

Lewin, G., 2010. Submission to inquiry into caring for older Australians. Productivity Commission, Canberra.

Lewin, G., Vandermeulen, S., 2010. A non-randomised controlled trial of the Home Independence Program (HIP): an Australian restorative programme for older home-care clients. Health and Social Care in the Community 18, 91–99.

Lewin, G., Vandermeulen, S., Coster, C., 2006. Programs to promote independence at home: how effective are they? Silver Chain, Perth, Western Australia.

Lin, H., Hsieh, C.L., Lo, S.K., et al., 2004. Preliminary study of the effect of low-intensity home-based physical therapy in chronic stroke patients. Kaohsiung Journal of Medical Sciences 20 (1), 18–23.

Mansell, J., 2006. Deinstitutionalisation and community living: progress, problems and priorities. Journal of Intellectual and Developmental Disability 31 (2), 65–76.

Mansell, J., Beadle-Brown, J., 2004. Person-centred planning or person-centred action? Policy and practice in intellectual disability services. Journal of Applied Research in Intellectual Disabilities 17 (1), 1–9.

McLeod, B., Mair, M., 2009. Evaluation of City of Edinburgh Council Home Care Re-ablement Service. Scottish Government Social Research, Edinburgh.

McMurray, A., 2007. Community health and wellness: a socio-ecological approach. Elsevier Australia, Sydney.

McWilliam, C., Diehl-Jones, W., Jutai, J., et al., 2000. Care delivery approaches and seniors' independence. Canadian Journal of Ageing 19 (1), 101–124.

Mead, N., Bower, P., 2000. Patient-centredness: a conceptual framework and review of the empirical literature. Social Science and Medicine 51 (7), 1087–1110.

National Ageing Research Institute & Bundoora Extended Care Centre. (NARI), 1999. Targeting in the Home and Community Care Program. Aged and Community Care Services Development and Evaluation Reports, No. 37. Department of Health and Aged Care, Canberra.

National Ageing Research Institute, 2006. What is person-centred care? A literature review. NARI and Victorian Government Department of Human Services, Melbourne. Online. Available: http://www.mednwh.unimelb.edu.au/pchc/downloads/PCHC_literature_review.pdf, 24 Apr 2013.

National Centre for Social and Economic Modelling. (NATSEM), 2004. Who's going to care? Informal care and an ageing population. Author, Canberra.

National Council on Disability (NCD), 2004. Consumer-directed health care: How well does it work? Author, Texas. Online. Available: http://www.ncd.gov/publications/2004/Oct262004, 24 Apr 2013.

National Health and Hospitals Reform Commission, 2009. A healthier future for all Australians. Author, Canberra. Available at http://www.health.gov.au/internet/nhhrc/publishing.nsf/Content/nhhrc-report, 24 Apr 2013.

O'Connell, H., 2006. The WATCH project: wellness approach to community homecare Perth. Community West Inc. and Western Australian Department of Health, Home and Community Care.

Ottman, G., Laragy, C., Haddon. M., 2009. Experiences of disability consumer-directed care users in Australia: results from a longitudinal qualitative study. Health and Social Care in the Community 17, 466–475.

Parker, M.G., 2001. Sweden and the United States: is the challenge of an ageing society leading to a convergence of policy? Journal of Aging and Social Policy 12 (1), 73–90.

Peel, N., Bartlett, H., McClure, R., 2004. Healthy ageing: how is it defined and measured? Australasian Journal on Ageing 23 (3), 115–119.

Pilkington, G., 2006. Homecare re-ablement workstream: executive summary. Care Services Efficiency Delivery Program, Department of Health Kingdom, United Kingdom.

Pilkington, G., 2010. Home care re-ablement. The experience of England. Available from http://www.health.vic.gov.au/hacc/projects/asm_seminar_2010.htm, 24 Apr 2013.

Productivity Commission, 2011. Caring for older Australians: Productivity Commission Inquiry report. Online. Available: http://www.pc.gov.au/projects/ inquiry/aged-care, 24 Apr 2013.

Productivity Commission, 2012. Report on Government Services 2012. Australian Government, Canberra. Online. Available: http://www.pc.gov.au/gsp/rogs/2012, 24 Apr 2013.

Retirement Villages Association, 2010. Caring for older Australians: submission to the Productivity Commission. Online. Available: http://www.pc.gov.au/__data/assets/ pdf_file/0008/102131/sub424.pdf, 24 Apr 2013.

Rowland, D., 2007. Historical trends in childlessness. Journal of Family Issues 28, 1311–1337.

Ryburn, B., Wells, Y., Foreman, P., 2009. Enabling independence: restorative home care provision for frail older adults. Journal of Health and Social Care in the Community 17, 225–234.

Seeman, T.E., Crimmins, E., 2001. Social environment effects on health and aging: integrating epidemiological and demographic approaches and perspectives. In: Weinstein, M., Hermalin, A.I., Stoto, M.A. (Eds.), Population health and aging: strengthening the dialogue between epidemiology and demography, vol. 954. Annals of the New York Academy of Sciences, pp. 88–117.

Silver Chain, 2007. Home independence program: user manual, Silver Chain Nursing Association. Silver Chain, Western Australia.

Someya, Y., Wells, Y., 2008. Current issues on ageing in Japan: a comparison with Australia. Australasian Journal on Ageing 27, 8–13.

Tennstedt, S., Harrow, B., Crawford, S., 1996. Informal care vs. formal services: changes in patterns of care over time. Journal of Social Policy and Aging 7 (3–4), 71–91.

Tilly, J., Rees, G., 2007. Consumer-directed care: a way to empower consumers? Alzheimer's Australia, Melbourne.

Trewin, D. (Ed.), 2001. 2001 Year Book Australia, No. 83. Australian Bureau of Statistics, Canberra.

Ware, Jr., J.E., 2002. Identifying populations at risk: functional impairment and emotional distress. Managed Care 11 (Suppl. 10), 15–17.

Weissert, W.G., Chernew, M., Hirth, R., 2003. Titrating versus targeting home care services to frail elderly clients: an application of agency theory and cost-benefit analysis to home care policy. Journal of Aging and Health 15 (1), 99–123.

Wittenberg, R., Comas-Herrera, A., Pickard, L., et al., 2004. Future demand for long-term care in the UK: a summary of projections of long-term care finance for older people to 2051. Joseph Rowntree Foundation, UK.

Wolfensberger, W., 1972. The principle of normalisation in human services. National Institute on Mental Retardation, Toronto.

World Health Organization, 2002. Active ageing: a policy framework. World Health Organization, Ageing and Life Course Programme, Madrid.

World Health Organization, 2007. Global age-friendly cities: a guide. WHO, Geneva. Online. Available: http://www.who.int/ageing/publications/age_friendly_cities_ guide/en/index.html, 24 Apr 2013.

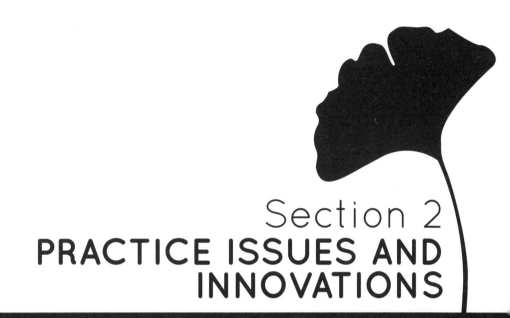

Section 2
PRACTICE ISSUES AND INNOVATIONS

CHAPTER 7

PERSON-CENTRED CARE

Rhonda Nay, Deirdre Fetherstonhaugh and
Margaret Winbolt

Editors' comments

*Person-centred care is the ideal approach to practice informing this book. It has its
roots in the work of Carl Rogers and his client-centred counselling. Understanding
how this approach differs from task- or disease-focused care is essential for contemporary health professionals. Although applicable to all care contexts, person-centred
care (or the lack of it) is perhaps best illuminated in care of people with dementia.
It is useful to have some way of deciding how you or your organisation is tracking
in terms of person-centred care and the chapter also provides a summary of
evidence-based tools that were developed by the authors for this purpose.*

INTRODUCTION

Healthcare has a long tradition of medicalising illness (Illich 1975). Parsons
(1951) wrote extensively on the 'sick role', which essentially placed the health
professional as the expert in a position of power over the patient. The patient[1]
was expected to hand over their body to the experts and unquestioningly be
compliant with 'orders' given in order to regain health. Noncompliance was
frowned upon and any patient behaving in this way was labelled as difficult.
The doctor determined healthcare goals for the patient and they were related to
curing disease. Care decisions were based on tradition and experience.

....
[1] The term 'patient' is used here in line with Parsons' sick role; however, elsewhere in the chapter, rather than
move between patient (in hospital), client (community) and resident (nursing home), the term 'person' will
be used as it is consistent with the person being more than the role they happen to be in relation to a health
professional.

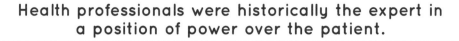

Health professionals were historically the expert in a position of power over the patient.

Nurses and other health professionals were also required to follow doctors' orders. There was a distinct hierarchy, with doctors at the pinnacle and patients at the bottom, and very clear boundaries determined who did what, who gave orders and who took them. The organisation of hospital and nursing home care reflected staff need and convenience—often to the extent that patients were dehumanised and deliberately stripped of identity (Goffman 1968). It was thought that objectified patients and detached staff facilitated good care in what could be otherwise distressing and embarrassing circumstances. Patients in hospital were typically referred to according to their disease or bed number (e.g. 'the stroke in bed 20') or the tasks health professionals did for them (e.g. 'she's a feed', 'he's a shower'). The emphasis was on the person's deficits and problems.

In these circumstances, older people were relegated to the backwards and side verandahs where a visit from the 'old man's friend'—pneumonia—would herald their demise. This was preferable to the 'usual care' production line of shivering, semi-naked bodies lined up awaiting a shower, the constant drug-induced state of confusion, or the abject horror of being manacled.

Some may argue the healthcare system has not changed much; others will not believe it was ever this bad. Nevertheless, expectations, policies and rhetoric now demand a very different approach to healthcare, and this chapter aims to outline current thinking on how health professionals should practise in partnerships with people to whom they provide treatment and care. A vignette (later in this chapter) will illuminate innovations, successes and failures.

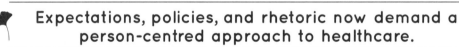

Expectations, policies, and rhetoric now demand a person-centred approach to healthcare.

SO WHAT IS PERSON-CENTRED CARE?

There are many definitions of person-centred care (PCC) and different terminology is used to describe what appears to be directed towards a similar outcome; such examples include demand-driven care, client-managed care and relationship-centred care. Carl Rogers (1961) is probably 'the father' of PCC. He coined the term and developed the notion of 'client-centred counselling'—and drew attention to the need for a rebalancing of the expert–client relationship to privilege the client and acknowledge their capacity for self-actualisation. Tom Kitwood (1997) adapted these ideas to the dementia care setting. The idea of person-centred and indeed client-directed care now have broad appeal; the rhetoric has crept into policy documents (Department of Human Services 2003) and the mission, visions and values statements of organisations. Essential to the definition of PCC we subscribe to is 'the need for a recognition of, and connection with, the *person*, a focus on the person's strengths and goals, an interdisciplinary approach, and recognition of the centrality of relationships' (Nay et al 2009 p 116).

> **Essential to the definition of person-centred care we subscribe to is the need for a recognition of, and connection with, the *person*, a focus on the person's strengths and goals, an interdisciplinary approach, and recognition of the centrality of relationships.**

Edvardsson and colleagues (2008), from a review of the literature on PCC of people with dementia, described the defining characteristics of the concept of PCC as:

- acknowledging the individual as an 'experiencing' person in spite of the disease
- offering and respecting the person's choices
- using the person's history and biography in care
- focusing on abilities rather than disabilities
- supporting individual rights, values and beliefs
- providing unconditional positive regard
- interpreting all behaviour as meaningful
- maximising potential and providing shared decision making.

Edvardsson et al also noted that much of the literature on PCC reports clinical experiences, personal opinions and anecdotal evidence and that there were few theoretically and empirically rigorous studies. The review therefore concluded that few valid reliable and clinically useful tools had been developed for measuring PCC. As a consequence associations between PCC and health outcomes have been relatively unexplored and strategies for clinical delivery and implementation of PCC are still in development. Nevertheless it does seem that physical and social environments play important roles in supporting or undermining PCC (see Ch 21).

> **Associations between person-centred care and health outcomes have been relatively unexplored and strategies for clinical delivery and implementation of PCC are still in development.**

PERSON-CENTRED CARE

Arguably, the care of people with dementia consists of the environment, the climate, the 'doing' and most importantly the *being*[2] needed to satisfy human needs. The environment can be frustrating and reduce the person's potential,

....

[2] We cannot begin to explain Heidegger's (1962) work on *being* here; however, of significance to PCC is his recognition of how the person is always historically situated and *being* is who or how we are in the world. To be human is to be connected temporally, spatially and historically. Humans are 'in the world' in a way objects are not.

or supportive of exercising maximum capacity. The climate may be likened to the ambient temperature: do we feel hot or cold; are we feeling drained and just wanting to lie in a cool place or full of energy? Similarly the care climate may be relaxed, fun, supportive of staff, welcoming of family or feel tense, be under- or over-stimulating, risk averse and conflict ridden. The latter is likely to increase confusion in the person with dementia. *Doing* consists of care tasks that need to be performed, for example, assisting with showering, toileting, and eating, and *being* is informed by all of these and the relationship (or lack thereof) that is formed between the staff member and the person with dementia. The *being* dimension of care can be understood as the way in which the tasks are performed. Have you ever been waiting in line at a shop while the staff member is on the phone totally ignoring you? It is likely you become frustrated, angry and may even leave. Or, same place, same person and he looks at you, acknowledges you are waiting and apologises, saying he will only be a moment. In the latter case, your frustration and anger probably evaporate and you are prepared to wait. In the second case you felt there had been a connection with you as a person. In the former you felt like an object getting in the way of his phone call! These examples are given to illuminate that PCC is not just about 'putting the person at centre of care' but is a total experience with all of the subtle qualities involved. The subtle qualities of connecting when carrying out tasks are of utmost importance to whether care is experienced as person-centred or task-oriented.

Language is also vital to connection. Let's look at the following vignette.

Vignette

At handover:

'Martha was a placement from hospital. She has to be restrained for now anyway. The family said she's used to it in the ward.

She is constipated, aggressive and a two-person transfer [failed rehab]. She is a feed, incontinent and be careful cos she makes balls of her faeces and throws them at you! She screams endlessly. Good luck with her!!'

or

'Martha comes from Kew; she spent her life working for charities. Martha is a very smart dresser and likes her hair plaited at night. She has the most beautiful smile and has been diagnosed with dementia. She has come to us from hospital very constipated and has been trying to self-evacuate. She is also reluctant to move and seems to be in pain. We have started her on an assessment and bowel regimen as well as immediate analgesia while we assess when the pain is occurring and what type of pain it is.

She loves you to make eye contact and joke with her. Her family brings in stewed fruit, which she eats with no trouble. Provided we ensure her hands are clean she also enjoys some finger foods.

They had bed rails at the hospital but we have settled her into a low bed and she seems very happy.'

What we see here in the first example is language objectifying: humans are not 'handed over' and they are not 'placed' like a book; and we do not speak of 'feeding' when it is time to eat! We certainly do not restrain unless life depends upon it. Constipation and refusal to 'cooperate' require assessment. 'Aggression' can mean different things to different people. Martha was not 'aggressive' but responding quite appropriately in trying to prevent staff from increasing her pain.

The alternative scenario demonstrates the recognition that Martha is not an object but a *being*—very much part of the world. How she is can only be understood by knowing how she is situated and what experiences ground her.

The environment, the *doing* and *being* of people therein interact and together form the climate of a care setting—a climate that can support or obstruct experiences of *being* a person, especially if one is frail, confused and dependent upon others (Edvardsson 2005, Rasmussen & Edvardsson 2007, Sandman et al 2006).

Now let's look at another situation where the author is a nurse, undertands PCC and reflects upon her own experience as a patient. As you read this vignette think about whether you have had similar experiences on either side of the 'bed'.

Vignette

Knowing the rhetoric and experiencing reality

Recognising and connecting with the person are the key elements of PCC (Nay et al 2009) but personal experience demonstrated to me how quickly and unintentionally a person can be stripped of what Kitwood (1997) described as their 'personhood'.

Through the noise of the crowded waiting room I hear my name. I look around and see a nurse in the doorway and rise to meet her. Without a glance or a word she turns and heads back through the doorway into the treatment room. I can only assume that I should follow her. We enter the large treatment room and I am instantly overwhelmed by the scene: four or five people scattered on chairs and couches, nurses and doctors rushing around, a radio screaming in the corner. As I hesitate, the nurse turns and shouts 'sit over there'. Obediently and without question or comment and feeling like a naughty child, I do as I'm told.

My feelings of anxiety, helplessness and isolation increase amid the business of the room and I long for someone to acknowledge my presence, if not me as a person. I look up and a doctor is standing across the room holding a medical file and seemingly searching the room. He turns to a nurse and shows her the file. The nurse glances at the file, looks around the room, points a finger in my direction and I hear her say 'the arm in the red chair'.

The words resonate through me and I fear I will cry: I am no one, nothing, dehumanised; just an injured arm.

I was then, and remain, surprised at the depth of my response to these words. I've spent all my working life in or around hospitals and know the nurse meant no harm and was only responding to the doctor's question as to my whereabouts. I have given much thought as to why this seemingly harmless situation had such an impact on me and can only conclude that it was because I was in pain, already feeling vulnerable and disempowered and these few words brought this to a head.

I have also reflected on what could have been different and believe changing the words slightly is all that would have been required. Using my name would have been ideal but simply saying 'she's in the red chair' would have sufficed as this at least acknowledged me as a person and as being more than an injured arm.

Time, resources and the physical environment are often cited as barriers to PCC but, from my perspective, the presence of these limitations would have been irrelevant and the whole experience different if staff had an awareness of the impact of the environment and their behaviour on the individual and exhibited a degree of empathy. Being greeted with a smile, by name and requests not orders are all that would have been required. This approach takes no more time and costs nothing yet their positive impact on the individual cannot be underestimated.

During this experience I met many health professionals who exemplified these aspects of PCC and whose clinical knowledge I admire but the feelings inspired by those few words remain with me; feelings I doubt I will ever forget.

It is incomprehensible to us that health professionals still behave this way. 'Everyone' is talking and writing about being person-centred. How can you know if they really are and if they are improving? How might you benchmark (National Ageing Research Institute 2006)? We need to be able to measure it.

 Environment, climate, *being* and *doing* are all mutually constitutive aspects of person-centred care.

PERSON-CENTRED CARE: MEASURING SUCCESS IN RESIDENTIAL AGED CARE

Measuring whether an organisation is person-centred or not, or whether care interventions, education or changes in philosophy make an organisation more person-centred, requires valid and reliable tools. In 2008–09 a search through the research and grey literature found that any existing tools were too long, not specific to residential aged care and didn't have explicit items related to people with dementia; some of the included items in the tools were not relevant to the residential aged care setting. After a process of: literature review; interviews with people with dementia, carers of people with dementia who lived in residential aged care and care staff who worked in residential aged care; and four drafts with several rounds with a international Delphi panel, two measuring tools were developed and validated. The first tool, the P-CAT (Person-Centred Assessment Tool), has 13 items and uses a five-point Likert-type scale for scoring purposes (ranging from 1 = 'disagree completely' to 5 = 'agree completely') (Edvardsson et al 2010a, 2010b). The P-CAT measures the extent to which residential aged care staff rate their settings to be person-centred. Specifically the P-CAT measures, from a staff perspective, the extent to which care of residents is personalised, the amount of organisational support for providing PCC and environmental accessibility for residents. Analysis of responses on the P-CAT will provide a score that can be used as a baseline before a care intervention, education or change in philosophy is implemented, and then afterwards to measure its/their effect. Since the development and validation of the P-CAT in English it has been translated into several languages and has been validated in Swedish (Sjogren et al 2012). Indicative of the increasing worldwide trend towards making PCC real and measurable, instead of being just rhetoric the Australian Centre for Evidence Based Aged Care (ACEBAC) has had numerous requests both nationally and internationally to use the P-CAT. Research published by Edvardsson et al (2011b) using the P-CAT showed how PCC can also improve job satisfaction.

The second measurement tool, the TURNIP (Tool for Understanding Residents' Needs as Individual Persons) has 39 items and also uses a five-point Likert-type scale for scoring purposes (ranging from 1 = 'disagree completely' to 5 = 'agree completely') (Edvardsson et al 2011a). Items on the TURNIP can be used to enhance the person-centredness of facilities by having reflective group discussions with staff to identify areas of improvement and areas where better practice is embedded.

 There are now tools available and in development that allow you to measure person-centred care.

A WHOLE-OF-ORGANISATION APPROACH

Effective implementation of PCC requires a whole-of-organisation approach, from the management structures, philosophies and systems through to direct care and ancillary care services. While an individual may be able to *be* person-centred and connected to the client, this experience can be undermined if the organisation is focused only on achieving the financial bottom line. Our research indicates that an organisation committed to PCC would have the following attributes (Nay et al 2009):

- leadership that models PCC in all actions and decisions—PCC is not just pulled out of the drawer for accreditation or something staff at the bedside have to enact
- a PCC philosophy that is understood by all staff—not just a framed piece of paper to hang on the wall
- relationships across the organisation that demonstrate valuing employees as 'people'—if staff are to be person-centred they need to see the philosophy modelled by management
- environments that value and support clients, families and staff and acknowledge the importance of supportive relationships to healing and wellbeing
- flexible systems and processes that enable—or indeed force—staff to move away from a task/disease orientation; for example, documentation focused on the 'doctor's orders' and 'nursing plan' and written about the client will invite medico-centric care, whereas PCC documentation that includes language such as the person's goals, strengths and values reflects and invites a focus on the human being and involvement in decision making about their life.

Effective implementation of person-centred care
requires a whole-of-organisation approach.

PRACTICAL APPROACHES TO FOSTER PERSON-CENTRED CARE AT A LOCAL UNIT LEVEL

When discussing PCC and its implementation with health professionals and care staff, they often perceive the following barriers:

- providing care in a person-centred way will take more time (in the longer term PCC may actually reduce time demands on staff)
- loss of autonomy, power or professional status by staff
- lack of clear understanding of what PCC is and how it can be applied in the health or care setting
- perception of greater challenges working in a person-centred way with people who have communication difficulties
- constraints of the physically and spiritually impoverished environments in some settings.

However, each of these perceived barriers can be worked through to achieve positive outcomes for staff or carers, older people and their families. Factors considered to facilitate or support PCC are:

- having skilled, knowledgeable and enthusiastic staff, especially with good communication skills, and supporting development and sustainability of these features
- providing opportunities for involvement by the older person and their carer/family
- providing the opportunity for staff to reflect on their own values and beliefs and express their concerns
- opportunities for staff training and education, including feedback from service users
- organisational support for this approach to practice
- working in an environment of mutual respect and trust
- providing physically and emotionally enriched care environments
- treating the environment as the older person's home.

There are a number of approaches to practice change (see Nolan et al 2006 and McCormack et al 2011 for examples). In the previous edition of this book Winbolt et al (2009) outlined Translating Evidence into Agedcare Methodology (TEAM), which we developed and evaluated.

CONCLUSION

PCC is an approach to care that places the older person and their carer central to all aspects of care and related decision making. We have argued that for it to be successful there needs to be an organisation-wide approach and PCC needs to be firmly embedded in policies, systems and relationships. Although, like any change, there are barriers to implementation; each barrier can be addressed and some useful examples have been identified.

This is an emerging area of both practice and research, and although there is growing appreciation of the value and need for this approach in health services and residential care settings, there is a need for a concerted, sustained and management-supported approach for the necessary changes to be achieved on a wide scale.

Reflective questions

1. Discuss with colleagues and/or other students the ways in which your experiences of healthcare reflect the 'old days' of doctor power or the new age of PCC.

2. What do you see as the barriers or enablers to having PCC?

3. In what ways could a health professional persuade a whole-of-organisation approach to PCC?

References

Department of Human Services, 2003. Improving Care of Older People. State Government of Victoria, Melbourne.

Edvardsson, D., 2005. Atmosphere in Care Settings. Towards a Broader Understanding of the Phenomenon, Umeå University Medical Dissertations, New Series No 941. Online. Available: http://www.diva-portal.org/umu/theses/abstract.xsql?dbid=406, 24 Apr 2013.

Edvardsson, D., Fetherstonhaugh, D., McAuliffe, L., et al., 2011b. Job satisfaction amongst aged care staff: exploring the influence of person-centered care provision. International Psychogeriatrics 23 (8), 1205–1212.

Edvardsson, D., Fetherstonhaugh, D., Nay, R., 2010a. Promoting a continuation of self and normality: person-centred care as described by people with dementia, their family members and aged care staff. Journal of Clinical Nursing 19, 2611–2618.

Edvardsson, D., Fetherstonhaugh, D., Nay, R., et al., 2010b. Development and initial testing of the Person-centered Care Assessment Tool. International Psychogeriatrics 22 (1), 101–108.

Edvardsson, D., Fetherstonhaugh, D., Nay, R., 2011a. The Tool for Understanding Residents' Needs as Individual Persons (TURNIP): Construction and initial testing. Journal of Clinical Nursing 20, 2890–2896.

Edvardsson, D., Winblad, B., Sandman, P.O., 2008. Person-centred care for people with severe Alzheimer's disease—current status and ways forward. The Lancet Neurology 7, 362–367.

Goffman, E., 1968. Asylums. Penguin, New York.

Heidegger, M., 1962. Being and time translated by John Macquarrie & Edward Robinson. Basil Blackwell, Oxford.

Illich, I., 1975. Medical nemesis. Lothian, London.

Kitwood, T., 1997. Dementia reconsidered: the person comes first. OUP, Buckingham.

McCormack, B., Dewing, J., McCance, T., 2011. Developing person-centred care: addressing contextual challenges through practice development. The Online Journal of Issues in Nursing 16 (2), 3.

National Ageing Research Institute, 2006. Benchmarking person-centred care statewide survey (2005): Victoria, Australia. Report to the Victorian Government Department of Human Services. Online. Available: http://www.mednwh.unimelb.edu.au/pchc/downloads/Survey%20report%20-%20Statewide%20Final.pdf, 24 Apr 2013.

Nay, R., Bird, M., Edvardsson, D., et al., 2009. Person-centred care. In: Nay, R., Garratt, S. (Eds.), Caring for older people: issues and innovations, third ed. Elsevier, Sydney, pp. 107–119.

Nolan, M.R., Brown, J., Davies, S., et al., 2006. The Senses Framework: improving care for older people through a relationship-centred approach. Getting Research into Practice (GRiP) Report No 2. Project Report. University of Sheffield.

Parsons, T., 1951. The social system. The Free Press, Glencoe III.

Rasmussen, B., Edvardsson, D., 2007. The influence of environment in palliative care: supporting or hindering experiences of 'at-homeness'? Contemporary Nurse 27, 119–131.

Rogers, C., 1961. On becoming a person: a therapist's view of psychotherapy. Constable, London.

Sandman, P.O., Edvardsson, D., Winblad, B., 2006. Care of patients in the severe stage of dementia. In: Gauthier, S. (Ed.), Clinical diagnosis and management of Alzheimer's disease, third ed. Taylor & Francis, London, pp. 233–246.

Sjogren, K., Lindkvist, M., Sandman, P.O., et al., 2012. Psychometric evaluation of the Swedish version of the Person-Centered Care Assessment Tool (P-CAT). International Psychogeriatrics 2012 Mar; 24 (3), 406–415.

Winbolt, M., Nay, R., Fetherstonhaugh, D., 2009. Taking a TEAM (Translating Evidence into Aged care Methods) approach to practice change. In: Nay, R., Garratt, S. (Eds.), Caring for older people: issues and innovations, third ed. Elsevier, Sydney, pp. 442–455.

CHAPTER 8

UPHOLDING RIGHTS AND MANAGING RISK WHILE IMPROVING QUALITY OF CARE

Joseph Ibrahim and Marie-Claire Davis

Revised from original authors Joseph Ibrahim, Susan Koch, Anne Holland and Linsey Howie

Editors' comments

The dilemma that arises from taking risks and protecting from harm is addressed well in this chapter. The governance issue is further discussed in Chapter 20, but the relationship to risk management cannot be overemphasised. The scenario in the vignette takes the risk management approach across all sectors of healthcare and raises many issues for the care of older people. Evidence-based practice can alleviate some of the decision-making dilemma posed as staff try to do what is considered safe—and right—for clients. The nature of chronic or acute disruptions to health experienced by older people often makes their contribution to decision making difficult for staff to understand. How people live with and manage their health problems is often very different from what the professional provider thinks should be the case. Depression and dementia also changes the way in which people make decisions. Managing risks in aged care is a complex matter and one in which quality outcomes are difficult to measure.

INTRODUCTION

Improving the quality of care is an important priority for all health and aged care services. The changes required for achieving better care are being actively addressed. Improving quality and safety for older people, while upholding their rights and managing risk, is a much more complex challenge. To meet this challenge requires an understanding of the theoretical concepts and constructs of quality, risk, stakeholder rights and evidence-based practice (EBP).

This chapter begins with a vignette that follows an older person's experiences as an individual citizen, an acute hospital patient, a community service client and a resident in an aged care service. The second section addresses the basic concepts of quality, risk, rights, EBP, and related constructs. The third and fourth sections explore, respectively, the broader quality and safety context in acute healthcare and the other settings in which older people receive healthcare.

The vignette provides a practical framework that assists in understanding the theoretical concepts and how these may apply in practice. Readers are asked to reflect on the vignette throughout the chapter.

Vignette

Individual citizen

Mr M is 75 years old and lives alone in a ground-floor unit; his daughter lives close by. Mr M has the active clinical conditions of Parkinson's disease, osteoporosis, diabetes mellitus and episodes of urinary incontinence. Mr M's daughter visits him almost every day and he pays for additional community services to assist with household cleaning and to have one meal delivered daily. Mr M is an enthusiastic rose gardener and is well known for growing vegetables, which he gives to family and neighbours.

After a number of falls at home, his general practitioner (GP) organises for a consultant physician in geriatric medicine (geriatrician) to assess him. The geriatrician explains the falls are related to a combination of factors and recommends wearing hip protectors at all times to prevent a serious injury.

Mr M purchases the hip protectors and wears them for only one week. He explains this to his GP at the next routine visit.

Inpatient acute hospital care

Several weeks later, on a Sunday, Mr M's daughter finds him is a state of confusion and disorientation. A visit to an emergency department leads to an admission to hospital with a urinary tract infection that is treated with antibiotics.

Assessment on the medical ward determines that Mr M is at high risk of falls. While in hospital, a multifaceted falls prevention plan is documented and implemented. This includes wearing hip protectors and using a low-low bed.

Mr M's daughter tells the nursing staff that the hip protectors are still at home. She explains that her father no longer uses the hip protectors because they are uncomfortable and make it difficult to go to the toilet, especially when he is in a hurry. The nursing staff explain that they will assist Mr M with the hip protectors during the hospital stay, and that, due to his delirium, the risk of falls is increased.

The hospital insists and ensures Mr M wears the hip protectors during his stay.

Community care

After several days, Mr M's confusion resolves and he is deemed ready for discharge home. His daughter expresses concern about his ability to cope at home, particularly with his reduced mobility and self-care. The multidisciplinary team agree that he is at risk and a package of community supports is put in place, including personal care, a continence nurse, physiotherapy and assistance with transport.

When the community-based nurse and physiotherapist visit Mr M at home, his daughter is present. Mr M still has an unsteady gait, even with a walking aid, and is unable to negotiate the two steps to his unit without significant assistance.

The discharge summary from the hospital doesn't mention the need for hip protectors, but his daughter asks the community clinical team whether he should be wearing these at home. The physiotherapist agrees this should occur and says he will ask the personal carer to assist.

Mr M agrees to wear the hip protectors to allay the concerns of his daughter. However, he only wears them on the two days of the week that the personal carer attends.

Residential care

Mr M's mobility does not recover to pre-morbid levels. The frequency of falls increases over the following months and this results in a number of hospital attendances for minor injuries. Eventually his daughter, GP and community clinical team agree that a move to a residential aged care facility (RACF) would be appropriate.

At the time Mr M enters the RACF the facility's policies include respecting the rights of the individual residents, adherence to healthcare recommendations, promoting quality improvement and reducing preventable harm. Falls are identified as a major source of preventable harm and there is an organisation-wide campaign to promote the use of hip protectors. This is supported by the facility's board of management, which had recently resolved a medico-legal dispute following the death of another resident from a fall.

Mr M reiterates his preferences and does not agree to wear the hip protectors.

RESEARCH EVIDENCE: HIP PROTECTORS

Although early studies indicated that hip protectors were a very effective strategy for preventing fractures in older people, more recent evidence is less conclusive (Gillespie et al 2010).

A Cochrane review of 13 studies comprising 11,573 participants found that hip protectors resulted in a small but significant reduction in the incidence of hip fractures among older people in nursing or residential care settings (risk ratio 0.81, 95% confidence interval 0.66 to 0.99). However, following exclusion of five studies (3757 participants) that were assessed as being biased this statistical significance was lost (Gillespie et al 2010).

Hip protectors also appear to have no beneficial effects for older people who are living in the community (Gillespie et al 2010, Parker et al 2005). The usefulness of hip protectors in hospital settings is unclear. Multifaceted falls prevention strategies in hospitals, which may include wearing hip protectors, result in a reduced rate of falls (relative risk 0.82, 0.68–0.997), but there is no effect on fracture rate (Oliver et al 2007).

All studies report that acceptance and adherence to hip protectors is poor (Gillespie et al 2010). It is common for 30% of eligible people to decline to participate in hip protector studies, while adherence is often as low as 30% by the end of the trial (Gillespie et al 2010, Parker et al 2005).

The main reasons given for poor adherence are discomfort, poor fit and skin irritation. In residential care it appears that those with a history of falls and those who are more physically dependent demonstrate greater adherence (Cryer et al 2008, O'Halloran et al 2007). Males and those with lower limb arthritis are less likely to comply (Cryer et al 2008, Hayes et al 2008).

QUALITY, RISK, RIGHTS AND EVIDENCE-BASED PRACTICE

QUALITY

The definition of quality is central to addressing these situations and is often taken for granted because it is a word used every day. Confusion arises because we do not provide an explicit statement to achieve a common understanding.

'Quality' is defined in the Oxford English Dictionary (Sykes 1982) as 'the degree of excellence'. A more explicit definition that can be used to measure performance requires specifying to whom and how the word is used.

Quality of healthcare and quality of life

The first step is to separate and recognise the differences between 'quality of healthcare' and 'quality of life'. Arguably this is an artificial distinction because our health and quality of life are interdependent. Nevertheless, a clear definition and separation of the two concepts enable us to understand why rational professionals who are committed to EBP may deliver seemingly contradictory approaches to individuals with the same disease.

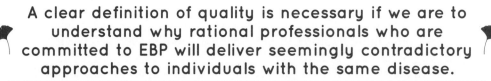

A clear definition of quality is necessary if we are to understand why rational professionals who are committed to EBP will deliver seemingly contradictory approaches to individuals with the same disease.

Quality of life is a concept that is typically applied to the individual, while quality of healthcare is a concept that is more applicable at the organisational level.

Importantly, the quality of healthcare provided does not necessarily equate to, or ensure, acceptable quality of life.

Health refers to 'a state of complete physical, mental and social wellbeing and not merely the absence of disease or infirmity' (World Health Organization 1946 p 1). By contrast, quality of healthcare refers to 'the degree to which health services for individuals and populations increase the likelihood of desired health outcomes and are consistent with current professional knowledge' (Lohr et al 1991 p 6).

The more amorphous concept of 'quality of life' incorporates mental and physical health and wellbeing as well as social and environmental aspects, and depends on subjective perception.

Quality of life means different things to different people, and changes with age. For example, older people have indicated that enjoying 'small things' takes on considerable importance later in life (Andersson et al 2008). Simple pleasures and even fleeting social interactions can carry significant meaning (Andersson et al 2008).

In making decisions that may affect an older person's quality of life we must remain cognisant that how we define quality of life for ourselves may differ considerably from how the person defines quality of life for themselves. While decreased quality of life associated with the inconvenience and discomfort of wearing hip protectors may not seem important to you or me, it may be untenable for someone whose quality of life is already poor.

Understanding the difference between quality of healthcare and quality of life are important if we are to successfully uphold a person's rights while managing risk.

RISK

Risk arises from exposure to a hazard, but exposure to a hazard may not necessarily result in negative consequences.

More specifically, risk is the 'effect of uncertainty on objectives … is often characterized by reference to potential events and consequences, or a combination of these' (Victorian Managed Insurance Authority 2010 p 9).

Risk is dynamic, context-specific and neutral in that it may relate to both positive and negative outcomes. We tend to focus on only the negative aspects of risk and forget that risk is a necessary and often beneficial part of everyday life (Morgan 2004).

If we consider the risk of both harmful and beneficial consequences associated with different decisions, we can see why sometimes contradictory yet equally reasonable approaches occur in care delivery.

Risk perception

Another factor contributing to variation in risk management approaches is how the individual or organisation perceives the hazards and associated levels of risk in each context.

The perception of risk is usually different from the actual or measurable level of risk. This is because an individual's perception of hazards and estimation of risk is influenced by past experiences, attitude, culture, inherent human frailties and biases in decision making as well as their ability to understand and interpret information (Slovic et al 2004).

 The perception of risk is usually different from the actual or measurable level of risk.

Consider what your advice to Mr M and his family would be if you had recently provided care for another older person who had fallen, fractured a hip and died. Your personal perception of the risk of negative consequences of not wearing hip protectors is likely to be exaggerated by this tragedy, therefore biasing your decision making.

Risks to different stakeholders

The other major factors to consider when examining risk are the different stakeholders involved and what each considers being a reasonable level of risk.

When we consider who is at risk we discover that it is all the people and organisations involved in providing care and not just the patient or resident.

Reflecting on the vignette, we see that Mr M is at risk of physical injury from falling but that he is also at risk of a decreased quality of life due to the discomfort and inconvenience associated with wearing hip protectors.

While Mr M may choose to accept the risk of harm and decline to wear hip protectors, on closer examination it becomes apparent that the hospital is at risk of damage to its finances and reputation if Mr M comes to harm under their care and later litigates. This may impact on the hospital's capacity to fund services in another part of the hospital.

The RACF is potentially caught in two ways. First, as mentioned, if they enforce wearing hip protectors they risk harm to their reputation and potential sanctions from regulators for failing to respect Mr M's right to accept the burden of risk.

Alternatively, if they respect Mr M's rights and he comes to harm, they risk damage to their reputation from negative media publicity, adverse professional assessment and potential sanctions for failing to foresee this outcome and reach a satisfactory compromise.

Mr M's daughter is at risk of social and emotional harm if her family and friends believe her actions are not in her father's best interests (i.e. either supporting her father's decision not to wear hip protectors or coercing him into wearing them).

Whenever we consider the risk of harm, it is important to consider the roles of all stakeholders, the potential consequences to each stakeholder and the risk or likelihood of each consequence occurring.

RIGHTS

Rights are basically a set of entitlements (e.g. legal, social, financial, health) that may apply to the individual or community (Department of Health and Ageing 2008). The nature of entitlements may vary between communities and alter with the passage of time. We consider the upholding of rights to refer to fair, just treatment and this includes the individual's entitlement to determine how they choose to live their life. As you will see, managing risk is intimately tied to the upholding or eroding of stakeholder rights.

The right to autonomy and 'dignity of risk'

Autonomy of thought and action is a fundamental human right. An individual's dignity is manifested, in part, by their autonomy. Without being permitted to take risks, an individual's autonomy and therefore their intrinsic dignity is eroded. The concept of 'dignity of risk' stems from the contribution of risk taking to an individual's dignity (Perske 1972).

Autonomy and decision-making capacity

Autonomous behaviour is predicated on the assumption that each individual possesses decision-making capacity. That is, that they understand the nature of the hazards and consequences associated with particular actions, the risk of these consequences occurring and alternative options available to them, thereby allowing them to make an informed decision.

However, decision-making capacity can be eroded or fluctuating due to mental illness or cognitive impairment.

Therefore, in balancing rights and risk we must also consider to what degree the person's decision-making capacity is affecting their ability to behave autonomously and how this will be accommodated (e.g. supported or substitute decision making). We also need to remember that individuals with severe cognitive impairments may contribute to decision-making processes, even if just by indicating their pleasure or displeasure (Darzins et al 2000).

Rights of the collective

Related to the various risks to different stakeholders is the tension between the rights of the individual and the rights of the collective.

In reflecting upon the vignette, most people would automatically focus on the rights of Mr M as the recipient of care. However, we must also consider the organisations and staff providing the care, other patients or residents, as well as those who live in the broader community who may be directly or indirectly impacted by Mr M's decisions.

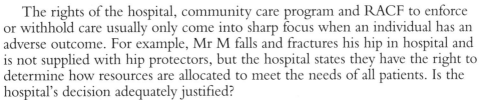

There is always a tension between respecting the rights of the individual and the rights of the collective.

The rights of the hospital, community care program and RACF to enforce or withhold care usually only come into sharp focus when an individual has an adverse outcome. For example, Mr M falls and fractures his hip in hospital and is not supplied with hip protectors, but the hospital states they have the right to determine how resources are allocated to meet the needs of all patients. Is the hospital's decision adequately justified?

Contrast this with the hospital enforcing the wearing of hip protectors against Mr M's wishes, arguing that research evidence supports the use of the equipment and that the hospital will be penalised by their regulator if they fail to apply EBP. Again, how do we judge the hospital's decision?

Our evaluation of care is often biased when we judge actions based only on outcomes. For example, let us assume Mr M receives identical treatment, be it with or without hip protectors, in residential care. He falls and sustains minor bruising and nobody gives the incident a second thought. Contrast this with the outcome of a fall causing a hip fracture that contributes directly to his death. The different outcomes completely change our judgment of the care providers' actions.

Rights and professional duty of care

Health professionals often refer to their 'duty of care' and fear of being found 'negligent' when faced with the challenge of upholding a patient's right to make autonomous decisions.

Duty of care refers to our responsibility to take reasonable care of a person and is subjugate to the broader definition of *negligence* (Department of Human Services 2000). *Negligence* involves a *breach of duty of care*—that is, when a person acts unreasonably either by commission or omission and causes injury (physical injury, 'nervous or emotional shock' or financial loss). Note that actions are only deemed unreasonable if they differ from what a hypothetically reasonable person (or professional) would do in the same situation (Department of Human Services 2000).

As health professionals we have the right to protect ourselves and our employers from legal sanction by ensuring we do not breach our duty of care. However, how can we accomplish this in a way that does not encourage an overly defensive approach to care and impingement on patient and resident rights?

EVIDENCE-BASED PRACTICE

The goal of EBP in the aged care sector is to translate clinical research into the best possible care for older people. It is highly unlikely that desired outcomes will be achieved if research evidence is applied without due regard for clinical expertise, the values and rights of the older person and/or their family, and the situational context in which the evidence needs to be implemented.

Appropriate EBP potentially reduces inconsistencies in care and supports clinical effectiveness. This supports health professionals in justifying and improving the quality of care provided.

Appropriate use of EBP potentially reduces inconsistencies in care and supports clinical effectiveness.

In evaluating research evidence on which to base our practice, we must ensure we use the best available resources. The best research evidence is:

> ... *methodologically sound, clinically relevant research about the effectiveness and safety of ... interventions, the accuracy and precision of ... assessment measures, the power of prognostic markers, the strength of causal relationships, the cost-effectiveness of ... interventions, and the meaning of illness or patient experiences.*

(DiCenso et al 2005 p 4)

PUTTING IT ALL TOGETHER

The diversity of our population who require care, and those who provide care, is a plurality of different religious and spiritual needs, socioeconomic circumstances and cultural background. Meeting the needs and expectations of those who require care presents an incredible challenge.

Blind application of clinical research evidence is insufficient to meet this challenge. EBP only provides a platform for professional decision making. Clinical practice requires research evidence to be considered in the context of an individual's right to autonomy and how healthcare affects the individual's quality of life.

Understanding and explaining the hazards and risks of harm (as well as benefit) to all concerned is a key step towards prudent and balanced decision making.

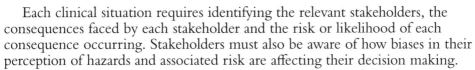

Understanding and explaining the hazards and risks of harm (as well as benefit) to all concerned is a key step towards prudent and balanced decision making.

Each clinical situation requires identifying the relevant stakeholders, the consequences faced by each stakeholder and the risk or likelihood of each consequence occurring. Stakeholders must also be aware of how biases in their perception of hazards and associated risk are affecting their decision making.

Box 8.1 proposes a step-by-step approach to decision making that attempts to balance the rights of different stakeholders while also managing risk of negative consequences.

THE BROADER CONTEXT: IMPROVING QUALITY OF CARE

Upholding stakeholder rights and managing risk occurs within broader quality of care systems. This broader context is explored in the following sections.

A SYSTEMS APPROACH

Success in improving the quality and safety of care is usually predicated on a systems approach to risk management—that is, the safety of an individual is improved by reducing the risk in a population (Corrigan et al 2001).

Healthcare is now recognised as a high-risk environment with significant levels of preventable patient injury and death. The United States (US) Institute of Medicine suggests that deaths due to healthcare are among the top 10 causes of death (Kohn et al 1999).

Most researchers agree that approximately 10% of hospital admissions are associated with an adverse event. These findings have been replicated throughout the Western world, including Australia (Wilson et al 1995), Canada (7.5%; Baker et al 2004), the United Kingdom (UK) (10.8%; Vincent et al 2001), New Zealand (10.7%; Davis 2001 et al), and the US (2.9% to 17.7%; Andrews et al 1997, Brennan et al 1991, Thomas et al 2000). These events cost billions of dollars each year and cause significant morbidity and mortality.

Box 8.1

Proposed step-by-step approach to balancing rights and risk in decision making

Step 1: Define the proposed action and reasons for the proposed action.

Step 2: List the stakeholders affected by the proposed action.

Step 3: Define hazards and reasonably foreseeable negative and positive consequences to each stakeholder if exposed to each hazard. What is the risk or likelihood of each consequence?

Step 4: Detail reasonable strategies that may be implemented in order to manage the risk of negative consequences occurring, along with strategies to minimise the harm experienced if negative consequences do eventuate.

Step 5: *Using this information:* Is each stakeholder willing and able to accept the burden of risk?

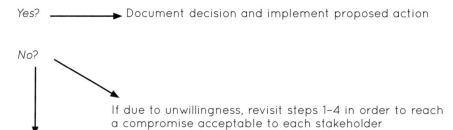

Yes? ⟶ Document decision and implement proposed action

No?

If due to unwillingness, revisit steps 1–4 in order to reach a compromise acceptable to each stakeholder

If due to a lack of decision-making capacity, determine if another party will accept the burden of risk on behalf of the person lacking capacity (i.e. a power of attorney, guardian or administrator). If nobody will accept the burden of risk, revisit steps 1–4 in order to reach a compromise acceptable to the patient or resident and their substitute decision maker.

The concept of a systems approach is a recent phenomenon in healthcare and draws from quality improvement efforts within the manufacturing industry and risk management strategies to reduce adverse events in the aviation industry.

SYSTEMS OF CARE

Improving care and preventing harm for patients requires a systems approach to care—that is, a shift from expecting individual health providers to be perfect in knowing and applying EBP to a situation where the working environment supports, trains and ensures EBP is the norm irrespective of the health professional delivering the care.

Improving care and preventing harm for patients requires a systems approach to care.

Although 60–80% of adverse events involve human error, the cause of the error does not lie with the individual (Kohn et al 1999); it lies with the structures and processes in place that are intended to support the provision of care. A core principle of the systems approach is that fallibility is part of being human and that the same situations provoke the same errors, regardless of who is involved.

The manufacturing industry was the first to develop the methods and statistical techniques to measure performance to ensure quality. It also developed the quality cycle (Plan-Do-Study-Act) that is now in widespread use throughout health.

The key components of quality systems in healthcare include clinical governance, a method of measuring or evaluating care and responding to improve care.

Evaluation of care occurs through a combination of clinical audit usually involving clinical record review, quality or performance indicators, patient experience surveys, medication prescribing and use of laboratory investigation, incident monitoring, credentialling, re-certification and accreditation.

Responses to improve care include developing policies, guidelines and clinical pathways, and improvements to work practice using systems thinking that simplify and standardise the approaches to care.

The most fundamental shift in developing quality systems in healthcare is the advent of clinical governance.

Governance

The concept of clinical governance is a recent phenomenon introduced into the healthcare system in the late 1990s and is the logical extension of the existing principles of corporate governance.

Corporate governance refers to the fact that the governing board of management has the ultimate responsibility or accountability for the standards and performance of the business; traditionally this focused on financial performance.

Clinical governance explicitly states that responsibility or accountability for standards and performance in clinical care rests at an organisation's board or senior management level and not at the clinician–patient level. This significant and radical shift in healthcare is now widely accepted.

The most commonly quoted definition of clinical governance is from the UK and arose as a consequence of the tragic situation at the Royal Bristol Infirmary where multiple preventable deaths following paediatric cardiac surgery occurred.

Clinical governance is 'the framework through which health organisations are accountable for continuously improving the quality of their services and safeguarding high standards of care by creating an environment in which excellence in clinical care will flourish' (Scally & Donaldson 1998 p 61).

The implication for health service boards is that they must now concern themselves with creating an environment for implementing and monitoring appropriate clinical and clinical support quality systems. This places an onus on the board to seek, review and act on their organisation's performance in the safety and quality of healthcare service.

The implication for those directly responsible for clinical services (e.g. directors of nursing) is that they have a responsibility similar to the chief financial officer of a corporation—that is, an obligation to monitor, identify, act and report on matters that impact on the overall performance of the organisation.

Effective clinical governance based on a partnership between clinicians and managers is required to address the major conditions that lead to systems that affect quality of care including: lack of senior leadership and management; poor communication and teamwork; diffusion of responsibility among multiple parties involved in the care of a patient; inadequately systematised and formalised procedures and protocols; and professional silos with entrenched hierarchies (Donaldson & Muir Gray 1998, Kohn et al 1999, West 2000).

While there may be limited evidence that good governance directly improves care outcomes (Phillips et al 2010), there is certainly evidence that poor care outcomes may arise because of poor governance (Kennedy 2001).

Measurement of care

The first two steps towards improving quality and safety of care is an understanding that we work in a complex system of care and have a functional clinical governance structure.

The third step is having a method for measuring and understanding the performance of a health service. Evaluating the quality of care begins by defining what aspects of care are to be examined. The components of the system are diverse, and it is common to focus carefully on a single component, although this often limits the amount of information available about the system as an integrated whole. To gain an understanding of the whole system requires deconstructing it.

To gain an understanding of the whole system requires deconstructing it.

The initial division is the site of service delivery: Is it inpatient hospital care, ambulatory or community-based care or within an RACF?

The next division reflects the individual or group accessing the service: the individual patient or resident, a specific patient group (e.g. people with dementia or at high risk of falls) or the entire population?

The final division is the nature of the service: Is it healthcare alone or healthcare as well as other aspects of functioning?

Reflecting on the vignette, it is obvious that measuring performance on the same component of care is both context- and setting- specific. Once the component of the system to be evaluated is determined, the next step is selecting the dimension of quality to be evaluated. A widely accepted model of quality evaluation refers to three dimensions: the structure of care, the process of care and the outcome of care (Donabedian 1966).

The structure of care refers to both the physical setting and the organisational setting in which care takes place. The process of care refers to the method of delivering care and includes the clinical history, physical examination, laboratory tests and treatment. The outcome of care refers to the wellbeing of the patient, and is usually expressed in terms of survival or restoration of function. Alternatively, the Institute of Medicine (Corrigan et al 2001) prefers a model based on multiple dimensions, and asks whether care is patient-centred, safe, timely, effective, efficient and equitable.

At present most of the work towards improving quality of care is focused on patient safety; this is especially the case in Australia, the UK and the US. Safety has achieved prominence because it is the most readily understood dimension of quality.

The principles of measuring clinical performance are well established and there are many 'quality of care indicators' available to assist in understanding and measuring care. An indicator is 'a measurable element in the process or outcome of care whose value suggests one or more dimensions of quality of care and is theoretically amenable to change by the provider' (Bernstein & Hilborne 1993).

The standards for determining the quality of care are currently defined through the use of evidence from clinical trials or peer review. However, there are still many barriers to achieving change through measurement, such as fear, cynicism and a lack of trust about the methods and purpose of measurement (Berwick 1989).

Responding to improve care

We should be cautious when interpreting the reports of performance measurements and success or failure of quality improvement initiatives from other settings. The size of an organisation, its resource base, the workforce and the role of external regulators and community expectations all play a role in the capacity, timeliness and nature of response.

Additionally, unlike other clinical interventions, improving quality and safety often require changes to our work practices, values and culture.

 Improving quality and safety often requires changes
to our work practices, values and culture.

Nevertheless, there are common situations across settings that contribute to the likelihood of human error occurring including time pressure, high workload, unworkable procedures, inadequate equipment, bad working conditions and supervisors turning a blind eye (Reason 1997).

There are also well-established principles that can assist in any quality improvement strategy. These are a systems approach with a clinical governance model, leadership, good team function, safe working conditions and work practices designed to reduce reliance on memory and increase standardisation and simplification of processes.

BALANCING RIGHTS AND RISK AT THE SYSTEMS LEVEL

The focus of quality and safety activity is often driven by service providers and based on the assumption that improving the quality of care will improve the care recipient's quality of life. Although the person and their fundamental disease afflictions remain the same, the different care settings alter the dynamics between the individual, the care provider and the organisation that employs the care provider. Understanding the underlying dynamics and tensions within and between settings clarifies why the approach to balancing rights and risk may engender quite divergent approaches.

A somewhat simplistic comparison of accreditation approaches between Australian RACFs and acute hospitals demonstrates this divergence. The accreditation requirements for an RACF are based on their performance against 44 outcomes within four standards: management systems; staffing and organisational development; health and personal care; resident lifestyle; and physical environment and safe systems (Aged Care Standards and Accreditation Agency 2008). Accreditation is mandated and is required in order to receive Australian Government funding. These accreditation standards reflect community expectations of the role of the facility as a home with direct effects on residents' quality of life and not as a healthcare service.

By contrast, the Australian accreditation requirements for healthcare organisations evaluate performance against 13 standards and 47 outcomes within the three topic areas of clinical, support and corporate (Australian Council on Healthcare Standards 2012). These accreditation standards focus on healthcare, not on quality of life.

SYSTEMS OF CARE AND AGED CARE

The need for more detailed evaluation of the care provision for older people is acknowledged, with the most obvious starting point being care in RACFs. Care of older people in acute and subacute hospital settings, as well as in general practice and community care settings, receives lower priority because of either the difficulty in measurement or a preoccupation with focusing on other patient groups.

RACFs are now an important component of the delivery of healthcare and, increasingly, the boundaries between quality of healthcare and consideration of quality of life are blurred. Measures are required for assessing quality of clinical care as well as the quality of the resident's life to ensure that quality of healthcare is not blindly pursued at the expense of quality of life.

By measuring both aspects, it is possible to gauge whether clinical risks for the population are being reduced while upholding an individual's right to decline evidence-based care if they perceive that it impinges on their quality of life.

The imperative for suitable healthcare measures continues to grow as the population ages and the health profile of older people becomes more complex.

Residents entering facilities are now more acute, with multiple comorbid chronic illnesses that include dementia, cancer, heart disease, diabetes mellitus, arthritis and depression. More than half of the residents of high-care facilities have dementia, and their age at the time of entering residential care is in the mid-80s (AIHW 2010).

The imperative for suitable healthcare measures continues to grow as the population ages.

There is increasing pressures for and reduced access to the hospital sector (including emergency departments) as innovations in the models of care such as 'hospital in the nursing home' continue to shift healthcare of older people into the community. The shift to (and expectation that GPs will provide) increasingly complex clinical care in the RACF—that is, traditionally provided in the acute or subacute hospital sector—is also contributing to the need to measure and monitor performance.

The increased therapeutic options and greater evidence knowledge base available now requires integrated care involving clinical nursing, medical care and allied healthcare within a collaborative model. This fundamentally alters the nature of aged care and health provision for older people. In an RACF this creates a contradictory blend of an acute clinical care setting for some, while others are living there because it is their home.

Ultimately, an integrated system of healthcare and aged care is required if substantial beneficial changes to the life and health of older people is to succeed. Understanding the different groups involved, their structure, workforce, method and purpose of delivering services and where they overlap and interface needs to be described, mapped and simplified. If we reflect on the vignette it is clear that there are different systems for acute, ambulatory and preventive healthcare as well as community and residential aged care.

MEASURING CARE IN AGED CARE

Limited information is readily available on the level and preventability of adverse events in community and residential aged care. The expectation is that there are similar issues as reported in the acute healthcare sector. Older people are likely to have similar rates of adverse events, particularly related to medication management, falls and wound and pressure care.

The quality of aged care is often measured by the quality of the healthcare provided to older people. However, this is a simplistic approach that does not consider that older people view healthcare as only one aspect of their lives.

Clinical risks that are applicable to all RACFs have already been identified. Recent examples include gaps in communication between acute health services and RACFs, workforce skills and training, specific resident issues including management of restraint, falls, medication (e.g. anticoagulants, sedatives), gastroenteritis and influenza outbreaks, and elder abuse. However, the selection of these risks assumes that clinical matters are more important than other aspects of a resident's life. It reinforces the paradigm of quality of care as the provision of care based primarily on the best available research evidence. It does not consider the individual or the community preference for living with risk to maintain dignity and an adequate quality of life.

A measurement approach is required that addresses the different settings in which healthcare is provided. There is a need to develop systems to measure the global health system performance as a society as well as individual health providers.

 A measurement approach is required that addresses the different settings in which healthcare is provided.

Societal responsibility for health may include measures that would reflect how well we identify and prevent an 'individual citizen' like Mr M falling and fracturing his hip at home, for example, the use of exercise groups for strengthening and balance.

Individual ambulatory care practitioner responsibility may include how well they identify and implement strategies to reduce falls risk and osteoporosis. For example, geriatricians and GPs may be asked to audit their practice for the diagnosis and management of osteoporosis and prescription of hip protectors.

Measurement of the healthcare delivered by providers of 'community care' is extraordinarily complex. The challenge lies in identifying the clinical governance and the actual healthcare being delivered. For example, is it the responsibility of the 'community care' provider to ensure the personal carer attends every day to ensure Mr M is wearing the hip protectors? Many would argue that community care services are providing assistance to protect a person's way of life (and therefore quality of life) rather than for healthcare.

The more complex questions for healthcare measurement for older people require an understanding of the relative contributions of health to quality of life. If we reflect on the vignette, this requires identifying and considering the merits of prevention, ambulatory care, acute care and healthy ageing programs alongside the current health and lifestyle of the individual.

How does our judgment alter when we consider these questions: 'What does the older person and their self-contained community value the most?', 'What benefits the majority of the community?' and 'Are resources better spent on non–clinical aspects?'.

Reflect on the vignette and ask yourself what your approach would be if Mr M and the other residents asked that instead of everyone being supplied with hip protectors the money be spent on better clinical treatment at end of life, or perhaps something that enhances quality of life in the short term, such as an entertainment system.

GOVERNANCE IN AGED CARE

In RACFs the diverse size, location, nature of services and existing board and managerial structures complicate the introduction of clinical governance. The major dilemma with clinical governance in an RACF is that the responsibility for clinical care is often a combined responsibility of the facility, GP, pharmacist and regional hospital.

Medical practitioners are not employed by the RACF and their formal relationship is with the resident and not the facility in which the resident lives.

Residents from low-care facilities usually organise their own contact with their GP, often visiting their GP's rooms for consultation.

Residents who require high care are usually seen by medical staff at the RACF. If a specialist is unable to visit a facility the resident may have to be transferred to a hospital emergency department or clinic. The resident, their representative or the facility staff may initiate this contact.

Further complicating the situation is the pharmacist who may or may not be the local community pharmacist but who supplies medications to the residents. The supplying pharmacist may not be the pharmacist who undertakes a medication review of the resident's medications.

Therefore, the GP and pharmacist, who are critical to good clinical practice, are independent and not legally answerable to the facility.

While the issues of clinical governance are clearest in acute healthcare institutions, they become considerably blurred in the RACF and other non-acute settings in which healthcare is provided.

THE BROADER CONTEXT

Reflect on the vignette. Although as a society we are responsible for the global health of the community, it is difficult to identify who is responsible for supporting the health and wellbeing for an 'individual citizen' like Mr M.

If Mr M falls and does not present to any healthcare provider or service the responsibility rests with him and his family. Is this appropriate for the needs of our society in the future?

An ambulatory care practitioner's responsibility for healthcare is clear and direct for their interaction with an individual (e.g. the GP and Mr M). However, the nature of the health system allows for diffusion of responsibility because patients have the freedom to choose, change or decline to attend a GP. This limits the capacity of health services to adequately address the needs of patients through continuity of care.

Lines of accountability are clearer for providers of 'community care' who are contracted to provide services to older people. However, their responsibility for identifying, implementing and monitoring healthcare is usually not a primary role. They are usually responding to requests from healthcare providers.

Much work is needed to define and explore the boundaries and lines of responsibility of all the health and way-of-life services provided to older people if effective improvements are to occur.

CONCLUSION

Each individual and organisation will consider and respond differently to risk management and quality and safety improvement due to variations in perceptions of hazards and associated risk and resource limitations.

Questions to consider when we want to respond to requests and concerns about improving quality of care and safety in aged care include: 'Do we have a common understanding of these concepts?'. We should check to see if we have agreed upon definitions of quality, risk, rights and EBP. Remember to consider and examine the rights and needs of all stakeholders involved by asking: 'What are we seeking to achieve?' and 'Why is this important to this person or organisation?'.

It is important to balance the health professional's clinical imperative of ensuring adherence to research evidence with an individual's right to make a decision about their quality of life that may also increase their risk of incurring harm.

Aged care is an important component for delivering healthcare, therefore the existing quality systems need to reflect and manage the complex organisational processes, clinical decision making and potential hazards.

Managing clinical risk in aged care, be it residential, community or hospital-based, is about identifying those circumstances where people are put at risk of harm and then acting to prevent or manage those risks while striving to uphold stakeholder rights.

Quality of care improvement also requires an interdisciplinary and intersectoral approach that is able to adopt a systems approach to work practice that serves the community as a whole, and reflects its values and expectations.

Reflective questions

1. What is your initial response to the care Mr M received in the different settings?

2. How do you judge the quality of care? Is it according to the level of adherence to EBP, the management of risks and rights, or the balance of all factors?

3. Does your judgment alter if:

   - As an 'individual citizen' Mr M falls and fractures his hip at home prior to any medical intervention?

   - As an 'individual citizen' Mr M falls and fractures his hip at home after the geriatrician's recommendation for hip protectors and the GP is told that Mr M stopped wearing the hip protectors?

   - As an 'inpatient in acute hospital care', Mr M falls and fractures his hip in hospital after being assessed as high risk, and hip protectors are not worn because the hospital does not supply the equipment?

   - As a 'client of community care', Mr M falls and fractures his hip at home and is not wearing the hip protectors because the personal carer did not attend that day?

   - As a 'resident of an aged care facility' Mr M is assessed as high risk and the facility staff comply with his request to decline to wear hip protectors—he subsequently falls, fractures his hip and dies?

   Considering and responding to these dilemmas in an ethical manner requires an understanding of the concepts and associated complexities involved.

References

Aged Care Standards and Accreditation Agency (ACSAA), 2008. Quality manual. ACSAA, Canberra.

Andersson, M., Hallverg, I.R., Edberg, A.-K., 2008. Old people receiving municipal care, their experiences of what constitutes a good life in the last phase of life: a qualitative study. Int J Nurs Stud 45, 818–828.

Andrews, L.B., Stocking, C., Krizek, T., et al., 1997. An alternative strategy for studying adverse events in medical care. Lancet 349, 309–313.

Australian Council on Healthcare Standards, 2012. EQuIP 5th edition. The Accreditation Standards. Online. Available: http://www.achs.org.au/publications-resources/equip5/, 2 Feb 2013.

Australian Institute of Health and Welfare, 2010. Residential aged care in Australia 2008–09: a statistical overview. AIHW, Canberra.

Baker, G.R., Norton, P.G., Flintoft, V., et al., 2004. The Canadian Adverse Events Study: the incidence of adverse events among hospital patients in Canada. Canadian Medical Association Journal 170, 1678–1686.

Bernstein, S.J., Hilborne, L.H., 1993. Clinical indicators: the road to quality care? Joint Commission Journal on Quality Improvement 19, 501–509.

Berwick, D.M., 1989. Codman and the rhetoric of battle: a commentary. Milbank Quarterly 67, 262–267.

Brennan, T., Leape, L., Laird, N., et al., 1991. Incidence of adverse events and negligence in hospitalized patients. New England Journal of Medicine 324, 370–376.

Corrigan, J.M., Donaldson, M.S., Kohn, L.T., et al., 2001. Crossing the quality chasm: a new health system for the 21st century. Committee on Quality of Health Care in America, Institute of Medicine. National Academy Press, Washington DC.

Cryer, C., Knox, A., Stevenson, E., 2008. Factors associated with hip protector adherence among older people in residential care. Injury Prevention 14, 24–29.

Darzins, P., Molloy, W., Strang, D., 2000. Who can decide? The six step capacity assessment process. Memory Australia Press, South Australia.

Davis, P., Lay-Yee, R., Schug, S., et al., 2001. Adverse events regional feasibility study: indicative findings. New Zealand Medical Journal 114, 203–205.

Department of Health and Ageing, 2008. Charter of Residents' Rights and Responsibilities. Australian Government Department of Health and Ageing. Online. Available at: www.health.gov.au/internet/main/publishing.nsf/Content/6CBC341074429321CA256F810018368C/$File/charter.pdf, 2 Feb 2013.

Department of Human Services, 2000. Duty of care. Online. Available: http://www.dhs.vic.gov.au/cpmanual/practice-context/duty-of-care, 2 Feb 2013.

DiCenso, A., Guyatt, G., Ciliska, D., 2005. Evidence-based nursing: a guide to clinical practice. Elsevier Mosby, St Louis.

Donabedian, A., 1966. Evaluating the quality of medical care. Milbank Memorial Fund Quarterly 44, 166–206.

Donaldson, L., Muir Gray, J., 1998. Clinical governance: a quality duty for health organisations. Quality in Health Care (Suppl), S37–S44.

Gillespie, W.J., Gillespie, L.D., Parker, M.J., 2010. Hip protectors for preventing hip fractures in older people. Cochrane Database of Systematic Reviews Issue 10. Art. No.: CD001255. DOI: 10.1002/14651858.CD001255.pub4.

Hayes, N., Close, J.C., Witchard, S., et al., 2008. What predicts compliance rates with hip protectors in older hospital in-patients? Age Ageing 37, 225–228.

Kennedy, I., 2001. Learning from Bristol: the report of the public inquiry into children's heart surgery at the Bristol Royal Infirmary 1984–1995. Cm 5207. The Stationery Office, London. Online. Available: http://webarchive.nationalarchives.gov.uk/20090811143745/http://www.bristol-inquiry.org.uk, 2 Feb 2013.

Kohn, L.T., Corrigan, J.M., Donaldson, M.S. (Eds.), 1999. To err is human: building a safer health system. Committee on Quality of Health Care in America, Institute of Medicine. National Academy Press, Washington DC.

Lohr, K.N., Harris Wehling, J., 1991. Medicare: a strategy for quality assurance, I: A recapitulation of the study and a definition of quality of care. Quality Review Bulletin 17, 6–9.

Morgan, S., 2004. Positive risk-taking: an idea whose time has come. Health Care Risk Rep 10 (10), 18–19.

O'Halloran, P.D., Cran, G.W., Beringer, T.R., et al., 2007. Factors affecting adherence to use of hip protectors amongst residents of nursing homes—a correlation study. International Journal of Nursing Studies 44, 672–686.

Oliver, D., Connelly, J.B., Victor, C.R., et al., 2007. Strategies to prevent falls and fractures in hospitals and care homes and effect of cognitive impairment: systematic review and meta-analyses. British Medical Journal 334, 82.

Parker, M.J., Gillespie, W.J., Gillespie, L.D., 2005. Hip protectors for preventing hip fractures in older people. Cochrane Database of Systematic Reviews Issue 3 Art No CD001255. DOI: 10.1002/14651858.CD001255.pub3.

Perske, R., 1972. The dignity of risk and the mentally retarded. Mental Retardation 10, 24–27.

Phillips, C.B., Pearce, C.M., Hall, S., et al., 2010. Can clinical governance deliver quality improvement in Australian general practice and primary care? A systematic review of the evidence. Medical Journal of Australia 10, 602–607.

Reason, J., 1997. Managing the risks of organizational accidents. Ashgate Publishing Ltd, Hampshire.

Scally, G., Donaldson, L.J., 1998. Clinical governance and the drive for quality improvement in the new NHS in England. British Medical Journal 317, 61–65.

Slovic, P., Finucane, M., Peters, E., et al., 2004. Risk as analysis and risk as feelings: some thoughts about affect, reason, risk, and rationality. Risk Analysis 24, 311–322.

Sykes, J.B. (Ed.), 1982. The Concise Oxford Dictionary of Current English, seventh ed. Oxford University Press, UK.

Thomas, E.J., Studdert, D.M., Burstin, H.R., et al., 2000. Incidence and types of adverse events and negligent care in Utah and Colorado. Medical Care 38, 261–271.

Victorian Managed Insurance Authority, 2010. Risk management: developing & implementing a risk management framework. Online. Available: http://www.vmia.vic.gov.au/Risk-Management/Guides-and-publications/Risk-Management-Guidelines.aspx#, 2 Feb 2013.

Vincent, C., Neale, G., Woloshynowych, M., 2001. Adverse events in British hospitals: preliminary retrospective record review. British Medical Journal 322, 517–519.

West, E., 2000. Organisational sources of safety and danger: sociological contributions to the study of adverse events. Quality in Health Care 9, 120–126.

Wilson, R.M., Runciman, W.B., Gibberd, R.W., et al., 1995. The Australian Quality in Health Care Study. Medical Journal of Australia 163, 458–471.

World Health Organization (WHO), 1946. Constitution of the World Health Organization, thirty-seventh ed. WHO, Geneva.

CHAPTER 9

HEALTH AND CARE OF OLDER ABORIGINAL AND TORRES STRAIT ISLANDER PEOPLES

Dina LoGiudice, Leon Flicker and Kate Smith

Editors' comments

Working with older Aboriginal and Torres Strait Islander peoples (collectively referred to as 'Aboriginal people' in this chapter) requires understanding, skills and knowledge not many health professionals possess. LoGiudice, Flicker and Smith are not armchair academics—this chapter is based on their extensive research with these groups. Importantly it also highlights the need for specific assessment tools and provides suggestions for what is appropriate, what is not and where the gaps remain. The first vignette is presented right at the beginning to immediately immerse you in the world of Aboriginal people—the authors then explain throughout the chapter the ideas introduced in the vignette, before taking you to another real-world situation in the second vignette.

Vignette

Mrs A

Mrs A is 72-year-old woman who presented to a local city-based Aboriginal health service. The appointment was initiated by her son, who was concerned that his mother was 'not like she used to be', particularly since a recent admission to hospital after a series of falls. At that time she was diagnosed with heart failure and noted to have been weak on the left side.

Her history is as follows: non-insulin-dependent diabetes mellitus with diabetic nephropathy and retinopathy, vitamin D deficiency, chronic pulmonary obstructive disease and atrial fibrillation.

Mrs A was born in rural Victoria but had lived in the city since she was a teenager. She was raised by her grandmother after her mother died when she was a child. She was educated in a 'mission' school until the age of 14 and enjoys reading and writing. She has been widowed for many years and has three children, one of whom (a son) died four years ago after a heart attack. Her children are supportive but work full time.

On assessment Mrs A appeared confused and slow in responses. Her gait was unsteady, requiring a walking frame, and noted to be dyspnoeic on minimal exertion. She denied symptoms of depression (scoring 2/9 on a patient health questionnaire), has a good appetite and sleeps well, apart from waking once or twice per night to pass urine. Her Kimberley Indigenous Cognitive Assessment (KICA) score was 25/39, with evidence of disorientation, poor recall (improved with prompts) and poor verbal fluency. Her heart rate was irregular and had scattered chest crackles, with mild pitting oedema of her ankles. She has poor hearing.

Investigations revealed poor diabetic control, mild renal failure and hyponatraemia. A recent computed tomography (CT) scan revealed significant white matter ischaemia and lacunar infarct in the right internal capsule.

A diagnosis of vascular dementia was made and medical review of cardiovascular risk factors and medication undertaken. The family were committed to caring for their mother and requested that the term dementia was not mentioned to her. Education about dementia was given to the family and referral to an Aboriginal health worker (AHW) to help link with local Health and Community Care (HACC) services, district nursing and discussion with an Aboriginal link person of the local aged care assessment service (ACAS) enabled/facilitated exploration of respite activities, nutrition and medication compliance. Regular review was organised and mood monitored for emerging depression. Information about Alzheimer's Australia and the Dementia Behaviour Management Assessment Service (DBMAS) was also given.

INTRODUCTION

Aboriginal and Torres Strait Islander peoples ('Aboriginal people') are a minority group in Australia, comprising 2.5% of the total Australian population; 25% live in remote areas. Approximately 50,000 (12.1%) Aboriginal people are over the age of 50 years (Australian Institute of Health and Welfare (AIHW) 2010). Recently much has been reported on the low life expectancy of Aboriginal people, with 'closing the gap' between the life expectancy of this population and other Australians being a key health priority of the Australian Government. The poor life expectancy of this population may lead to the unfounded assumption that health conditions usually associated with ageing, such as dementia, falls and incontinence, are not highly prevalent and therefore should not be a priority of research and service provision in Aboriginal and Torres Strait Islander communities. This chapter reviews the research available on common 'aged care' syndromes, including depression, to discuss the pathways leading to these highly prevalent conditions and to inform prevention and management strategies that meet the needs of Aboriginal people. An approach to care is described in the setting of a person with dementia, as a guideline to good practice.

BACKGROUND

Australian Aboriginal culture is considered to be one of the oldest in the world. Prior to contact with the European world, it was thought there were more than

500 'tribes' living throughout Australia, with close relationship to their respective 'countries' (Flood 2006). The land was a source of food and spirituality, with obligations, kinship systems, languages and social processes that were complex and varied throughout communities. The diversity of Aboriginal people continues, with a multitude of languages and cultural traditions in use (Dudgeon et al 2000).

Currently Aboriginal people have the worst health status of any population in Australia (Hill et al 2007), with life expectancy more than 10 years less than the non-Aboriginal population. There is some discrepancy between states and territories, but for Aboriginal people born between 1998 and 2001, the life expectancy at birth of a male is approximately 67.2 years and for a female approximately 72.9 years (AIHW 2010). Standardised mortality rates indicate that the number of deaths is four times higher than expected for all age groups but particularly so for young and middle adult years, with 75% of Aboriginal men dying before the age of 65 years (compared with 26% in non-Aboriginal men). These statistics reflect lower life expectancy than other indigenous populations, with all-cause mortality twice that of indigenous New Zealanders or those in North America. Aboriginal males live eight to 13 fewer years than indigenous males in Canada, New Zealand and the United States (Ring & Brown 2003).

Despite the Aboriginal population having a younger age structure than the wider Australian community, both ends of the age spectrum are growing rapidly, with a large young population (0–24 years) and an ageing group, particularly led by the young–old (45–64 years) group (Australian Bureau of Statistics (ABS) 2007, AIHW 2010) (see Fig 9.1). Regardless of the damning mortality statistics, the Aboriginal population is ageing. Significant numbers of older Aboriginal people (aged 75 years or older) live in all areas of Australia, including remote areas. The young–old (45–64 years) continue to display a higher burden of morbidity and disability (Broe & Jackson-Pulver 2007). The majority of Aboriginal people live in cities and non-remote areas (75%), but one-quarter live in remote (15%) or very remote areas (9%) (ABS 2007, AIHW 2010).

The Aboriginal population is ageing and demographically appears similar to non-Aboriginal Australians more than 50 years ago.

Culturally appropriate approaches to clinical care require health professionals to understand the impact of history, including European colonisation and government policies enforced during their lifetime (Flood 2006). Awareness of these issues is important in providing holistic care (Vicary & Andrews 2001). Some of this history includes introduction of diseases at the time of colonisation, with resulting deaths of many even without direct exposure to non-Aboriginal people. Subsequent appropriation of land and water resources occurred, often by force, as rural lands were converted for farming. Ongoing dispossession from land, culture and forceful removal of children from their families highlighted many injustices and lack of access to human rights. From

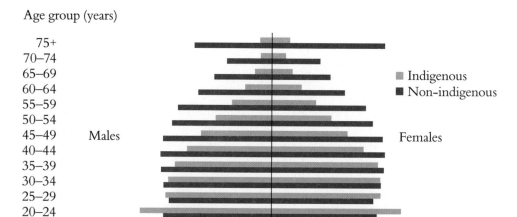

Figure 9.1

Age structure, by sex and Aboriginal status
Source: ABS 2008a

the 1960s onwards, awards for equal pay, the right to vote and declaration of the invalid nature of 'terra nullius' heralded some improvements in human rights; however, the ongoing discrepancy continues with an aim to 'close the gap' relating to life expectancy, infant mortality, early childhood development, education and employment (Broe & Jackson-Pulver 2007, Dudgeon et al 2000, Flood 2006).

> **Awareness of the impact of history, including colonisation and government policies enforced during their lifetime, is required for providing holistic care to older Aboriginal people.**

Broe and Jackson-Pulver (2007) identified five key areas that contribute to health disparity in Australia: historical; social and political; socioeconomic and environmental factors; lack of access to quality primary healthcare; and specific health risk factors. Issues such as: low income; low employment and education; poor health linkages and financial barriers associated with substandard housing and sanitation on a background of years of social and political changes including separation from families; lack of trust with governmental bodies; and other factors contribute to the continued poor statistics.

Traditionally Aboriginal people perceive health not only in physical terms but more generally encompassing social, economic and cultural wellbeing of the whole community. Aboriginal health is intrinsic to Aboriginal spirituality. This is a whole-life view and includes a cyclical concept of life-death-life. Healthcare services should strive to achieve the state where 'every individual can realise their full potential as human beings and thus bring about the total well being of their communities' (Swan & Raphael 1995 p 14). These differences in cultural knowledge and worldview, in addition to language differences, impact on communication with non-Aboriginal health service providers (Trudgen 2000).

CHRONIC DISEASE AND RISK FACTORS

The discrepancy in health status of Aboriginal people is primarily due to chronic disease and injury, which also contribute to the development of functional disability at a younger age (Marmot 2005). Consequently, Aboriginal people are experiencing life changes at an earlier age than other Australians, and the Commonwealth Department of Health and Ageing recommends that Aboriginal people aged older than 50 years are eligible to access aged care services (ABS & AIHW 2008).

The Australian Commonwealth states the age of 50 years or older for Aboriginal people to qualify for aged care health programs and services.

Risk factors such as hypertension and diabetes contribute significantly to functional disability. In northern Australia hypertension was found to be more prevalent in Aboriginal Australians (27%) than in other Australians (9%) aged 25–54 years (Wang et al 2006). A study by Smith et al (1992) reported that the prevalence of hypertension in the Kimberley Aboriginal population aged older than 50 years was 45% in men and 50% in women, with obesity and alcohol being primary risk factors. Poor adherence with medications may also be a factor, and Wang et al (2006) found that only 25% of those with hypertension reported taking antihypertensive medication and only one-third of those with antihypertensive medications had their hypertension adequately controlled. Similarly, Aboriginal rates of diabetes are nearly four times higher than in non-Aboriginal Australians (ABS & AIHW 2008, O'Dea et al 2007). In a study of Kimberley and Pilbara Aboriginal Australians over the age of 35 years, 58% of the men and 59% of the women had diabetes (Gracey et al 2006).

Other conditions that lead to an increased burden of disease for Aboriginal people compared with non-Aboriginal Australians, as measured by disability-adjusted life years (DALYs), include cardiovascular disease (4.6-fold), chronic respiratory disease (2.7-fold), cancer (1.7-fold) and mental disorder (1.6-fold). One in three Aboriginal people have eye problems (including cataract, trachoma and diabetic retinopathy), and chronic otitis media can increase the risk of hearing impairment. Other factors such as high levels of obesity, poor activity levels and higher rates of smoking and alcohol use contribute to poor health status (ABS & AIHW 2008).

Functional disorders commonly seen in older age include dementia, depression, falls, urinary incontinence and stroke; however, limited research exists in the extent of these problems among Aboriginal people.

High rates of risk factors among Aboriginal people are associated with higher rates of common causes of disease burden compared with non-Aboriginal Australians.

DISABILITY

The ABS defines a disability as impairment that has lasted or is likely to last at least six months. Assistance from carers, aids or equipment may be required to perform tasks, ranging from using a hearing aid to requiring constant supervision for advanced dementia (ABS 2004a).

Approximately 20% of all Australians have a disability. The most common health conditions leading to a disability are physical; however, mental or behavioural disorders are the most common conditions, leading to profound or severe limitations. Fifty-six percent of people classed as having psychoses or mood affective disorders (including dementia and depression) have a profound or severe core activity limitation, compared with 33% of people with circulatory conditions such as heart disease and stroke (ABS 2004a). Fifty-one percent of Australians aged older than 60 years have a disability. People with a disability in this age group most commonly require assistance with property maintenance, healthcare and transport (ABS 2004a). For Aboriginal people the first collection of disability rates was in the 2002 National Aboriginal and Torres Strait Islander Social Survey, which reported that 77% of Aboriginal males and 69% of Aboriginal females over the age of 65 years had a disability or long-term health condition (ABS 2004b). Of those Aboriginal people over the age of 15, 37% had a disability or long-term health condition and 8% had a profound activity limitation requiring assistance with at least one activity of daily living.

Zhao et al (2004) reported that premature mortality was the main contributor to the large discrepancy between levels of disease burden (measured as DALYs) in the Aboriginal and non-Aboriginal Northern Territory population. Aboriginal people experience DALY rates at the level of non-Aboriginal people who are 20–30 years older, with DALY rates in Aboriginal people aged 45–54 years exceeding those of non-Aboriginal people aged 65–74 years (see Fig 9.2). Years lost due to disability (YLD) is also more prevalent in Aboriginal people than in their non-Aboriginal counterparts, with a gap existing in both fatal and non-fatal health outcomes. Much of the discrepancy is due to preventable and environmental factors such as diet, lifestyle, education and physical activity, which are potentially modifiable as communicable diseases decrease.

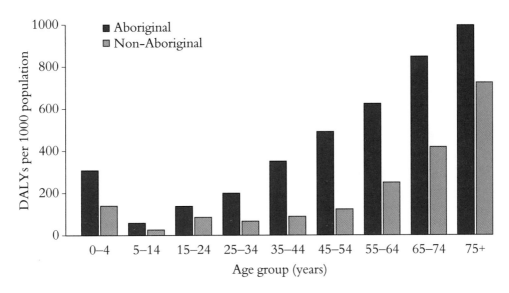

Figure 9.2

Age-specific disability age-adjusted life years lost per 1000 population, Northern Territory, 1994–98

Source: Zhao et al 2004

GERIATRIC SYNDROMES IN OLDER ABORIGINAL AUSTRALIANS

Geriatric syndromes refer to multifactorial health conditions usually seen in older frail people. These syndromes are characterised by features such as immobility, falls, incontinence and dementia, and result in functional decline, disability and mortality (Inouye et al 2007). The interrelationships between aged syndromes, disability and activity restriction are often affected by environmental and social conditions (World Health Organization 2010). A number of theories have been described that may explain these complex interactions. Drachman (2006) states that accumulated insults from multiple pathways may increase the risk of chronic disease, with physiological differences (partly due to genetic variations) affecting each individual's susceptibility to the disorder. This is an example of the stochastic ageing phenomenon (Rockwood & Mitnitski 2007). Research indicates that significant childhood stresses (e.g. family abuse) are strongly associated with poor adult health outcomes and that social disadvantage and other factors in early childhood may have a negative effect on cognitive function (Arkles et al 2010). Aboriginal people exposed to multiple environmental and endogenous insults may, therefore, have an elevated prevalence of geriatric syndromes at an earlier stage of life, such as dementia, falls, urinary incontinence and chronic pain.

Multiple physical, social and psychological stressors and risk factors at an early age (including childhood) likely contribute to multifactorial syndromes with poorer health outcomes at a younger 'old age'.

Recent research is uncovering the significant problem of dementia in Aboriginal communities, but there is limited data on the prevalence of other syndromes (Smith et al 2008). High levels of chronic disease and injury may contribute to the development of functional disability at a younger age. During 2005–06 a community survey of 363 people in six communities of the Kimberley and one town demonstrated a high level of dementia in those aged older than 45 years at 12.4%—up to five times those of non-Aboriginal Australians of the same age. At the same time of this survey, self- or carer-reported rates of multifactorial syndromes appeared high—31% for falls, 50% for poor mobility and 55% for pain—although urinary problems and urinary incontinence had lower rates of 20% and 9% (LoGiudice et al 2012a). Currently there are no validated culturally appropriate screening tools to assess falls, urinary continence or pain in older Aboriginal people. Each of these syndromes will now be discussed in further detail, in the context of older Aboriginal people.

DEMENTIA

Cultural understanding of dementia may vary within societies and communities, and may impact on the presentation and experience of dementia for the person, their carers, families and communities. For health professionals this cultural context of understanding dementia is essential for appropriate assessment, provision of care and education.

> *Dementia is a sick spirit, a lost spirit looking for help … It may not need to get fixed as long as the individual is safe and the family and the community is safe … Other causes of a sick spirit … is the past history of the stolen generation, dispossession, physical, social and emotional trauma, child abuse, drug and alcohol abuse, poor diet, a lack of traditional healers and herbal medicine being understood and used …*

(Arkles et al 2010)

A recent qualitative survey explored community members' and workers' knowledge of dementia, giving examples such as head injury, lack of family visits and ageing as reasons for developing dementia. '*Ah talk like um silly and … yeah walk around everywhere … sometimes he used to get lost*' (Smith et al 2011). Other issues such as a high tolerance of behavioural issues within the community setting, and fear of being admitted to care facilities away from their 'country', may impact on seeking assessment and assistance (Smith et al 2011). Factors such as low levels of literacy and languages spoken other than English confound cognitive assessments (Smith et al 2007). The overall level of understanding of dementia is poor in Aboriginal communities, particularly younger people, and misconceptions about dementia and Alzheimer's disease are common (Garvey et al 2011).

Our knowledge of the burden of dementia in Aboriginal populations is increasing in recent times, improved by development of culturally appropriate cognitive assessment tools such as the Kimberley Indigenous Cognitive Assessment tool (KICA-Cog) for remote and rural Aboriginal Australians (LoGiudice et al 2006). The KICA-Cog was assessed and validated in three different populations (and there appears to be no education bias found) and is most reliable at a cut-off point of 33/39 with sensitivity 93.3%, specificity 98.4% and Area Under Curve (AUC) 0.98 (95% CI 0.97, 0.99) (Smith et al 2009). The KICA-Cog is a screening tool that measures recall (visual) with prompting, verbal fluency, graphomotor perseveration, dyspraxia and other domains. It is not a comprehensive cognitive assessment and does not assess capacity. Instructions on its use are available on the WA Centre for Health and Ageing (WACHA) website (www.wacha.org.au), as is a video on its use with interpreters. The KICA-Screen is a shorter version, with a cut-off point of 21/25 and a sensitivity of 82.4% and specificity of 88.5%, and the area under the Receiver Operating Characteristic (ROC) curve was 0.94 (95% CI 0.87– 1.0). The shorter screen version was developed and validated in the northern area of Queensland, including people of Torres Strait Islander background (LoGiudice et al 2011).

The KICA not only includes a cognitive assessment section but also has subsections that address informant assessment, emotional wellbeing, function and behavioural symptoms. Prompts for medical history such as diabetes and hypertension, vision, alcohol use, smoking, falls and incontinence are included. The tool (including KICA-Screen) can be viewed with an instruction manual (and DVD) on the WACHA website. A modified form is being assessed for its utility in urban regions of Sydney. Previous tools have been for younger age groups, particularly addressing executive dysfunction (Dingwall & Cairney 2010). The KICA is recommended by aged care assessment teams (Sansoni et al 2010) as is most suitable for the cognitive assessment of older Aboriginal people.

The Kimberley Indigenous Cognitive Assessment scale is the recommended screening tool for cognitive assessment of Aboriginal people.

Utilising the KICA, Smith et al (2008) conducted a study to determine the prevalence of dementia in an Aboriginal population. The study was conducted in six remote communities and one town in the remote Kimberley region of Western Australia with a sample of 363 Aboriginal participants over the age of 45 years. In this group only 40% had any formal schooling, and many spoke two or three non-English languages. The prevalence of dementia in this sample was 12.4%, approximately five times greater than reported for the corresponding age group in the wider Australian population (2.4%), and 26.8% of participants aged older than 65 years had dementia. These figures are among the highest reported worldwide. Alzheimer's disease accounted for 24% on clinical assessment; vascular dementia 13% and dementia related to alcohol abuse was only 4%. Limited access to brain imaging complicated adequate classification of subtypes of dementia.

The high comorbidity of health risk factors, occurring at a relatively young age, is thought to have led to the high prevalence of dementia in this population. Factors associated with dementia included older age, male gender (OR 3.1) and no formal education (OR 2.7). And after adjusting for age, sex and education, dementia was associated with current smoking (OR 4.5), previous stroke (OR 17.9), epilepsy (OR 33.5), head injury (OR 4.0), poor mobility, incontinence and falls (Smith et al 2010).

The prevalence of dementia in remote areas of Australia appears to be five times more than non-Aboriginal Australians; the presence of dementia is associated with older age, male gender, poor education and history of head injury, stroke and epilepsy.

Some developing countries have a similarly high prevalence of dementia, notably Venezuela (10.3% among those aged over 65 years) (Molero et al 2007), Argentina (12.2% aged over 65 years) (Larraya et al 2004) and an Arab community in Israel (21.1% over 65 years) (Bowirrat et al 2002). Kalaria et al (2008) have collated a number of international studies on risk factors for dementia including these countries. The results from this Australian study have been compared with the international studies in Table 9.1. The factors that are associated with dementia in both this study and studies in other regions are increasing age, gender, head injury, lack of education, vascular disease and smoking. Emerging evidence of risk factors that were initially thought to predict vascular cognitive impairment is also associated with Alzheimer's disease. These include midlife hypertension (Skoog et al 1996), obesity, diabetes (Arvanitakis et al 2004) and decreased physical activity (Flicker 2010, Vaynman & Gomez-Pinilla 2006). Another intriguing hypothesis is that exposure to conditions related to poverty in utero (such as poor nutrition) may lead to chronic disease in later life (Barker et al 1993). This latter factor is also likely to be an underlying factor in developing countries and Aboriginal populations and indicates possible interventions that could reduce the rate of dementia in vulnerable populations. The importance of the early life cycle to the later development of dementia is currently being explored (Arkles et al 2010).

Prior to this study the prevalence of dementia in Aboriginal people was unknown. A Commonwealth report had estimated that the prevalence of cognitive impairment was 20% among the 133 Aboriginal people aged older than 65 years sampled in northern Queensland, but the assessment procedures were not validated for this population and there was no clear-cut sampling strategy. Of the 20% with dementia, medical records were used to identify half of the cases, with the other half derived from the use of a modified version of the Psychiatric Assessment Scale that was not standardised for Aboriginal and Torres Strait Islander people (Zann 1994). A study investigating the prevalence of aged care conditions in Aboriginal people referred to the Kimberley Aged Care Assessment Team (ACAT) reported that 40% had dementia (Bruce et al 1998). As the patients had been referred for aged care assessment this sample

Table 9.1

Comparison of Aboriginal Kimberley study and international dementia risk factors

	DEVELOPED REGIONS	ASIA	AFRICA	LATIN AMERICA	AUSTRALIAN ABORIGINALS
Increasing age	Positive	Positive	Positive	Positive	Positive
Female sex	Positive	Positive	Unclear	Unclear	Negative
Head injury	Positive	–	–	Positive	Positive
Lack of education	Positive	Positive	Positive	Positive	Positive
Vascular disease	Positive	Positive	Positive	Unclear	Positive
Smoking	Positive	Positive	–	Unclear	Positive
Epilepsy	Unclear	–	–	–	Positive

Adapted from Kalaria et al 2008 p 6

did not reflect the wider Kimberley population and the age range was not stated. Current research is addressing the uncertain prevalence of dementia in urban regions of Australia and among Aboriginal people (Forster et al 2010).

DEPRESSION

Depression comprises 13% of the total burden of disease in Australia (AIHW 2009, 2010). As mentioned, Aboriginal Australians perceive health not only in physical terms but also the social, economic and cultural wellbeing of the whole community. Aboriginal health is intrinsic to Aboriginal spirituality. Aboriginal coping mechanisms rely on expression and communication of feelings and reliance on collective coping responses. Loss and fragmentation of their group will lead to mental illness (Dudgeon et al 2000, Sheldon 2001).

Symptoms of depression must be considered in the context of cultural, social and spiritual wellbeing.

There have been various explanations of the concept of depression, with one developed by Joseph Roe based in the Kimberley region (Roe 2000). He indicated that the Ngarlu is place of inner spirit (stomach) and the centre of emotions and wellbeing. This can be weakened by the colonisation process, and associated changed lifestyle, dispossession and disempowerment (see Fig 9.3). Older people can connect with Ngarlu and work with it through cultural initiation and laws. When the Ngarlu is suppressed this can lead to poor self-esteem and illness. Serious sickness (including mental health) is often attributed to *external forces or reasons, or may be due to 'doing something wrong culturally'*. It is often unnoticed unless visible, such as being seen crying, engaging in high-risk behaviour or suicidal tendencies. The aim is to build resistance against harmful spirits and work with Ngarlu. But how does this fit into modern criteria of depression? How do we measure *longing for, crying for or being sick for country* (Vicary & Westerman 2004)? There is limited agreement on data definition, collection and standards, making it difficult to know how to measure depression accurately in Aboriginal people.

Jorm et al (2012) performed a survey of 11 meta-analyses and noted that six surveys of Aboriginal adults revealed a higher prevalence rate of high or very-high levels of psychological distress score (50% to three times more) but little difference in adolescents. Aboriginal people are more likely to be hospitalised for mental health conditions than non-Aboriginal people, with mental-illness-related mortality twice as prevalent. A recent AIHW (2009) report indicated 27% of Aboriginal adults reported high or very-high levels of psychological distress, twice that of non-Aboriginal Australians. Life stressors was measured by a 15-item list seeking positive or negative responses to experiences such as bereavement, job losses and alcohol problems over the preceding year, and quantified by frequency. In relation to life stressors, four in 10 Aboriginal adults indicated that they, or their family or friends, had experienced the death of a family member or close friend in the previous year and 28% reported serious illness or disability. Yet over half of adults reported feeling calm and

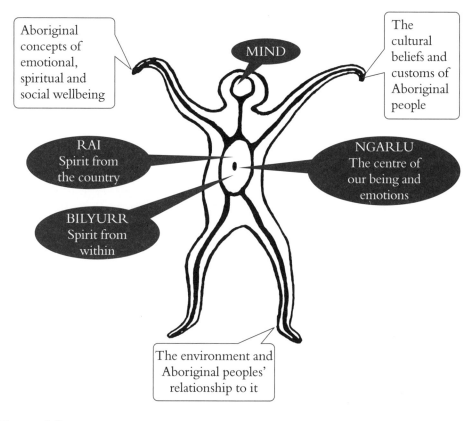

Aboriginal concepts of emotional, spiritual and social wellbeing

MIND

The cultural beliefs and customs of Aboriginal people

RAI
Spirit from the country

NGARLU
The centre of our being and emotions

BILYURR
Spirit from within

The environment and Aboriginal peoples' relationship to it

Figure 9.3

Ngarlu assessment model
Source: Roe 2000 p 396. With kind permission of Joe Roe Broome

peaceful (51%) and/or full of life (55%) all or most of the time. More recently the nine-item Patient Health Questionnaire (PHQ) (Esler et al 2008) was modified and tested in a small number of Aboriginal people with heart disease and validated against psychiatric interview by a medical practitioner. For the detection of depression the PHQ demonstrated specificity and sensitivity of 80% and 71.4% respectively. The terminology of the PHQ was modified specifically for Aboriginal people, although it requires further investigation of its psychometric properties.

Guidelines on cultural understandings of mental health in Aboriginal people are available (Eley et al 2006, Vicary & Westerman 2004), but specific information on the assessment and unmet needs for older people with mental health issues is lacking, particularly for those living in remote communities. In a recent study questions eliciting symptoms of depression were administered to 363 people over the age of 45 years in remote communities, with 10 questions and responses of 'sometimes' or 'all of the time'. Surprisingly only 11 people from the total cohort of 363 indicated a score of three or more positive responses of 'all of the time' (Smith 2008). The authors' clinical experience indicates that many older Aboriginal people living in remote and rural areas complain of 'worry and anxiety' related to their family and community. The levels of major depression and subsyndromal depression and anxiety have not been accurately described. Resilience of older people may be playing a part, but effective ways of assessment and management in this older group requires clarification.

FALLS

Falls may lead to disability, decreased quality of life and even death. The consequences of falls are severe, with 10% of falls causing serious injuries such as fractures requiring hospitalisation with other sequelae such as minor injuries and loss of confidence. A number of risk factors have been identified in the general population including impaired cognition, sensory problems, impaired gait and home environmental hazards as well as alcohol, obesity and polypharmacy and some medications leading to postural hypotension (Hill et al 2000, Mitra et al 2007).

In Aboriginal populations, data on falls pertain mainly to younger people, being the second most common cause of injury leading to hospitalisation following assault (National Public Health Partnership 2006). Further information on the prevalence of falls in Aboriginal populations can be obtained from hospital morbidity data. There is a rapid increase in fall-related hospitalisations in Aboriginal people from the age of 45 years, which does not occur in non-Aboriginal Australians until approximately 60 years of age (Helps & Harrison 2006). In this population, deaths due to falls are at lower rates than other injuries but are still two and a half times higher in this population than for non-Aboriginal people (Peel et al 2008). Hip fracture injury is thought to be uncommon due to lower life expectancy, and MacIntosh and Pearson (2001) showed that Aboriginal people have a lower incidence of these fractures than might be expected on an overall population basis and that Aboriginal females develop osteoporotic-type fractures of the femoral neck at a later age than non-Aboriginal females (Peel et al 2008). A recent Western Australian (WA) study indicated that Aboriginal people admitted with a hip fracture were significantly more likely to have diabetes and renal disease and to report high alcohol use but significantly less likely to have a low vitamin D level and polypharmacy, after adjustment for age, sex and rural residency. Aboriginal people may have risk factors that contribute to fracture through diabetes-related complications such as visual impairment, stroke and peripheral neuropathy and osteoporosis related to renal dysfunction. Excessive alcohol intake at a young age among Aboriginal people may affect peak bone mass and secondary effects on mobility and cognition (Lai & Waldron 2011). It appears that older Aboriginal people may be more at risk for hip fracture than similarly aged non-Aboriginal people and, unfortunately for Western Australia, the age-standardised rates increased by an average of 7.2% per year over the period 1999–2009 among Aboriginal adults, whereas non-Aboriginal rates fell by an average of 3.4% per year (Wong et al 2012).

Little data is available on falls and associated factors among older Aboriginal people, but a prevalence study that included self- or carer-reported falls indicated 31% of Aboriginal people over the age of 45 years in six remote communities experienced a fall, responding positively to 'Do you fall down sometimes?'. Twelve percent of participants had been injured by a fall, responding positively to 'Did you hurt yourself?'. The odds of falling in this cohort increased with poor mobility, drinking alcohol, stroke, epilepsy, head injury and poor hearing (LoGiudice et al 2012a). Although there are a number of screening tools and recommendations for diminishing risk of falls in the general population, these have not been validated or proven in Aboriginal communities. A multifactorial approach to falls prevention has been successfully trialled in the general population; for example, injury minimisation is possible when hip protectors or vitamin D are used (Hill et al 2000). Many of these approaches will have little relevance to an Aboriginal population, highlighting the need to assess the rate of falls in this population and the associated circumstances and morbidity. Recent guidelines for best practice in falls prevention highlight the key role for primary care clinicians in improving 'case finding'. The guidelines recommend that older people be periodically asked whether a fall was sustained in the preceding 12 months (Hill et al 2000, Peel et al 2008). For Aboriginal people living in remote areas, other factors may be important including overcrowding of housing, high rates of impaired vision, diabetic peripheral neuropathy, stroke, cognitive impairment and limited allied health input to assess mobility aids and provide exercise programs. These may all contribute to increase the risk of falls and their morbid consequences. To date, there has been no systematic study documenting the extent and impact of falls in older Aboriginal populations.

Further research is required to determine the prevalence of falls in Aboriginal and Torres Strait Islander communities, and associated risk factors that are likely to be diverse in this population.

URINARY INCONTINENCE

It is estimated that more than two million Australians have some degree of urinary incontinence, being more prevalent in women and the older population (Chiarelli et al 2005). There is a dearth of published studies on incontinence in Aboriginal populations. However, it is plausible that the high rates of diabetes, cerebrovascular and kidney disease, obesity, smoking, urogenital infections and male ceremonial surgical procedures are likely to contribute to a higher prevalence of incontinence in this population. In one of only two epidemiological studies of this nature available, a female doctor interviewed 151 rural Aboriginal women aged 16–69 years (Benness & Manning 1997). In this survey 56% of women reported urinary incontinence, 46% reported being troubled by their symptoms, 87% had one or more children and 35% had had five or more deliveries. Incontinence was more likely to be stress incontinence (48%), although urge (30%) and mixed (23%) were also common. A review of Kimberley Aboriginal people referred to the Kimberley ACAT reported that

43% of clients were incontinent; however, the age range of this older sample was not stated (Zann 1994). Underreporting seems likely because of gender and kinship issues and limited availability of continence diagnostic procedures and aids to remote areas.

In a recent survey of 363 Aboriginal people over the age of 45 years, 20% self-reported urinary problems of some kind (LoGiudice et al 2012a). The latter is probably an underrepresentation related to possible reluctance and embarrassment to disclose symptoms and only more severe episodes of urinary incontinence were reported, despite using gender-specific interpreters. Reporting of the generic term 'urinary problems' seemed more accepted, and included episodes of urinary tract infections, difficulty with urination, urinary incontinence and others. A follow-up study of this cohort is addressing both male and female urinary symptoms to a greater degree, and explores appropriate questions for screening. In remote areas continence nurses and services are available but are likely to be underutilised. There are many education resources available on the continence.org website, such as *Leaking pee—let's yarn about women's business* and others (Continence Foundation Association 2012). Awareness of cultural issues that might contribute to underreporting, such as gender issues where women are unlikely to feel comfortable discussing issues with males and vice versa, need to be considered. Education on management is important. Advice from Aboriginal health or liaison workers may assist to determine the best approach.

 Urinary incontinence is likely underreported, considering numerous risk factors that contribute to this condition. A culturally sensitive approach is essential.

CHRONIC PAIN

The prevalence of chronic pain in general community studies varies considerably between 2% and 40% (Blyth et al 2001) but in older people rises steadily with age, often reaching 50% in community studies and 80% in those living in residential care (Helme & Gibson 1999). Few studies among Aboriginal people have focused on the prevalence of pain in the community, yet those performed suggest that musculoskeletal pain is underreported and undertreated (Vindigni & Perkins 2003). Injury, psychological morbidity, as well as lifestyle and cultural factors, appear to mediate the presentation of pain to health professionals.

One previous study based in an Aboriginal community in New South Wales conducted by Vindigni and Perkins (2003) documented 68% of those interviewed reporting high levels of pain, most commonly related to musculoskeletal disorders (Honeyman & Jacobs 1996, McGrath 2006). Underreporting of pain is considered common, and in one community one-third of the community acknowledged the presence of long-term back pain only when closely questioned, preferring not to show pain publicly in the community (Honeyman & Jacobs 1996).

In the Kimberley survey described above, pain was reported in half of those surveyed across all age groups, being consistently present in 67 (18%) participants, and appeared to decrease with age. The odds of chronic pain were increased for women and those with poor mobility or hearing. This study's estimate of prevalence of pain may be an underestimate, especially in the older groups, and gender and cultural differences may contribute to lack of disclosure of pain (LoGiudice et al 2012a). The issue of pain is particularly pertinent in the setting of end-of-life or palliative care. McGrath (2006) has addressed the issue of palliative care in this group and found many cultural practices and beliefs need to be understood and respected before appropriate care can be delivered. This includes discovering the cultural relationships regarding who should be directly involved with care and decision making—a reluctance to disclose pain, particularly among men, and other factors relating to blame and 'pay back'. A fear of Western medicines that may inhibit passing on traditional knowledge at end of life may impact on adequate management of pain. Guidelines on palliative care in this setting are available and are an important resource.

Chronic pain is likely underreported in Aboriginal people, who are likely to suffer chronic musculoskeletal conditions. Knowledge of local cultural traditions and beliefs are necessary for an appropriate approach to pain relief, particularly at end of life.

COMMUNITY AND RESIDENTIAL CARE

The importance of older people remaining in their community close to family and country is well documented.

It is still important for them to feel connected to their country and taking them away like I am sure that they want to die and pass in their country. You know that's their spirituality that's their connection.

(Smith et al 2011)

Residential facilities are often seen as a place where people are sent to die, and this perception is compounded by the fact that the facility may be in a town or city a long distance from their country (Smith et al 2011).

The National Aboriginal and Torres Strait Islander Flexible Aged Care Program was introduced to assist with providing culturally appropriate care, and in June 2011 there were 28 aged care facilities through this funding to deliver 645 aged care places and community aged care services to meet the needs of the community at a cost of $25.3 million (AIHW 2012). The program was aimed at establishing a combination of community and residential care services in rural and remote Aboriginal communities and are funded outside the regulatory framework of the *Aged Care Act 1997*. Aboriginal people can still access services through mainstream providers. Since the initiative began, quality standards were set to improve infrastructure, including professional support, increased quality in facilities and strengthening crisis and emergency care. A review of the aged care standards was recently prompted at the recommendation of a coroner's case resulting from an elder falling into a pit fire during a ritual ceremony in the Northern Territory (Brooke 2011).

Services throughout Australia are widespread and varied, ranging from small non-government packages or outreach services to state and nationally funded care. The provision of mainstream aged care packages is based on population estimates of people aged around 70 years. Significantly, this age criteria are altered for Aboriginal people, with provision based on populations aged 50 years or older, due to the high mortality gap and prevalence of chronic disease.

Nationally, in comparison to the proportion of the target population as a whole, Aboriginal people are underrepresented in access to HACC, Extended Aged Care at Home—Dementia (EACH-D) and residential care but overrepresented in access to Community Aged Care Packages (CACPs). These results for Aboriginal people should be interpreted with caution due to varying means of measurement. HACC services are measured in terms of target population that are based on the number of households with moderate or severe disability. In 2011 the proportion of Aboriginal clients aged over 70 years receiving HACC services was 28.9% compared with non-Aboriginal older Australians where uptake was 70.8%, reflecting differing patterns of morbidity and mortality. Comparison of other services includes Aboriginal people aged 50–69 years as a target proxy group compared with all people aged over 70 years. Nationally, the number of Aboriginal people receiving CACPs aged over 50 years was 24.6 per 1000, compared with 18.8 per 1000 of the target population aged over 70 years (Steering Committee for the Review of Government Service Provision 2012). In June 2011, 1127 residents in aged care facilities (0.7%) identified as Aboriginal, tending to be younger (24% aged under 65 years compared with 4%), with more male residents and slightly higher use of respite (AIHW 2012).

The provision of culturally appropriate care in these facilities and programs requires addressing principles and concepts of 'cultural comfort' and 'community control' and recognising mutual competence between traditional and mainstream services. Other essentials for remote health models include adequate funding, consultation, participation, leadership and quality assurance, with the aim to enhance cultural resiliency, empowerment and assistance with education and advocacy. Areas that require further development include the importance of local workforce engagement, and the need for appropriate education and training (Brooke 2011, Carroll et al 2010).

APPROACH TO CARE

A holistic, person-centred approach supported by knowledge of the local culture, perceptions and norms are needed for adequate assessment and management of conditions of older Aboriginal people, their family and community. Keeping in mind that the cultural, language and spiritual differences vary enormously, for example, Koori people living in urban areas (Aboriginal people from Victoria, parts of New South Wales and Tasmania) compared with remote and rural Aboriginals living in the Kimberley desert region. Knowledge can be gained through interpreters, Aboriginal liaison officers, local community members, elders and experienced local service providers. There are many references that can be used to assist (Dudgeon et al 2000, Sheldon 2001) including local cross-cultural training workshops.

In the next section we will outline an approach to dementia assessment, management and care in broad terms, as adapted from a recent report developing pathways to care for Aboriginal people with dementia living in the Northern Territory (Jensen et al 2012). As with the assessment of all older people, consideration of other 'geriatric syndromes' is necessary as they often co-exist; risk factors may be similar and therefore need to be documented. This template is a basis for all possible conditions among older people.

Awareness, recognition and referral

This begins with community education and awareness to increase understanding of symptoms of dementia and the benefits of timely diagnosis. In communities and families, behavioural symptoms are often tolerated and changes are considered part of ageing. There are numerous educational resources available that are specific for Aboriginal clients and families such as Alzheimer's Australia's *Looking out for dementia*. Adequate knowledge of dementia is also required by health professionals and aged care workers. There are guidelines for primary care (Couzos & Murray 2008), manuals (e.g. Central Australian Rural Practitioners' Association manual) and vocational certificates for health workers and others. For those over 55 years of age the 'older person's health check' is recommended in primary care, which includes a cognitive screen, and also general assessment for osteoporosis, vision, etc. Carers provide valuable information and need to be taken seriously when raising concerns about their family members.

Initial assessment and diagnosis and post-diagnosis support

In the setting of possible cognitive impairment the KICA is the recommended tool of choice, and is included in the ACAS tool kit guidelines. Interpreters should be used if English is not the client's first language and they should be briefed both prior and after assessment to discuss any potential cultural issues that may arise during the consultation, and that may impact on the outcome. Table 9.2 outlines guidelines for the KICA.

As with anyone with a potential diagnosis of dementia, depression/delirium must be excluded, medications reviewed (particularly those with anticholinergic side effects) and other conditions (such as metabolic conditions, thyroid disorder and B12 and folate deficiencies) ruled out. Imaging may be useful; however, availability may be an issue in remote areas. Where possible a specialist review is helpful to confirm the diagnosis (e.g. Alzheimer's disease, vascular cognitive impairment) and determine suitability for cognitive-enhancing medications or a review of behavioural and psychiatric signs of dementia symptoms, and this is increasingly being conducted through telehealth. Informing the person and their family about the diagnosis should be performed with the assistance of an interpreter and/or AHW, and in the presence of appropriate family members and health professionals who are familiar with the person and their family.

Table 9.2

Kimberley Indigenous Cognitive Assessment guidelines

	GUIDELINE
WHEN TO BE USED	• When a family member or other carer expresses concern about cognitive decline • As part of an older person's health check (as per standard treatment manual) • After checks have been done for possibility of delirium (and depression) • No more than every three months
WHO SHOULD DO KICA	• Acute setting—doctors, occupational therapists, speech pathologists, ACAT/psychogeriatric service • Urban community—ACAT staff, allied health professionals (AHPs), DBMAS • Residential care registered nurses, AHPs • Remote communities ACAT staff, AHPs, remotes area nurses, AHWs, aged care team leaders
USE OF INTERPRETERS	• For all clients who do not have English as a first language • Best practice is use of trained interpreters from the Aboriginal interpreter service • Alternative may be an AHW or aged care worker • Family member is unsuitable • Interpreter will need education about dementia (e.g. KICA DVD)
PHYSICAL ENVIRONMENT	• Somewhere that client feels comfortable • Distraction-free • Preferably no family members
PHYSICAL DISABILITY	• KICA-Cog can be altered for people with a disability • Should be wearing hearing aids and glasses if they have them • For those with visual impairment, objects can be given to them for recognition and naming • Enlarged pictures can be used for visual naming and recall. If not able to see them, these questions can be eliminated and the score adjusted accordingly
KICA CARER	• This is as important as the KICA-Cog and must be completed • If a family member is not available, aged care workers can be used or someone who knows the person well

Table 9.2

Kimberley Indigenous Cognitive Assessment guidelines—cont'd

	GUIDELINE
KICA-COG	• Adaptations can be made for regional differences • Inclusion of collection of bush tucker in places where there are not many animals to hunt • Use of alternative pictures if not easily recognised
CHECKLIST	• Important to complete all sections • Score is only part of assessment • Observations form important part of decision-making process

Management, care, support and review

All areas of Australia, including remote areas, have access to ACATs and HACC services. Services are administered through a variety of governance structures. A comprehensive care plan should be drawn up to assist to match the patient's and their family's needs (Table 9.3).

Services available in varying degrees include home care, meals, laundry services and personal care through HACC or private services, or they may be supplemented through CACPs and others. Case conferences with local service providers help coordinate services; the presence of a 'key worker' or case manager is often helpful. Information about support services is needed to assist families. There are many innovative respite programs such as the Troopy respite program, which is culturally appropriate in remote areas. Newer models of culturally appropriate care are being evaluated based on principles of community consultation, collaboration and inclusion (LoGiudice et al 2012b).

Carer education about dementia can be supported by Alzheimer's Australia and DBMAS, with a number of culturally appropriate resources. Discussion of future care planning, for financial and medical issues and end of life, are required in a timely manner.

CONCLUSION

The conditions of dementia, chronic pain, falls, incontinence and depression are common among older Aboriginal Australians. We need to acknowledge that cultural, social and environmental factors play a role in the prevalence, assessment and management of these conditions if we are to 'close the gap' in a population already greatly affected by many disabling and costly conditions.

The access and quality of local health services need to be improved for older Aboriginal people to decrease the prevalence, severity and likelihood of recurrence of these conditions. This is in line with the policy of the Australian

Table 9.3

Issues addressed by a comprehensive care plan

ISSUE	COMMUNITY CARE	VISITING SERVICES AND ASSESSMENTS AS REQUIRED
Food	Meals on Wheels Sufficient drinking water	Dietitian if required Speech pathologist swallowing assessment if required
Personal hygiene	Personal care Laundry	Occupational therapy assessment and equipment Continence advice and equipment
Mobility	Transport around community	Physiotherapy assessment and equipment Driving assessment if required Transport into regional centre as required
Day activity	Centre-based day respite Recreation Home-based respite	Advice regarding activities from AHPs or DBMAS
Behavioural and psychological issues	Assess for depression	Support from DBMAS if required
Carer support	Information and support from aged care service and clinic to build resilience Day/home-based respite Carer pension as required	Residential respite Centrelink
Accommodation	Appropriate housing	Occupational therapy assessment and home modifications as required Advocacy if required
Finances	Centrelink Advocacy if abuse suspected	Guardianship if required Advocacy if abuse suspected
Health	Medication for dementia if appropriate Treatment of comorbidities by clinic	Dental care Medication review if required from pharmacist

Government, which has bipartisan political support, that Aboriginal Australians should have at least equivalent access to health services.

There is a shortage of Aboriginal people employed in health and aged care at all levels. In particular, Aboriginal people are required in positions of aged care policy development and decision making. Aboriginal-specific aged care training and best practice guidelines are required for all health professionals who work with Aboriginal people. All health services need to encourage the use of professional interpreter services because of differences in health concepts and communication contributing to poor Aboriginal health outcomes.

Further research is required on the prevalence and cause of disabling conditions in Aboriginal and Torres Strait Islander populations, and on the needs of Aboriginal people affected by them. Conducting methodologically sound research into these areas would expand the knowledge of the mechanisms of these conditions, which may in turn inform appropriately delivered and sustainable models for management and support in Aboriginal and Torres Strait Islander communities.

Vignette

Billy is an old man who lives with his family in a remote community of the Northern Territory. He is unsure of his age because he travelled to the community from the desert many years ago. He worked as a stockman, which he enjoyed, riding horses and mustering. He recalls falling off his horse a number of times and was told he 'blacked out for quite a while' on one occasion. He is a traditional elder who underwent the community law rituals and is respected in the community. He has many children and grandchildren and was widowed three years ago. His daughter, who looks out for him, is concerned because his pants are often soiled with urine, but he refuses to discuss it when she tries to approach him about it. He is withdrawn, avoiding visiting family, playing cards and traditional lore time rituals. He has never been a drinker, and chews tobacco. He walks with a limp and his daughter notes that he grimaces, particularly when getting up from the ground. He often talks about his wife who has died.

Reflective questions

1. In undertaking a holistic assessment of an older Aboriginal person, discuss how you would approach gathering and understanding the possible cultural and traditional issues that may impact on this.

2. Discuss how you might address developing an education program on falls, dementia or incontinence in an Aboriginal community. What might be the difference in your approach between an urban and remote community?

3. How might you determine whether a currently utilised assessment tool is suitable for Aboriginal Australians?

References

Australian Bureau of Statistics, 2004a. Disability, ageing and carers: a summary of findings 2003. ABS, Canberra.

Australian Bureau of Statistics, 2004b. National Aboriginal and Torres Strait Islander social survey 2002. ABS, Canberra.

Australian Bureau of Statistics, 2007. Population distribution, Aboriginal and Torres Strait Islander Australians. 2006. ABS, Canberra, Contract No.: ABS cat. no. 4705.0.

Australian Bureau of Statistics, Australian Institute of Health and Welfare, 2008. The health and welfare of Australian Aboriginal and Torres Strait Islander peoples. Commonwealth Australia, Canberra.

Australian Institute of Health and Welfare, 2009. Measuring the social and emotional wellbeing of Aboriginal and Torres Strait Islander peoples. Commonwealth Australia, Canberra.

Australian Institute of Health and Welfare, 2010. The Health and Welfare of Australia's Aboriginal and Torres Strait Islander Peoples. Commonwealth Australia, Canberra.

Australian Institute of Health and Welfare, 2012. Residential aged care in Australia 2010–11: a statistical overview. Aged care statistics series no. 36. Cat. no. AGE 68. AIHW, Canberra.

Arkles, R., Pulver, L.J., Broe, G., et al., 2010. Ageing, cognition and dementia in Australian Aboriginal and Torres Strait Islander Peoples. Neuroscience Research Australia and Muru Marri Indigenous Health Unit.

Arvanitakis, Z., Wilson, R.S., Bienias, J.L., et al., 2004. Diabetes mellitus and risk of Alzheimer's Disease and decline in cognitive function. Archives Neurology 61, 661–666.

Barker, D., Gluckman, P., Godfrey, K., et al., 1993. Foetal nutrition and cardiovascular disease in adult life. Lancet 341, 938–994.

Benness, C., Manning, J., 1997. Urinary dysfunction in Australian Aboriginal women. International Urogynaecology Journal (8), S65.

Blyth, F., March, L., Brnabic, A., et al., 2001. Chronic pain in Australia: a prevalence study. Pain 89, 127–134.

Bowirrat, A., Friedland, R., Korczyn, A., 2002. Vascular dementia among elderly Arabs in Wadi Ara. J Neurol Sci 203, 73–76.

Broe, A., Jackson-Pulver, L., 2007. Aboriginal ageing: is there such a thing? University of NSW, Sydney.

Brooke, N., 2011. Needs of Aboriginal and Torres Strait Islander clients residing in Australian residential aged-care facilities. Aust J Rural Health 19, 166–170.

Bruce, D.G., Baird, M., Saddler, A.H., et al., 1998. A preliminary survey of patients seen by the Kimberley Aged Care Assessment Team. Australasian Journal on Ageing 17 (2), 95–97.

Carroll, E., Smith, K., Shadforth, G., et al., 2010. Indigenous Services Study: Lungurra Ngoora Community Care Final Report. Online. Available: http://www.wacha.org.au/docs/misc/IDSS-Final-Report.pdf, 12 Sep 2012.

Chiarelli, P., Bower, W., Sibbritt, D., et al., 2005. Estimating the prevalence of urinary and faecal incontinence in Australia. Australiasian Journal Ageing 24, 19–27.

Continence Foundation Association, 2012. Leaking pee—let's yarn about women's business. Online. Available: www.continence.org, 12 Sep 2012.

Couzos, S., Murray, R., 2008. Aboriginal primary health care: an evidence-based approach, third ed. Oxford University Press, South Melbourne.

Dingwall, K.M., Cairney, S., 2010. Psychological and cognitive assessment of Indigenous Australians. Australian and New Zealand Journal of Psychiatry 44 (1), 20–30.

Drachman, D., 2006. Ageing of the brain, entropy and Alzheimer's disease. Neurology 67, 1340–1352.

Dudgeon, P., Garvey, D., Pickett, H., 2000. Working with Indigenous Australians. A handbook for psychologists. Gunada Press, Curtin Indigenous Research Centre, Perth.

Eley, D., Hunter, K., Hannah, D., et al., 2006. Tools and methodologies for investigating the mental health needs of Indigenous patients: it's about communication. Australian Psychiatry 14 (1), 33–37.

Esler, D., Johnston, F., Thomas, D., et al., 2008. The validity of a depression screening tool modified for use with ATSI people. Australian NZJ Public Health 32 (4), 317–321.

Flicker, L., 2010. Modifiable lifestyle risk factors for Alzheimer's disease. Journal Of Alzheimer's Disease: Journal Alzheimers Disaese 20 (3), 803–811.

Flood, J., 2006. The original Australians. Story of the Aboriginal people. Allen & Unwin, Crows Nest NSW.

Forster, S., Wall, S., Roberston, H., et al., 2010. Aboriginal Ageing, Growing old in Aboriginal Communities, Linking services and research. A report of the 2 National Workshop of the Australian Association of Gerontology Aboriginal and Torees Strait islander Ageing Committee. Darwin.

Garvey, G., Simmonds, D., Gorman, D., et al., 2011. Making sense of dementia: understanding amongst indigenous Australians. International Journal of Geriatric Psychiatry 26 (6), 649–656.

Gracey, M., Bridge, E., Martin, D., et al., 2006. An Aboriginal driven program to prevent, control and manage nutritional related 'lifestyle' diseases including diabetes. Asia Pacific Journal of Clinical Nutrition 15, 178–188.

Helme, R., Gibson, S., 1999. Pain in older people. IASP, Seattle.

Helps, Y., Harrison, J., 2006. Hospitalised injury of Australia's Aboriginal and Torres Strait Islander people: 2000–02. AIHW, Adelaide. (AIHW cat no. INJCAT 94).

Hill, K., Barker, B., Vos, T.. 2007. Excess Indigenous mortality: are Indigenous Australians more severely disadvantaged than other Indigenous populations? International Journal of Epidemiology 36, 58–89.

Hill, K., Smith, R., Murray, K., et al., 2000. P. An analysis of research on preventing falls and falls injury in older people: Community, residential care and acute care settings: Commonwealth Australia.

Honeyman, P., Jacobs, E., 1996. Effects of culture on back pain in Australian Aboriginals. Spine 21, 841–843.

Inouye, S., Studenski, S., Tinetti, M., et al., 2007. Geriatric syndromes: clinical, research and policy implications of a core geriatric concept. Journal American Geriatric Society 55 (5), 780–791.

Jensen, H., Smith, K., Flicker, L., et al., 2012. Development of pathways to care and education for Aboriginal people living with dementia. Dementia Collaborative Research Centre website.

Jorm, A.F., Bourchier, S.J., Cvetkovski, S., et al., 2012. Mental health of Indigenous Australians: a review of findings from community surveys. The Medical Journal Of Australia 196, 118–121.

Kalaria, R., Maestre, G., Arizaga, R., et al., 2008. Alzheimer's disease and vascular dementia in developing countries: prevalence, management, and risk factors. Lancet Neurol 7, 812–826.

Lai, M., Waldron, N., 2011. Hip fracture risk profiles in older Indigenous Australians. Med J Aust 195 (3), 159–160.

Larraya, F., Grasso, L., Mari, G., 2004. Prevalence of dementia of Alzheimer's type, vascular dementia and other DSM-IV and ICD-10 dementias in the Republic of Argentina. Revista Neurologica Argentina 29, 148–153.

LoGiudice, D., Smith, K., Flicker, L., et al., 2006. Kimberley Indigenous Cognitive Assessment tool (KICA): development of a cognitive assessment tool for older indigenous Australians. International Psychogeriatrics 18 (02), 269–280.

LoGiudice, D., Strivens, E., Smith, K., et al., 2011. The KICA screen: the psychometric properties of a shortened version of the KICA (Kimberley Indigenous Cognitive Assessment). Australian Journal Aging 30 (4), 215–219.

LoGiudice, D.C., Smith, K., Flicker, L., et al., 2012a. A preliminary evaluation of the prevalence of falls, pain and urinary incontinence in remote living Indigenous Australians over the age of 45 years. Internal Medicine Journal 42 (6), e102–e107.

LoGiudice, D.C., Smith, K., Shadforth, G., et al., 2012b. Lungurra Ngoora—a pilot model of care for aged and disabled in a remote Aboriginal community—can it work? Rural and Remote Health 12, 2078. Online. Available: www.rrh.org.au, 12 Sep 2012.

Macintosh, D.J., Pearson, B., 2001. Fractures of the femoral neck in Australian Aboriginals and Torres Strait Islanders. Australian Journal of Rural Health 9 (3), 127–133.

Marmot, M., 2005. Social determinants of health inequalities. The Lancet 65, 1099–1104.

McGrath, P., 2006. 'The biggest worry …': research findings on pain management for Aboriginal peoples in Northern Territory, Australia. Rural and Remote Health 6 (549), Online. Available: www.rrh.org.au, 12 Sept 2012.

Mitra, B., Cameron, P., Gabbe, B., 2007. Ladders revisited. Medical Journal Australia. 186, 31–34.

Molero, A., Ramirez, G.P., Maestre, G., 2007. High prevalence of dementia in a Caribbean population. Neuroepidemiology 29, 107–112.

National Public Health Partnership, 2006. The National Aboriginal and Torres Strait Islander Safety Promotion Strategy. NPHP, Canberra.

O'Dea, K., Rowley, K., Brown, A., 2007. Diabetes in Indigenous Australians—possible ways forward. Med J Aust 186 (10), 494–495.

Peel, N., Bell, R., Smith, K., 2008. Queensland Stay on your Feet: Community Good Practice guidelines–preventing falls, harm from falls and promoting healthy active ageing in older Queenslanders. Queensland Health, Brisbane.

Ring, I., Brown, N., 2003. The health status of indigenous peoples and others. BMJ 327 (7412), 404–405.

Rockwood, K., Mitnitski, A., 2007. Frailty in relation to the accumulation of deficits. J Gerontol A Biol Sci Med Sc 62 (7), 722–727.

Roe, J., 2000. Ngarlu: A cultural and spritual strengthening model. In: Dudgeon, P., G, D., Pickett, H. (Eds.), Working with Indigenous Australians: a handbook for psychologists. Gunada Press, Curtin Indigenous Research Centre, Perth, pp. 395–402.

Sansoni, J., Marosszeky, N., Fleming, G., et al., 2010. Selecting Tools for ACAT Assessment: A Report for the Aged Care Assessment Program (ACAP) Expert Clinical Reference Group. Australian Government Department of Health and Ageing, Canberra, Report for the Aged Care Assessment Program.

Sheldon, M., 2001. Psychiatric assessment in remote Aboriginal communities. Australian & New Zealand Journal of Psychiatry 35, 435–442.

Skoog, I., Nilsson, L., Persson, G., et al., 1996. 15-year longitudinal study of blood pressure and dementia. The Lancet 347 (9009), 1141–1145.

Smith, K., 2008. Assessment and prevalence of dementia in Indigenous Australians (thesis). University of Western Australia, Perth.

Smith, K., Flicker, L., Dwyer, A., et al., 2010. Factors associated with dementia in Aboriginal Australians. Aust N Z J Psychiatry 44 (10), 888–893.

Smith, K., Flicker, L., LoGiudice, D., et al., 2009. Assessing cognitive impairment in Indigenous Australians: re-evaluation of the Kimberley Indigenous Cognitive Assessment in Western Australia and the Northern Territory. Australian Psychologist 44 (1), 54–61.

Smith, K., Flicker, L., LoGiudice, D., et al., 2008. Dementia and cognitive impairment in remote Indigenous Australians—evidence of different patterns of risk factors and increased prevalence. Neurology 71 (19), 1470–1473.

Smith, K.F.L., Shadforth, G., Carroll, E., et al., 2011. Gotta be sit down and worked out together': views of Aboriginal caregivers and service providers on ways to improve dementia care for Aboriginal Australians. Rural and Remote Health 11, 1650.

Smith, K., LoGiudice, D., Dwyer, A., et al., 2007. 'Ngana minyarti? What is this?'Development of cognitive questions for the Kimberley Indigenous Cognitive Assessment. Australasian Journal on Ageing 26 (3), 115–119.

Smith, R., Spargo, R., King, R., et al., 1992. Risk factors for hypertension in Kimberley Aborigines. Med J Aust 156, 562–566.

Steering Committee for the Review of Government Service Provision (SCRGSP), 2012. Report on Government Services 2012, Indigenous Compendium, Productivity Commission, Canberra. Chapter 13. Aged Care Services 290–306.

Swan, P., Raphael, B., 1995. Ways Forward: National Aboriginal and Torres Strait Islander Mental Health Policy National Consultancy Report. Commonwealth of Australia, Canberra.

Trudgen, R., 2000. Why warriors lie down & die: towards an understanding of why the Aboriginal People of Arnhem Land face the greatest crisis in health and education since European contact: Djambatj Mala. Aboriginal Resource & Development Services Incorporated, Darwin.

Vaynman, S., Gomez-Pinilla, F., 2006. Revenge of the 'sit': how lifestyle impacts neuronal and cognitive health through molecular systems that interface energy metabolism with neuronal plasticity. J Neurosci Res. 84, 699–715.

Vicary, D., Andrews, H., 2001. A model of therapeutic intervention with Indigenous Australians. Australian and New Zealand Journal of Public Health 25, 349–351.

Vicary, D., Westerman, T., 2004. 'That's just the way he is': Some implications of Aboriginal mental health beliefs. Advances in Mental Health 3 (3), 103–112.

Vindigni, D., Perkins, J., 2003. Identifying musculoskeletal conditions among rural Indigenous peoples. Australian Journal Rural Health 11, 187–192.

Wang, Z., Knight, S., O'Dea, K., et al., 2006. Blood pressure and hypertension in ATSI people. European J Cardiovascular Prevention and Rehabilitation 13, 438–443.

Wong, Y., Flicker, L., Draper, G., et al., 2012. Hip fractures among Indigenous people from Western Australia from 1999–2009. Internal Medicine Journal Nov 23 Epub; doi.1111/imj.12040.

World Health Organization, 2010. International Classification of Function, Disability and Health. WHO, Geneva.

Zann, S., 1994. Identification of support, education and training needs of rural/remote health care service providers involved in dementia care. Rural Health, Support, Education and Training (RHSET), Project Progress Report. Northern Regional Health Authority, Townsville.

Zhao, Y., Guthridge, S., Vos, T., et al., 2004. Burden of disease and injury in Aboriginal and non-Aboriginal populations in the Northern Territory. Medical Journal Australia 180, 498–502.

CHAPTER 10

WORKING WITH FAMILIES: EVIDENCE, TOOLS, IMPLEMENTATION AND EVALUATION

Michael Bauer, Rhonda Nay, Wendy Moyle and Deirdre Fetherstonhaugh

Editors' comments

Older people benefit when staff and families work harmoniously together—so do staff and families. This chapter takes the situation of staff conflict with families and reframes it as a person-centred partnership in which all stakeholders are recognised as 'people' whose goals need to be negotiated to ensure the best outcome for the older person at the centre of care and support. It outlines research undertaken by the authors as well as a number of tools that have been developed to implement and audit constructive staff/family relationships in residential aged care.

INTRODUCTION

Most older people want to remain in their own homes for as long as possible; this is very often made possible by an unpaid carer—usually spouse or daughter. The Australian Government and state/local governments currently provide support to keep people at home through such means as Community Aged Care Packages (CACPs), Extended Aged Care at Home (EACH) and Extended Aged Care at Home—Dementia (EACH-D) for older people assessed as requiring high-level care that would otherwise need to be provided in residential aged care facilities (RACFs). Home and Community Care (HACC) provides in-home support such as ironing, shopping and personal care. District nursing assists with more complex care needs. Transition care, in-reach and various other forms of care are provided by local hospitals. Nevertheless, whether at home, living with family or in hospital/aged care, the role of the family is almost always vital in quality person-centred care provision.

Whether at home, living with family or in hospital/aged care, the role of the family is almost always vital.

Anyone who has been involved with, and wants to remain involved with, an older person in a care setting can be defined as family. This can include friends (Haigler et al 2004). The importance of family in the lives of older people who are in a care setting is widely acknowledged since they can play a significant role in maintaining the person's wellbeing, not only because of their relationship to the person but because they have often been the primary caregiver prior to the person's transition to the health or supportive care service. In addition many families want to continue to be involved in some aspect of care provision following admission or in preparation for discharge (Bauer 2006, Bauer et al 2009, Gaugler & Kane 2007).

Families are known to hold unique knowledge and expertise that can inform the care of older people and both families and staff share a common goal of preserving health and identity through providing individualised high-quality care (Marziali et al 2006). The support of family carers through promoting a relationship-centred approach to care is now a policy priority throughout the developed world (Nolan et al 2009). It is therefore important that the dynamics between staff and family (in addition to the care recipients), the reciprocal exchange of information, collaboration in decision making and a recognition of the role of family carers and relationship quality are at the forefront of the care planning process (Nolan et al 2009). For family, the most positive care experiences are those where they can work in partnership with the staff, knowing there is open communication, involvement in care decisions and that their views will be taken into account (Wilson et al 2009). It is vital that health professionals have a good understanding of the issues that impact on family involvement, as well as the strategies to best support it. The beneficial outcomes of positive staff–family relationships have been observed from the perspective of staff (Moyle et al 2003, Utley-Smith et al 2009), family members (Bauer & Nay 2003, Legault & Ducharme 2009) and by older people in care (Brown-Wilson et al 2009, Gaugler 2006).

Developing and maintaining positive relationships with families is nonetheless often difficult for staff in care settings because the role of the family is sometimes seen as ambiguous in terms of the degree and nature of their involvement, with some staff viewing family members as a disturbance or a hindrance (Bauer 2006, Bauer & Nay 2011, Bauer et al 2009). Conflict can often occur when staff and family have differing expectations for care (Lindgren & Murphy 2002, Utley-Smith et al 2009) or when there is a lack of mutual understanding of roles (Specht et al 2000). A significant source of tension is often an 'us versus them' way of thinking that can develop between staff and families. This can be caused by staff and families having differing opinions as to what is in the care recipient's best interests (Austin et al 2009).

The implications of not fostering positive staff–family relationships can be significant. Majerovitz et al (2009) found that when staff–family relationships lacked trust and communication, family caregivers felt that staff were criticising them directly. This exacerbated existing feelings of guilt at placing their relative into care, as well as increasing family distress and confusion. Chen et al (2007) found that perceived conflict between family caregivers and staff directly correlated with levels of caregiver stress and depression. Staff–family friction can also have a negative effect on staff. Abrahamson et al (2010) found that conflict between staff and families led to increased staff dissatisfaction and burnout. Utley-Smith et al (2009) noted that negative interactions with family members had made staff want to quit their employment. Park (2010) found that relationships with families were worse, and stress levels higher, in nursing assistants compared with nurses, and suggests that this is due to nursing assistants being 'so acutely focused on accomplishing the many physical tasks of care that they fail to interact with residents and families in appropriate ways' (p 139).

Twenty-five years ago Bowers (1987) argued that family caring comprises several interrelated components including:

- anticipatory care—seen as 'just in case' in which family members engage in speculation about what they would do 'if' an older family member were to need care
- preventative care—whereby support is subtly provided to prevent potential difficulties from arising
- supervisory care—more overt support that is nevertheless, as far as is possible, kept 'hidden' from the recipient
- instrumental care—the form of support typically associated with the caring role
- protective care—whereby family members try to 'protect' their relative from becoming aware of their increasing frailty.

Based on her grounded theory study, Bowers (1987) contended that family carers see protective care as the most important and stressful of their roles. In a later study Bowers (1988) argued that care continues after admission to a nursing home but that then the most important type of care becomes 'preservative' care, which involves family carers in attempts to 'preserve' the identity and individuality of their relative. Nolan et al (1996) suggested that (re)constructive and reciprocal care are important components that involve both the carer and the cared-for person as active participants in maintaining reciprocity in their relationship and reconstructing roles and relationships over time.

It is now widely acknowledged that to develop and maintain constructive staff–family relationships a reciprocal approach to caregiving, where families and staff are partners rather than competitors, is required (Dijkstra 2007, Kemp et al 2009, Legault & Ducharme 2009, Majerovitz et al 2009). Such an approach sees family support helping staff provide the best level of care (Kemp et al 2009) and a collaborative attitude from staff ensuring that family members are kept up to date about the wellbeing and care needs of the person in care (Legault & Ducharme 2009).

> Family carers see protective care as the most
> important and stressful of their roles.

A BRIEF HISTORY OF OUR WORK

The role of family was highlighted in Nay's (1994) doctoral research, which led to further qualitative work on family experience of nursing home entry (1996, 1997). In the interviews for the latter research family members said 'placing' a loved one in a nursing home was the hardest thing they had ever done. Such a view was also confirmed in further Australian research (Moyle et al 2002) that identified the grief families developed as their role changed from sole carer, to one where they felt they had no role in the care of their family member once the person was 'placed' into care.

Recent Australian research using a mixed-method approach explored the effect of a family involvement in care (FIC) partnership intervention on family and staff wellbeing in long-term dementia care (Bramble et al 2009, 2011). This partnership model derives from the premise that the family is also a client and families are a valuable resource for improving quality of care. Bramble et al (2009, 2011) utilised a FIC intervention developed in an American study (Maas et al 2004). The intervention involved three staff education sessions that aimed to improve staff knowledge of care of people with dementia as well as an understanding of the role of the family in this care. The third session, delivered only to the intervention site, presented information on how to negotiate with family caregivers to increase their involvement in care. The families were given a resource manual that provided information on how they could become involved in the care of their family member as well as information about dementia. A written partnership contract of care was developed and agreed upon by the family and staff. The study findings indicate the importance of education for both staff and families as a means to enable an understanding of each other's role, as well as the partnership contract as a clear means of operationalising this understanding. Although the FIC intervention was successful in changing practice, the study also highlighted the challenge of this intervention and its role in increasing stress for staff involved in negotiations with families. The care facility manager was acknowledged as being crucial in 'making or breaking' the success of a staff–family intervention.

As a means of designing an intervention suitable for families of people with dementia in acute care settings a large team of Australian researchers (Moyle et al 2010) conducted an exploratory study of family carer involvement, their role and needs, in the care of a person with dementia staying in an acute care setting. Initial analysis of this data demonstrates the importance of health professionals engaging families in the decision-making process related to the care of the person with dementia, families feeling their role is valued by staff members and the important role families play in helping staff to understand the needs of the person with dementia.

Bauer (2003, 2006, Bauer & Nay 2003), in his doctoral research exploring how RACF staff construct working with residents' families, found that there was still a great deal of rhetoric around participatory family care when it came to the attitudes and practices of many care staff. Bauer found that while many RACF staff had developed a substantive family orientation and adopted practices that were inclusive of the needs of the family, it was equally evident that care staff also had attitudes that suggested they cast family into a competitive and adversarial role. Bauer's research highlighted a number of questions that needed to be answered regarding how care practices could better establish and support collaborative partnerships with families in residential aged care.

In 2006 the Australian Centre for Evidence Based Aged Care (ACEBAC) began a systematic program of research that has involved reviewing the research evidence and developing several measurement tools. These tools measure the constructiveness of staff family relationships from both an individual attitudinal level and that of facility support and current facility practice, with the aim of identifying areas for improvement and developing implementation strategies.

SYSTEMATIC REVIEW OF THE RESEARCH EVIDENCE

Haesler et al (2006) examined the research over the previous 15 years that reported on staff–family relationships in the care of older people in hospital, subacute, rehabilitation and long-term care. This systematic review and a subsequent update (Haesler et al 2010) highlighted a number of key areas that are critical to supporting the relationship with family carers.[1] These include: acknowledging the uniqueness of the older person; providing information and emotional support; facilitating open, two-way communication that is responsive to the family's needs; and recognising that some families place great value on collaboration in care, and that conflicting staff and family perspectives on their role will ultimately lead to competitive relationships that are detrimental to care. The organisational practices that underpin and inform care delivery are of paramount importance because they will support or impede the role of family carers. Specifically the review found that:

> Family members' perceptions of their relationships with staff showed that a strong focus was placed on opportunities for the family to be involved in the patient's [resident's] care. Staff members also expressed a theoretical support for the collaborative process, however, this belief often did not translate to the staff members' clinical practice.

(Haesler et al 2010 p 289)

Five key factors, listed next, have emerged from this collection of research that are essential to interventions designed to support a collaborative partnership between family members and healthcare staff.

....
[1]The findings from the systematic review were also developed into a consumer booklet for families of older people living in residential care (Fetherstonhaugh et al 2012).

Communication

- Being able to create a caring friendly environment where family feel safe and heard is essential to developing constructive staff–family relationships. To do so staff must have the ability to:
  - be good active listeners
  - communicate openly and honestly
  - work in partnerships
  - provide information
  - promote the uniqueness of the resident.

Information

- Family expect staff to share information about the older person living in the facility with them and, furthermore, expect to be able to share information they possess to preserve the individuality of the older person.
- Interventions designed to promote constructive staff–family relationships should address strategies to increase the flow and exchange of information.

Education

- Incorporation of staff and family education into interventions designed to promote constructive staff–family relationships is highly recommended.
- Education should include relationship development, power and control issues, communication skills and negotiating techniques.

Administrative support

- Support from administration and management staff is more likely to result in sustained positive effectiveness from interventions designed to promote constructive interactions.
- Support should include addressing workloads and staffing issues, practical support or education and introduction of care models focused on collaboration with families.

Familiarity, trust, respect and empathy

- Familiarity, trust, respect and empathy are essential building blocks for developing constructive relationships between staff and family members.

Many of these themes have continued to be reflected in the more recent literature, suggesting that the translation of the research into practice remains an issue.

 Family members' perceptions of their relationships with staff showed that a strong focus was placed on opportunities for the family to be involved in the resident's care.

IMPLEMENTING RESEARCH EVIDENCE INTO PRACTICE

Having some clear findings to work with, ACEBAC then began the work of translating the research findings into real-world practice with a pilot in three residential care facilities in Melbourne. The methodological approach to this 'translation', now defined as TEAM (or Translating Evidence into Aged care Methodology), comprised the following components but can be easily modified to the context and specific evidence of the implementation project (Winbolt et al 2009):

- establishing what needs to be changed and why
- establishing a 'community of practice' that comprises advisors and users
- ensuring organisational readiness and organisational sponsorship and engagement
- co-opting the enthusiasts/opinion leaders as change fellows and champions
- establishing what research evidence exists
- developing audit indicators
- developing an appropriate sample and how audit data will be collected, analysed and managed
- conducting an audit of current practice and comparing this with the research evidence
- developing evidence-based guidelines or modifying an existing contextualised guideline
- educating and supporting fellows and champions to lead, encourage and monitor the practice change process
- developing a change plan with stakeholders
- embedding change in usual practice
- re-auditing practice
- selling the practice change by focusing on the benefits (not blame) and rewarding success.

In line with TEAM, the recommendations from the systematic review of the evidence (Haesler et al 2010) were developed into a guideline that included measurable indicators that a residential aged care service could audit their current practice against (Table 10.1). Each of these indicators were then broken down further into the criteria that were needed for each indicator to be met. *Structure criteria* are those that are necessary in the system/service/facility in order to meet the indicator. For instance, if you wanted staff and family to be educated then there needs to be an education program available in the service/facility. *Process criteria* are those actions/decisions/behaviours that are taken in order to meet the indicator. For example, there may be a staff–family education program in existence, but if staff and family do not attend the education program they will obviously not be educated. *Outcome criteria* are what you expect to achieve, the results for which in this instance may be from the perspective of staff, family or the resident. An example may be that following from the structure and process criteria, *all* staff and/or families have been educated. However, while you may want a target of 100% compliance in

Table 10.1

Guideline recommendations and indicators for building staff–family relationships

EVIDENCE-BASED GUIDELINE RECOMMENDATION	AUDIT INDICATOR(S)
Incorporate into staff development programs education designed to promote constructive staff–family relationships	• Permanent staff participate in an education/training program covering the four areas of: (1) relationship development and conflict resolution; (2) power and control in relationships; (3) communication skills and negotiation techniques; and (4) reflection and self-knowledge • Families receive information about developing and maintaining constructive staff–family relationships
Establish policies and procedures that enable and support family involvement in decision making and/or care planning	• Families that wish to be involved in decision making and/or care planning, and that have the resident's permission to be involved in such decision making and/or care planning, are involved and supported in doing so
Establish formal communication channels for both staff and families	• Families are provided with information on the facility's formal communication channels • Families have been given the opportunity to participate in regular resident–family meetings (as agreed and defined by the facility in consultation with families) • Permanent care staff provide detailed information about each resident's health, care, facility policies, procedures and the aged care industry (within their scope of practice) as requested by the family • Where a complaint has been made, the complaints policy is followed
Informal communication channels are embedded to encourage staff–family interaction	• Families report satisfaction with information sharing by staff at the facility
Environments that support staff/families in promoting constructive relationships exist (e.g. a person-centred approach to the involvement of families exists)	• The facility has a procedure to guide staff in the management of family anger/aggression • The facility has a procedure for dealing with distressing staff–family communication incidents • Staff and families have the opportunity to participate in formal peer support/debriefing following distressing staff–family communication incidents

education, this may not be achievable and so outcome results/targets should be determined specifically for each service/facility and judged relative to those measured at baseline (Morrell & Harvey 2003).

As part of the evaluation process we used a tool modified for our contexts that was being developed by Nolan et al (unpublished). The recommendations from this phase (Bauer et al 2009) were:

- Facilities should examine their practices in relation to family care and adopt the audit tool as a means of benchmarking those practices.
- Facilities should distribute the consumer booklet to all family carers of residents.
- To facilitate cross-cultural communication, translating the consumer booklet into the identifiable languages spoken by residents and their families/carers in RACFs should be pursued.
- The survey tool is further contextualised and tested for use in the Australian residential aged care context.
- A key staff member at each aged care facility should be designated as the point of contact for other staff and families and be responsible for driving the adoption and implementation of the clinical guideline and audit tool.
- The research should be replicated in a wider range of facilities.

MEASURING STAFF-FAMILY RELATIONSHIPS

The literature and our own research has highlighted the existence of both active and more subtle tension between health professionals and family members as a significant barrier to the participation of older people's families in their care. To realise the benefits that family involvement offers the older person, their family and the care professional, there needs to be an understanding of the relationships that exist between staff and family and the strategies that will be most effective in promoting positive interaction and collaboration. While the important components of constructive staff–family relationships were identified by the two systematic reviews and therefore could be defined theoretically, gauging the views of staff and what activities are actually occurring in an aged care setting that support establishing and maintaining constructive staff–family relationships remained a challenge in the absence of adequate measurement tools.

Although a number of instruments that assess nurses' perceptions of and attitudes towards families are available, these tools are either not validated, not developed for the aged care setting, or are very generic measures of the importance of involving the family in nursing care (see Benzein et al 2008). To build on the previous work of ACEBAC, context-specific measurement tools to assess how residential aged care staff understand staff–family relationships, the factors they perceive to be important to a relationship, their attitudes towards family and how well they engage with them were required.

Two tools—the Family and Staff Relationship Implementation Tool (FASRIT) (Bauer et al 2012a) and the Family and Staff Relationship Attitude Tool (FASRAT) (Bauer et al 2012b)—were developed to make it possible for residential services to measure, evaluate and improve the quality of care they provide. The 25-item FASRIT helps identify and implement interventions aimed at improving staff–family relationships by enabling facilities to appraise current practice against what is known to be best practice in promoting constructive staff–family relationships. The 26-item FASRAT allows facilities to measure the attitudes and beliefs of care staff with respect to the factors that are known to promote constructive staff–family relationships.

Tool items were derived from the best available research evidence on the factors that make up a constructive staff–family relationship (the systematic reviews), were verified by care staff and residents' families and confirmed by an expert panel. The psychometric properties of both tools supports their use in the Australian residential aged care setting as a means to identify gaps that impact on the quality of staff–family relationships, identify areas where further education may be required and evaluate and monitor facility practice over time.

CONCLUSION

Being the family carer of an older person can be difficult and at times stressful. Even when health professionals have taken over the primary caregiver responsibility, however, many family members wish to continue to play a significant role. There is widespread recognition that family involvement in the life of older people in care, which may include input into the planning and execution of the care itself, is essential to person–centred care and, more importantly, can improve care outcomes. Establishing positive staff–family relationships is nevertheless not without its challenges. Instituting relationship-centred care requires a commitment from organisations and individuals to ensure their practices genuinely underpin, inform and support the establishment and maintenance of relationships. There are a number of tools and other resources available that allow aged care services to appraise their practices, identify gaps and support positive staff–family relationships. The use of evidence-based measures and resources to promote and support quality are recommended.

Vignette

Mary has been admitted to 'Golden Treetops' aged care facility following a six-week hospital stay for a fractured hip after falling over at home. While in hospital Mary is also diagnosed with dementia, albeit in its early stages. Her daughter, Joan, is naturally devastated about all that has happened and she is very worried that the facility staff won't be able to take care of her mother as well as she did, especially now that she also has dementia. In addition to these concerns, Joan has been left with selling the family home and organising everything herself.

The registered nurse at the facility carries out the standard admission procedure with Mary. The nurse assures Joan that her mother will be fine and that she will gradually settle into life there. As part of the admission process Joan and Mary are asked many questions about the sorts of things that Mary has enjoyed throughout her life and these are ticked off on the form used. Mary is also asked a few questions about her proudest moments, but neither she nor her daughter can remember anything because both were very tired.

Joan is very stressed the first few days after Mary's admission because things are going not at all as she had expected. Joan knows that her mother can't sleep without the talkback radio playing softly throughout the night, so she stays at the facility longer to make sure the radio is turned on each evening. The staff also don't get her mother out of bed till after 9 am and her mother has always been dressed and ready for the day by 7 am. Her mother never used to complain about anything so Joan is afraid that she might not 'stick up for herself' in the facility if she herself isn't there to keep an eye on things and protect her. During the day Joan sits in the lounge with her mother just watching everything, noticing all of the things that are not right about the place.

Over the next few weeks Joan comes in every day at 7 am to make sure the staff look after her mother properly in the mornings. She stays at the facility until 7 pm when her mother is settled in bed. The staff try to avoid both Joan and Mary as much as possible. Joan's constant presence in the facility and her monitoring of everything staff do is causing the staff to become increasingly stressed. Her presence and frequent comments to staff about how they could improve her mother's care also become annoying for staff. Many staff start to see Joan as demanding and difficult—a constant 'complainer'. The one time that staff took Joan's mother to a gardening group (this was one of the interests that she had mentioned in the initial life history assessment), Mary told her daughter that she had a terrible time and 'never wants to do that again'. Joan has stopped looking after herself. Because Joan spends all her time at the facility; she can't bear to take time out for herself as it involves leaving her mother in the hands of staff who don't know or understand her.

One day a new nurse at the facility, Dan, who had read the ACEBAC *Consumer booklet for families of older people living in residential care* and the ACEBAC staff-family assessment tools as part of the new staff member's orientation program, decided to sit and talk with Mary and Joan for a while and find out more about them—more than had been captured in the standard admission documentation. Dan finds out that Mary had been a hard worker all of her life, and had always been up early to make breakfast for the family and then leave the house to go to work herself. He discovers that Mary had a love of gardening ... but that her love of gardening was not so much about doing the gardening but about doing gardening with her husband—who had died some years ago. As they spoke, Joan told Dan many stories about her mother, and described in detail the last few years of her life where she had looked after her mother all by herself. Joan missed parts of that life very much and felt 'useless and helpless' now that the care of her mother was in the hands of 'strangers'. From Dan's conversation with Mary and Joan it becomes apparent that Joan does not have much understanding of dementia or its trajectory and could probably benefit from some education and contact with organisations such as Alzheimer's Australia.

Dan shares all this information with the rest of the care team and over the next month both Joan and Mary are invited to attend a coffee and chat club with some other relatives and families. Joan finds out that there are other families that are going through very similar things to what she is. The nurse notes the times that Mary likes to be up and dressed, and suggests to the lifestyle staff that gardening might hold more of a 'spiritual' meaning for Mary than actually joining a 'gardening group'. So, each day staff assist Joan and Mary to a shady place in the courtyard where they can share morning tea together. Joan is encouraged to lay out Mary's clothes for the next day each night—this is found to be very important to Joan because she knows exactly what her mother likes to wear. Joan also begins taking her mother's clothes home so she can wash them herself, just as she had always done. Joan is also given information about dementia and put into contact with consumer organisations that can provide education and support for people who care for loved ones with dementia.

Being involved in her mother's care in a meaningful way, and knowing that the staff better understand her mother, allows Joan to relax and gives her a renewed sense of purpose in life. It gives Joan 'permission' to take more time out for herself. Joan also develops trust in the knowledge that the staff are able to meet her mother's needs in a more person-centred way. The facility's efforts to support the continuation of her pre-existing relationship with her mother and emphasise the establishment of positive relationships with the staff, provides comfort and confidence in the facility and Joan becomes more involved in the life of the facility, other residents and their families.

Reflective questions

1. Think of an older person in care who has a family member that visits. How have you encouraged positive relationships with the family?

2. Working through the guideline recommendations how do you/your organisation fare?

3. How is the promotion of staff–family relationships demonstrated in the day-to-day work practices of your organisation?

4. What education and other support do you receive from your organisation to encourage more relationship-centred care with families?

5. Can you imagine what support interventions you would like if you were to provide care for an older person and their family member with dementia at home or in care? Make a list and share this with your work colleagues.

References

Abrahamson, K., Anderson, J.G., Anderson, M.M., et al., 2010. The cumulative influence of conflict on nursing home staff. Research in Gerontological Nursing 3 (1), 39–48.

Abrahamson, K., Suitor, J., Pillemer, K., 2009. Conflict between nursing home staff and residents' families: does it increase burnout? Journal of Aging and Health 21 (6), 895–912.

Austin, W., Goble, E., Strang, V., et al., 2009. Supporting relationships between family and staff in continuing care settings. Journal of Family Nursing 15 (3), 360–383.

Bauer, M., 2003. Collaboration and control: a naturalistic study of nurses' constructions of the role of family in nursing home care. [Doctor of Philosophy], La Trobe University, Melbourne.

Bauer, M., 2006. Collaboration and control: nurses' constructions of the role of family in nursing home care. Journal of Advanced Nursing 54 (1), 45–52.

Bauer, M., Fetherstonhaugh, D., Lewis, V., 2012a. Assessing the quality of staff–family relationships in the Australian residential aged care setting: development and evaluation of the Family and Staff Relationship Implementation Tool (FASRIT) as a contribution to person-centered healthcare. The International Journal of Person-Centered Medicine 2 (3), 564–567.

Bauer, M., Fetherstonhaugh, D., Lewis, V., 2012b. Attitudes towards family-staff relationships in Australian residential aged care settings: development and psychometric evaluation of the 'Family and Staff Relationship Attitude Tool' (FASRAT). Australasian Journal on Ageing. doi: 10.10.1111/ajag.12006.

Bauer, M., Nay, R., 2003. Family and staff partnerships in long term care: a review of the literature. Journal of Gerontological Nursing 29 (10), 46–53.

Bauer, M., Nay, R., 2011. Improving staff–family relationships in assisted living facilities: the views of the family. Journal of Advanced Nursing 67 (6), 1232–1241.

Bauer, M., Nay, R., Bathgate, T., et al., 2009. Final report to the Department of Health and Ageing: constructive staff/family relationships in residential aged care. Australian Centre for Evidence Based Aged Care, La Trobe University, Melbourne.

Benzein, E., Johansson, P., Arestedt, K., et al., 2008. Families' importance in nursing care: nurses' attitudes—an instrument development. Journal of Family Nursing 14 (1), 97–117.

Bowers, B., 1988. Family perceptions of care in a nursing home. The Gerontologist 28 (3), 361–368.

Bowers, B.J., 1987. Intergenerational caregiving: adult caregivers and their ageing parents. Advances in Nursing Science 9 (2), 20–31.

Bramble, M., Moyle, W., McAllister, M., 2009. Seeking connection: family care experiences following long-term dementia care placement. Journal of Clinical Nursing 18 (22), 3118–3125.

Bramble, M., Moyle, W., Shum, D., 2011. A quasi-experimental design trial exploring the effect of a partnership intervention on family and staff well-being in long-term dementia care. Aging & Mental Health 1–13.

Brown-Wilson, C., Davies, S., Nolan, M.R., 2009. Developing relationships in care homes—the contribution of staff, residents and families. Ageing and Society 29, 1041–1063.

Chen, C., Sabir, M., Zimmerman, S., et al., 2007. The importance of family relationships with nursing facility staff for family caregiver burden and depression. Journals of Gerontology Series B: Psychological Sciences & Social Sciences 62B (5), 253–260.

Dijkstra, A., 2007. Family participation in care plan meetings. Journal of Gerontological Nursing 33 (4), 22–29.

Fetherstonhaugh, D., Garratt, S., Bauer, M., 2012. Suporting families and friends of older people living in residential aged care Consumer monograph. ACEBAC.

Gaugler, J., 2006. Family involvement and resident psychosocial status in long-term care. Clinical Gerontologist 29 (4), 79–98.

Gaugler, J., Kane, R., 2007. Families and assisted living. The Gerontologist 47 (Suppl. 1), 83–99.

Haesler, E., Bauer, M., Nay, R., 2006. Factors associated with constructive staff–family relationships in the care of older adults in the institutional setting. International Journal of Evidence-Based Healthcare 4 (4), 288–336.

Haesler, E., Bauer, M., Nay, R., 2010. Recent evidence on the development and maintenance of constructive staff–family relationships in the care of older people—a report on a systematic review update. International Journal of Evidence-Based Healthcare 8 (2), 45–74.

Haigler, D.H., Bauer, L.J., Travis, S.S., 2004. Finding the common ground of family and professional caregiving: education agenda at the Rosalynn Carter Institute. Educational Gerontology 30, 95–105.

Kemp, C.L., Ball, M.M., Perkins, M.M., et al., 2009. 'I get along with most of them': direct care workers' relationships with residents' families in assisted living. Gerontologist 49 (2), 224–235.

Legault, A., Ducharme, F., 2009. Advocating for a parent with dementia in a long-term care facility: the process experienced by daughters. Journal of Family Nursing 15 (2), 198–219.

Lindgren, C.I., Murphy, A.M., 2002. Nurses' and family member's perceptions of nursing home residents' needs. Journal of Gerontological Nursing 28 (8), 45–55.

Maas, M., Reed, D., Park, M., et al., 2004. Outcomes of family involvement in care intervention for caregivers of individuals with dementia. Nursing Research 53 (2), 76–86.

Majerovitz, S., Mollott, R., Rudder, C., 2009. We're on the same side: improving communication between nursing home and family. Health Communication 24 (1), 12–20.

Marziali, E., Shulman, K., Damianakis, T., 2006. Persistent family concerns in long-term care settings: meaning and management. Journal of the American Medical Directors Association 7 (3), 154–162.

Morrell, C., Harvey, G., 2003. The clinical audit handbook. Oxford, Bailliere Tindall.

Moyle, W., Edwards, H., Clinton, M., 2002. Living with loss: dementia and the family caregiver. Australian Journal of Advanced Nursing 19 (3), 25–31.

Moyle, W., Nay, R., Bauer, M., et al., 2010. Family involvement in care of older people with dementia in acute care. Unpublished work.

Moyle, W., Skinner, J., Rowe, G., et al., 2003. Satisfaction and dissatisfaction in Australian long-term care. Journal of Clinical Nursing 12, 168–176.

Nay, R., 1994. Benevolent oppression: lived experiences of nursing home life. PhD.

Nay, R., 1996. Nursing home entry: meaning making by relatives. Australian Journal on Ageing 15 (3), 123–126.

Nay, R., 1997. Relatives' experiences of nursing home life: characterised by tension. Australasian Journal on Ageing 16 (1), 24–29.

Nolan, M., Bauer, M., Nay, R., 2009. Supporting family carers: implementing a relational and dynamic approach. In: Nay, R., Garratt, S. (Eds.), Older people: issues and innovations in care, third ed. Elsevier, Sydney, pp. 136–152.

Nolan, M., Grant, G., Keady, J., 1996. Understanding family care. Open University Press, Buckingham.

Park, M., 2010. Nursing staff stress from caregiving and attitudes toward family members of nursing home residents with dementia in Korea. Asian Nursing Research 4 (3), 130–141.

Specht, J.P., Kelley, L.S., Manion, P., et al., 2000. Who's the boss? Family/staff partnership in care of persons with dementia. Nursing Administration Quarterly 24 (3), 64–77.

Utley-Smith, Q., Colon-Emeric, C., Lekan-Rutledge, D., et al., 2009. Staff perceptions of staff–family interactions in nursing homes. Journal of Aging Studies 23, 168–177.

Wilson, C.B., Davies, S., Nolan, M., 2009. Developing personal relationships in care homes: realising the contributions of staff, residents and family members. Ageing & Society 29, 1041–1063.

Winbolt, M., Nay, R., Fetherstonhaugh, D., 2009. Taking a TEAM (Translating Evidence into Aged care Methods) approach to practice change. In: Nay, R., Garratt, S. (Eds.), Older people: issues and innovations. Elsevier, Sydney, pp. 442–455.

CHAPTER 11

OLDER PEOPLE AND ACUTE CARE

David Ames and Rhonda Nay

Editors' comments

This chapter raises the importance of the nature of the environment, skill in assessment and appropriate healthcare intervention for older people who are admitted to an acute hospital. The focus on differential diagnosis, correct use of medication, hydration, nutrition and safety issues should be part of the initial admission process and undertaken within a few hours. Once issues are identified the matter of discharge and ongoing intervention should begin as soon as possible. Older people respond to interventions better in their home environment and are less likely to develop further complications.

Prof. Ames gives you his thoughts, particularly on dementia, in Session 3 of Evolve.

INTRODUCTION

Older people, and especially those with dementia, are often best kept out of acute care hospitals. Is this discrimination? We would argue quite the opposite; in fact, *not* admitting is often the best clinical judgment, based on the best available evidence. If given the opportunity to discuss their goals many older people will also state this as their choice.

The previous edition of this book provided a good overall discussion of acute hospital care, here our aim is to highlight and emphasise some of the major current issues and what health practitioners can and must do should the decision be made that hospital admission is appropriate. Risk management is essential to ensure older people are not discharged with a decreased health status.

SHOULD OLDER PEOPLE BE IN ACUTE CARE?

Modern hospitals are home to antibiotic-resistant pathological bacteria (Yoshikawa 2002), subject to intense cost pressures, have few (if any) staff interested/qualified in geriatric care/medicine and do not provide the kind of calm, reassuring environment that is likely to enhance the cognitive or affective status of an older person (Edvardsson & Nay 2009). There are many specialists who are expert in various parts of the body, but often there is little interdisciplinary teamwork. Care remains largely disease- and task-driven and problem-focused. Acute care is designed to deal quickly with emergencies, undertake major surgery and expensive diagnostics such as magnetic resonance imaging (MRI).

Adverse events are common; for example, a 2007 Australian Institute of Health and Welfare (AIHW) report noted that in 2004–05 there were 14,000 admissions to 28 hospitals in New South Wales (NSW) (16.6% associated with accident and emergency departments), of which (AIHW & ACSQHC 2007):

- 51% were considered preventable
- 13.7% resulted in permanent disability and 4.9% died
- 53 operations were undertaken on a wrong body part
- 27 patients had instruments and so forth left inside their bodies
- seven died from ingesting the wrong medication.

According to Melbourne Health's Clinical Epidemiology & Health Services Evaluation Unit (Clinical Epidemiology & Health Services Evaluation Unit on behalf of the AHMAC 2004), leading reported complications for hospitalised older people are:

- pressure sores
- decreased mobility
- delirium
- incontinence
- malnutrition.

Modern hospitals are the site of many adverse events.

Some investigations and some treatments, especially those requiring surgery or intravenous access, can be done only in hospital. However, just because something can be done does not necessarily mean that it should be done. An individual with profound dementia who enters a coma, a person with incurable bowel cancer who is vomiting, or someone who is breathless with end-stage cardiac failure unsuitable for a cardiac transplantation may well be sent to hospital for further assessment and management. Whether they should be is another matter entirely. Families should talk about their desires for treatment and care in late life well in advance. Children should know what their parents may want in certain common situations. Advance care directives and medical powers of attorney are useful documents which, if prepared in calm and rational times, can be of great use in guiding decisions made in a crisis (Silvester & Detering 2011). Residential care facilities should have clear policies on when to refer their residents to hospital. Individual case notes should be very clear in indicating the person's current quality of life, their family's desires in respect to acute treatment and hospital transfer, and the degree to which their current care is considered palliative or terminal.

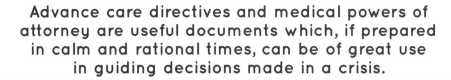

Advance care directives and medical powers of attorney are useful documents which, if prepared in calm and rational times, can be of great use in guiding decisions made in a crisis.

If an older person is sent to hospital in an emergency situation, it is likely they will spend time in the emergency department. Examples of conditions likely to benefit from a trip to hospital include suspected fractures, infections requiring intravenous antibiotics, suspected subdural haematomas and acute abdominal pain (unless the older person is receiving a palliative approach to care).

The environment is particularly important when caring for older people, especially those with dementia. The noise, foreign odours, lighting, indeed any aspect of the environment that over or under stimulates, can increase confusion. Frequent moves within the hospital and discontinuity in staffing can also increase confusion and have associated adverse outcomes. Ideally, at the very least there will be continuity of staff who have the necessary geriatric and person-centred expertise.

The environment is particularly important when caring for older people, especially those with dementia.

Most hospitals are hard to find your way around; we would argue that if you get it right for people living with dementia, others will also find the environment more accommodating. Parking is a major first challenge for families and people with dementia.

Vignette

Emmy and her son arrive at the emergency entrance of The City Hospital … *but* Emmy cannot be left alone, she cannot walk very far and the hospital parking staff tell her son 'You cannot park here!'. Emmy is becoming increasingly confused. She is screaming that she wants to go home, trying to remove the seatbelt and banging on the car door.

Reflection question

What could The City Hospital have done to prevent this situation?

Chapter 23 provides information on the significance of environments and you can find more on dementia-friendly environments at <www.health.vic.gov.au/dementia/changes>.

Vignette cont ...

Luckily Bob is quite assertive and tells the parking staff to 'bugger off'. They then report him for verbal aggression and fine him for not moving his car, but at least he gets Emmy into emergency and the staff realise she needs immediate attention (if only so they can have some peace).

Emergency department

Emmy is situated on a trolley in the hallway to try to reduce the disturbance while the staff deal with other people using emergency. She continually tries to climb over the trolley rails until they use soft manacles to protect her from falling. Now she bangs constantly on the rails. After 24 hours of her screaming and the staff reaching zero tolerance she is admitted to the medical ward. The handover has basic demographic information: *a past history of emphysema (she brought it on herself by smoking); ?demented; arthritis; and becoming more aggressive. She is doubly incontinent and a two-person transfer. Unable to contact her GP but assume she has epilepsy and major depression as she is prescribed pregabalin and duloxetine. In the toilet bag there is also some tramadol, which was administered a couple of times in emergency without calming effect.*

Reflection questions

1. What could/should have occurred in emergency?
2. What could be the reason(s) for Emmy constantly screaming?
3. For what other reasons might pregabalin and duloxetine be given?

Emergency department presentations among older people are often non-specific (e.g. confusion, fall, 'gone off her feet') and it is common for multiple pathologies to be present. If it is expected that assessment will take some time, pressure care should commence immediately, as pressure sores develop rapidly and are largely preventable if appropriate measures are taken. As with all admissions, it is essential to obtain a history, and because many older people in the emergency department will have either acute or chronic cognitive impairment, it is vital to obtain a history from somebody who knows the person well.

Older people often present with non-specific symptoms and likely comorbidities; comprehensive assessment is vital.

Before commencing the assessment it is important to ensure the person is wearing glasses and hearing aides if used routinely, and that if the person's first language is not English, some form of interpreter service (face-to-face or telephone) is available.

Among the many things to be assessed are: medication use and history; cognitive status; pain; temperature; heart rate; state of hydration; respiratory rate and evidence of consolidation; evidence of heart failure; hypo/hypertension; and mobility.

Investigations, if ordered, should be targeted towards diagnosing the presenting complaint and should not be requested if the results are unlikely to contribute meaningfully to managing the presenting complaint within a short time.

Emergency departments are busy, noisy, disorienting environments and older people should be sent to them only when essential (e.g. to assess hip pain after a fall) and should be assessed and moved through (either to be admitted or to go home) in a timely fashion. If permitted to languish for a lengthy time, it is likely that the older person will leave the department in worse shape than they entered it.

Emmy actually was taking pregabalin and duloxetine as together they have been found to reduce neuropathic pain. Chapter 15 provides extensive information on pain management.

> **If permitted to languish for a lengthy time, it is likely that the older person will leave the department in worse shape than they entered it.**

Vignette cont ...

Emmy is 'reassured' and admitted to the ward. (If transferring to acute care it is a good idea to tell a family member that the person is to be transferred and why this decision has been taken.)

The rails are raised to prevent falls. She finds it very hard to walk and dress so she is nursed in bed. Meals are left on her table, which she cannot reach, and then taken away uneaten. Her incontinence results in pressure wounds, and despite the staff constantly 'reassuring' her, she continues to scream and try to climb over the end of the bed. Several times staff find her caught between the rails and the mattress. They call the junior doctor who adds a sedating antipsychotic immediately with oral routinely.

Reflective questions

1. What should you be concerned about in terms of nursing a person in bed?
2. Was the decision to prescribe these additional medications wise?
3. What does it mean to 'reassure'?

The language of 'reassurance' is so embedded in healthcare and yet what reassures one person may make another very angry, for example, rubbing their arm. People have very different personal space needs. Also 'reassured' does not tell the next staff member anything! Documentation is more helpful if it is specific and individualised: 'Emmy stops screaming if she has Panadol six-hourly and her favourite rug from home on her lap'. New staff can readily see what it is that works for this person.

The risk of malnutrition and deconditioning in hospital is high. Older people are far less likely to leave hospital worse than when they came in if they are supported to eat and walk to the toilet rather than be wheeled, have any aids they use nearby and if there is no clutter for them to fall over in the corridors. A recent systematic review (Hemple et al 2013) indicated that while a gold standard remains elusive multiple interventions such as risk assessments using validated tools, visual risk alerts, direct observation, post-fall assessment, regular audits and care rounds are all used with some promise.

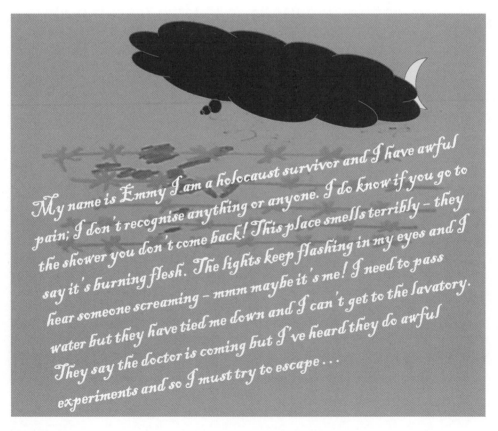

Figure 11.1

Emmy's experience

The nurse's experience:

Ward X is very busy; the junior doctor has been up all night; the phones have not stopped ringing; two nurses have rung in sick and the bathroom's flooding.

Emmy has been aggressive, verbally abusive, impossible to shower and trying to get out of bed all night—we had no option but to restrain her to stop her hurting herself.

She nearly strangled herself in the rails so we sedated her. She then fell over the end of bed and now has a major bump on her head. The family is furious and said we should have called them earlier but we just didn't have time. NOW the great Prof—who has nothing to do but read books—is here asking for a personal profile, pain chart, behaviour chart or a … who had time for that? By the time the shift's over we feel like we've been hit by a truck!

Emmy's son's response

I'm Emmy's son—I have told them and told them to call me if Mum has a problem—now I get here and find her all banged up and bleeding! They wonder why I shout at them or indeed why Mum does. She is never angry at home but they rush her and don't listen. She has bloody pain that's why she is here, but they don't give her anything. She is very dignified and would be mortified to wet the bed BUT they don't care! Will someone answer that bloody buzzer!

Reflective questions

Thinking about the significance of staff–family relationships, how could this have been better handled? See Chapters 7 and 10 for some ideas.

1. Could Emmy's behaviour be due to dehydration, pain and/or constipation? What assessment tools are suggested in Chapter 14 that you should use?

2. How could you assess for delirium?

3. What side effects would you expect from a cocktail of these drugs?

4. Are restraints an appropriate option to stop falls?

5. Apart from pressure ulcers, what conditions may result from prolonged nursing in bed?

6. What alternatives could you use to reduce falls?

7. How might the staffing situation be addressed? (see Ch 23 on innovative staffing)

A major risk for older people is polypharmacy. This is likely to increase confusion, falls and sleep disturbances, which then leads to more falls and greater confusion. Any drug prescribed must be considered in light of other possible interventions and the purpose for which it is given. If the staff are stressed by 'disruptive behaviours' perhaps it is better to give them the drugs! Drugs should never be prescribed without full assessment and for behaviours; this means assessing for any unmet needs such as pain, constipation, infection and boredom. Antipsychotics do not aid any of these conditions. Sedation is rarely a treatment of choice.

Restraint should only be used when all other alternatives have been tried and failed and the person is likely to injure themselves or another person. Restraint increases the risk of serious injury and even death. McCusker et al (2013) found evidence to suggest environmental factors may be able to assist to predict delirium in long-term care such as the sensory impairment and the absence of aids such as reading glasses, signs to assist orientation, use of restraints including bed rails and the addition of two or more medications.

Not surprisingly, having dementia increases sensitivity to these factors.

Vignette cont ...

Finally a specialist interdisciplinary aged care team is called in; staff are provided with appropriate assessment tools and advised to get Emmy up and walking. The family brings in her favourite food and a glass of wine to go with meals. They know she will eat if she is watching her favourite television shows. These are provided and her diet and hydration improve markedly. A comprehensive assessment reveals deafness due to wax and her ears are syringed with remarkable effect. The restraints are removed and a high/low bed used so that Emmy can get out of bed without strangulation or falls. Her footwear and capacity to 'get up and go' are assessed and found to be fine. She is offered an in-home occupational therapy (OT) assessment to support her independence. The medications are reviewed and the tramadol and olanzapine ceased. The pregabalin and duloxetine are continued for pain. She is found to be severely constipated and, after this is treated, her faecal incontinence stops and the family is advised about fibre products, diet and social continence products. Emmy is eventually discharged home. By now they are using the electronic care plan, which alerts the GP and district nursing that she will be home and requiring ongoing care of her pressure wound and risk of constipation.

ACUTE HOSPITAL INPATIENT CARE

Whether admissions are elective or the result of some emergency, the prime purpose of admission to hospital is for the person to receive treatment and care that can be delivered nowhere else (e.g. surgery for a fracture, intravenous antibiotics for an infection, electroconvulsive therapy for severe depression). In addition to treating the condition that caused the admission as well as is possible (e.g. ameliorating congestive heart failure, pinning a fractured neck of femur, replacing a terminally osteoarthritic knee), it is essential that both incidental conditions that may complicate the admission (e.g. dementia, depression, ingrowing toenails) be detected and quantified and that potentially preventable conditions that often emerge during hospital stays (e.g. delirium, pressure sores) be prevented where possible.

On admission a thorough history and examination should be performed and appropriate investigations undertaken. A clear picture of the person's social arrangements is essential. Who (if anyone) lives with the person, who will take them home and what other responsibilities (e.g. care of a husband with dementia) will the person resume on discharge? Is the person competent to administer their own medications or will this need to be supervised? Is the home environment safe and what emergency help is available?

As well as physical assessment it is important that cognition and mental state be assessed in detail and recorded. Rates of depression are higher among older people admitted to hospital than in those living at home (Ames & Tuckwell 1994), so some form of depression screening (e.g. Geriatric Depression Scale) is useful. The results need to be interpreted and acted upon and any well-run hospital should have the facility to call upon specialist psychiatry liaison services to assess and help manage people with pre-existing or emergent psychiatric disorders. Cognitive assessment should use a reliable reproducible tool, such as the Mini-Mental State Examination (MMSE) or Montreal Cognitive Assessment (MoCA), that produces a numeric score that can be interpreted and acted upon, and that can be repeated in future to see if the person's cognitive state has changed. What scale is used is far less important than assessing and recording cognitive function for comparison against future function with the same instrument.

Dementia care in hospitals: costs and strategies, the 2013 publication by the AIHW (2013), reports that 'simple measures taken in the hospital setting that appear to reduce length of stay for dementia patients and improve outcomes include staff training, discharge planning, dementia-friendly ward adaptations, and mental health and ageing liaison services' (Kalish 2013).

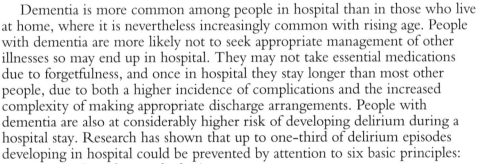

As well as physical assessment it is important that cognition and mental state be assessed in detail and recorded.

Dementia is more common among people in hospital than in those who live at home, where it is nevertheless increasingly common with rising age. People with dementia are more likely not to seek appropriate management of other illnesses so may end up in hospital. They may not take essential medications due to forgetfulness, and once in hospital they stay longer than most other people, due to both a higher incidence of complications and the increased complexity of making appropriate discharge arrangements. People with dementia are also at considerably higher risk of developing delirium during a hospital stay. Research has shown that up to one-third of delirium episodes developing in hospital could be prevented by attention to six basic principles:

- ensuring adequate hydration
- giving repeated orientation cues
- ensuring adequate sleep
- providing appropriate correction of visual and hearing impairment
- ensuring early mobilisation after any period of bed rest
- treating the underlying cause(s) (e.g. infection, medication toxicity etc. should commence at once).

Delirium is a distressing condition to experience; it has a high rate of associated complications and mortality and should be prevented wherever possible (Milisen et al 2005). If it develops, treating the underlying cause(s) (e.g. infection, medication toxicity) should begin at once and the use of any sedating treatment to control associated behavioural challenges should be kept to an absolute minimum. Research has shown that sedation in older people rarely has good outcomes and frequently increases the risk of falls, incontinence, non-restorative sleep (caused by sedation reducing REM sleep), confusion and other adverse events (Pagel & Bennett 2001).

Research has shown that up to one-third of delirium episodes developing in hospital could be prevented by attention to six basic principles.

Some valuable work undertaken by the Victorian Government for the Council of Australian Governments (COAG) focused on preventing functional decline in older people. The initial report (2004) outlines interventions that address the areas of cognition and emotional health, mobility, vigour, self-care, continence, nutrition and skin integrity. More recently this was progressed, with health services taking responsibility for an area and the implementation of evidence-based practice. Another useful document is that produced some years back for the Australian Government (Dorevitch et al 2004), which provides information on evidence-based assessment tools that are recommended for use in acute care environments. Chapter 12 also discusses geriatric assessment in detail. There is evidence to indicate that older people enjoy better outcomes in units specific to their needs such as geriatric assessment units (Baztan et al 2009).

DISCHARGE PLANNING

Discharge planning should commence preferably before admission (Bauer et al 2011, Nay et al 2003), but in emergency admissions, almost as soon as the older person enters the ward. As noted above, a clear picture of the person's social matrix, home environment and previous level of functioning are essential. Assessment of functional abilities (e.g. cooking, banking) by an OT (often including a home visit) can be invaluable in determining if a person can be sent home safely. A social worker can coordinate provision of necessary services and ensure that arrangements to offer necessary support are in place. Many hospitals now have transition care teams or nurses dedicated to providing some form of follow-up (e.g. liaison between the older person, family and general practitioner to diminish the risk of recurrent stroke in those discharged after a cerebral infarction) and this can be helpful in reducing the chances of readmission. Having endured a period of hospital care, the last thing most people want to do is to come back any time soon!

Discharge planning should commence preferably before admission.

CONCLUSION

Where possible, people living with dementia and older people (especially those with multiple comorbidities) should be treated without acute hospital admission. If they are admitted, a comprehensive assessment is required to tease out what issues led to the presentation and potential discharge destinations. The environment, including parking support, require the attention of health service/ hospital boards and management. Clinical governance and risk management strategies are preferable to adverse event reporting and are more cost-effective. As the population of people with comorbidities, dementia and risk of delirium increases, any service that treats older people (the majority) and ignores the issues outlined in this chapter can expect damage to their reputation, bottom line and, most especially, increased adverse outcomes for clients. All staff require some gerontological knowledge because of the percentage of older people using health services; all services require access to interdisciplinary expertise in the care of older people.

References

Ames, D., Tuckwell, V., 1994. Psychiatric disorders among elderly patients in an acute general hospital. Medical Journal of Australia 160, 671–675.

Australian Institute of Health and Welfare (AIHW), 2013. Dementia care in hospitals: costs and strategies. Online. Available: http://www.aihw.gov.au/publication-detail/?id=60129542746, 26 Mar 2013.

Australian Institute of Health and Welfare (AIHW) & Australian Commission on Safety and Quality in Health Care, 2007. Sentinel events in Australian public hospitals 2004–05. AIHW, Canberra.

Bauer, M., Fitzgerald, L., Koch, S., et al., 2011. How family carers view hospital discharge planning for the older person with a dementia. Dementia 10 (3), 317–323.

Baztán, J.J., Suárez-García, F.M., López-Arrieta, J., et al., 2009. Effectiveness of acute geriatric units on functional decline, living at home, and case fatality among older patients admitted to hospital for acute medical disorders: metaanalysis. BMJ 338, b50 doi:10.1136/bmj.b50.

Clinical Epidemiology & Health Services Evaluation Unit on behalf of the AHMAC, 2004. Best practice approaches to minimise functional decline in the older person across the acute, sub-acute and residential aged care settings. Department of Human Services, Melbourne.

Dorevitch, M., Davis, S., Andrews, G., 2004. Guide for assessing older people in hospital. Published by Metropolitan Health and Aged Care Services Division, Victorian Government Department of Human Services. Victoria on behalf of Australian Health Ministers' Advisory Council, Melbourne.

Edvardsson, D., Nay, R., 2009. Acute care and older people: challenges and ways forward. Australian Journal of Advanced Nursing 27 (2), (Dec 2009–Feb 2010).

Hemple, S., Newberry, S., Wang, Z., et al., 2013. Hospital fall prevention: a systematic review of implementation, components, adherence, and effectiveness. Journal of the American Geriatrics Society Online. Available: http://onlinelibrary.wiley.com, 26 Mar 2013.

Kalish, D., 2013. Media Release: Dementia care in hospitals: costs and strategies. 14 Mar 2013 Online. Available: http://www.aihw.gov.au/publication-detail/?id=60129542746, 26 Mar 2013.

McCusker, J., Cole, M., Voyer, P., et al., 2013. Environmental factors predict the severity of delirium symptoms in long-term care residents with and without delirium. Journal of the American Geriatrics Society Online. Available: http:// onlinelibrary.wiley.com/, 26 Mar 2013.

Milisen, K., Lemiengre, J., Braes, T., et al., 2005. Multicomponent intervention strategies for managing delirium in hospitalized older people: systematic review. Journal of Advanced Nursing 52 (1), 79–90.

Nay, R., Fetherstonhaugh, D., Pitcher, A., et al., 2003. Improving the admission and discharge practices of acute and sub-acute facilities in relation to people with dementia. Department of Human Services, Melbourne.

Pagel, J.F., Bennett, L.P., 2001. Medications for the treatment of sleep disorders: an overview. The Primary Care Companion to the Journal of Clinical Psychiatry 3 (3), 118–125.

Silvester, W., Detering, K., 2011. Advance care planning and end-of-life care. Med J Aust 2011; 195 (8), 435–436.

Yoshikawa, T.T., 2002. Antimicrobial resistance and aging: beginning of the end of the antibiotic era? Journal of the American Geriatrics Society 50 (S7), 226–229.

CHAPTER 12

PERSON-CENTRED COMPREHENSIVE GERIATRIC ASSESSMENT

Sally Garratt and Dimity Pond

Revised from original authors Sandra Davis, Michael Dorevitch and Sally Garratt

Editors' comments

In the authors' opinion, assessment is the cornerstone of contemporary care of older people. Such assessment must be comprehensive and requires an interdisciplinary approach to be effective. Person-centred assessment is the foundation for delivering person-centred care. If the person is the focal point of the team involved in care then the culture and philosophy of the team is fundamental for successful outcomes. Sharing information, collaborative decision making and involving the person is essential. The value of comprehensive assessment is to improve diagnostic accuracy, improve planning to reduce the need for long-term residential care, reduce short-term mortality, improve functioning and reduce healthcare costs. Selecting the right tools for assessment is very important, as many tools are not age-specific nor do they cater for cultural differences. This chapter offers some sample tools for consideration but does not prescribe any in particular because the selection of an assessment tool depends on the reason for its use and the competence of the assessor. Good clinical skills, observation, listening and judgment are also necessary to inform decision making.

You can see and hear Sally in Session 2 of Evolve.

INTRODUCTION

Although the majority of older people have a positive view of their health status and are free from disability, the proportion with more intensive care and assistance needs rises with age (Australian Institute of Health and Welfare

(AIHW) 2007). Traditional healthcare service provision, which is largely task-oriented and procedurally based, is not always well suited to meet the needs of older people (Hickman et al 2007). Frail older people with multiple problems and comorbidities, particularly those not under the direct care of geriatric services, are at risk of adverse outcomes. Appropriate assessment is required to address the complexities of health needs. Hence, the cornerstone of contemporary care of older people is assessment (Dorevitch et al 2004). If health is viewed as a multidimensional construct, then it follows that assessing health status should address the physical, social, psychological and other dimensions as well as the medical.

Person-centred care (PCC) is considered the optimum way of delivering healthcare and has been defined simply as 'valuing people as individuals' (Winefield et al 1996). Further exploration of this concept has led to defining 'the person as the centre of care' or client-directed care (Edvardsson et al 2008). Chapter 7 discusses PCC in detail. Yet, there has been limited discussion of person-centred assessment. Given that assessment sets the scene and the approach to an episode of care and the working relationship that follows, person-centred comprehensive assessment would be a crucial step to delivering PCC. The older person should be the focal point of the assessment in a partnership that is both respectful and reciprocal, and the person should feel empowered by the process (Heath 2000). It is the significance of the relationships between health professionals and the older person, as well as the relationships between health professionals themselves, that is often overlooked as a result of misconceptions about the concept of person-centredness. The culture and philosophy of the care team that underpins the context of assessment should be given consideration (Beers & Berkow 2000).

Some research has been done on the nature of the relationship that works best in primary care between health professionals and their clients. It would seem that a relationship works best when the client's autonomy is respected and the health professional and the person work towards goals that are in line with that person's values. There is a tension between this approach and the need for safety in older people as their physical and mental capacities are challenged by age.

THE IMPORTANCE OF AN INTERDISCIPLINARY APPROACH TO COMPREHENSIVE GERIATRIC ASSESSMENT

In health terms, comprehensive assessment is the detailed evaluation of health status. This involves a more detailed review than screening and leads directly to diagnostic conclusions and assignment to intervention strategies if necessary. It is important to understand that comprehensive assessment is a process that identifies both residual functional capacities and limitations of function in order to plan and deliver the most appropriate care. Furthermore, it represents a critical information-gathering phase, without which effective decisions regarding health-promoting interventions cannot be made, or the monitoring of changes in health status cannot be undertaken (Dorevitch et al 2004).

Although interdisciplinary teams have evolved from multidisciplinary teams, they are indeed different. Multidisciplinary teams tend to assess their own area of expertise and create discipline-specific care plans and deliver care that may be fragmented with overlapping assessment. An older person who is subjected to repeat questioning by various health professionals becomes confused and irritated by a seemingly endless repetition of similar information gathering (Rubenstein 2004). An interdisciplinary approach means that a team works together to assess and share information before care planning is completed. The team collectively set goals for assessment and share resources and responsibilities. A number of barriers to multidisciplinary teamwork have been identified that include differing perceptions of teamwork, different levels of skills that impact on how teams function, the dominance of medical power impacting on team interactions, and conflict arising from the tension between role boundaries and perceived control (Atwal & Caldwell 2006, Jones 2006). The latter is of particular importance because the hierarchical structure of a multidisciplinary team can frequently undermine its effectiveness. If a team is led by the perceived specialist knowledge of one person the other members will follow the directions given by the specialist, and day-to-day knowledge of care from frontline care providers may be missed or not given the attention it deserved. Given that follow-up, implementation of assessment recommendations, and patient adherence to recommendations are likely to be factors impacting on the effectiveness of comprehensive geriatric assessment (Bogardus et al 2004, Wolfs et al 2007), an approach that alienates frontline care staff is problematic.

An interdisciplinary approach, on the other hand, specifically refers to integration through active coordination. Therefore, interdisciplinary comprehensive assessment is more than sharing information across disciplines involved in the process of assessment. As a result of a much higher level of collaboration, an assumed equality across the team fosters a shared responsibility for effectiveness and team functioning to maximise the care outcomes for the older person (Zeiss & Thompson 2003). Interdisciplinary geriatric assessment and intervention is a proven model for the care of frail older people that is appropriate across community and institutional settings (Fenton et al 2006). Specifically, interdisciplinary team approaches to assessment and care have been shown to facilitate adherence to recommendations, prevent functional decline and decrease hospitalisations and nursing home placement (Somers et al 2000). Payne et al (2002 p 110) note that 'patients require alliances and effective partnerships across professional boundaries to support continuity of care and adequate information transfer'. The implications, then, for comprehensive geriatric assessment are clear; an interdisciplinary approach to assessment provides important alliances and partnerships that underpin person-centred care plans and maximise health outcomes.

Interdisciplinary comprehensive geriatric assessment and intervention is a proven model for the care of frail older people that is appropriate across community and institutional settings.

WHAT IS THE VALUE OF COMPREHENSIVE GERIATRIC ASSESSMENT?

Comprehensive geriatric assessment programs across a range of care settings have been shown to play an important role in improving the quality of life for older people and their informal caregivers (Aminzadeh et al 2005). For example, in the acute hospital setting poor outcomes can be a result of three main factors: 'age-related physiological changes that afford less resiliency in responding to acute illness; diseases that precipitated hospitalisation, pre-existing co-morbidities and newly acquired disorders; and the healthcare delivery system that renders care' (Reuben et al 1999 p 274). Inpatient comprehensive geriatric assessment has the potential to reduce short-term mortality, increase the chances of living at home at one year, and improve physical and cognitive function (Ellis & Langhorne 2004). Comprehensive geriatric assessment in appropriate cases can lead to improved patient outcomes including better diagnostic accuracy and treatment planning, reduced need for long-term residential care, improved physical and mental functioning, prolonged inpatient survival and reduced healthcare costs (Scanlan 2005). Reduced medication use and improved quality of life and mental health, improved client/carer satisfaction and a reduction in carer burden have also been identified as positive benefits stemming from comprehensive assessment (Dorevitch et al 2004). Therefore, prompt and early assessment is critical in identifying and preventing complications among many older people and, in turn, affects the quality of care (Koch & Garratt 2001). A fundamental component of the various successful models to enhance the care of older people has been appropriate assessment with interdisciplinary input (Harari et al 2007). Research has shown that shorter length of stay, better maintenance of existing functionality and fewer hospital readmissions are just some of the benefits experienced by older adults with complex problems if an interdisciplinary geriatric team assesses and actively manages their healthcare (Harari et al 2007, Landefeld 2003). Comprehensive assessment is most effective when targeted to older people who are at risk for functional decline (physical or mental), hospitalisation or residential care placement (American Geriatrics Society 2006). Not all older people require comprehensive assessment and screening; targeting those most likely to benefit is common practice. Selection criteria may include the following: advanced age (75 years or older); living alone; recent hospitalisation; multiple comorbidities; polypharmacy; regular use of health services; difficulty managing in the home environment; domiciliary nursing; home care; carer stress; poor balance; falls; confusion; incontinence; limited performance in two or more instrumental activities of daily living; and inability to independently perform personal activities of daily living, bed or chair transfers or mobilisation (with or without a gait aid).

Comprehensive assessment is most effective when targeted to older people who are at risk for functional decline (physical or mental), hospitalisation or residential care placement.

THE STRUCTURE OF A COMPREHENSIVE ASSESSMENT

The main reason for carrying out comprehensive assessment of older people is to identify unreported and unmet healthcare needs that can potentially be positively impacted upon. Comprehensive assessment informs the development of healthcare plans that are framed in terms of recommended health-promoting interventions that are both acceptable to the person and their carers and readily accessible. Such assessment demands a detailed and exhaustive evaluation of the older person's health status. While the format of comprehensive geriatric assessment may vary, there are a number of specific domains under the fundamental dimensions of medical health and physical, psychological and social functioning.

MEDICAL HEALTH

Assessing medical health is primarily concerned with identifying symptoms and signs. Usual clinical medical practice requires the assessor to:

- ask about the presenting or main problem(s) and past medical history
- undertake a detailed systems review (including cardiorespiratory, gastrointestinal, urogenital, musculoskeletal and neurological symptoms; hearing and vision; pain; falls and dizziness; appetite and recent weight loss or gain; fatigue and exercise tolerance; swallowing and communication problems; bladder and bowel function; sleep habits; sexual functioning; and problems with feet and footwear)
- perform a physical examination with a focus on areas of concern uncovered by the history and particularly those areas known to be of concern for older people (e.g. gait, balance)
- list prescription and 'over-the-counter' medications (name, dose and frequency), including complementary or alternative therapies and recreational drugs and any known allergies
- take a smoking and alcohol consumption history
- take a dietary, dental and immunisation history (including influenza, pneumococcus, tetanus and zoster virus live vaccine)
- establish if there has been any advance care planning (nomination of any agent or proxy decision maker, recording of advance care directives)
- take a sexual health history. Older people do engage in sexual intimacy and even though impotence, diminished libido and dyspareunia (pain with intercourse, usually related to vaginal dryness) are common in older adults, it is seldom discussed but can be of concern to individuals. Asking straightforward, closed questions in a non-judgmental way is the best approach (e.g. 'Are you currently sexually active?' as opposed to 'Are you still sexually active after all these years?').

PHYSICAL FUNCTION

At the heart of comprehensive assessment is a review of functioning, as reflected in terms of everyday activities that cover self-care, managing household affairs and mobility (Wieland & Hirth 2003). This dimension contains the domains of personal care or activities of daily living (ADLs). The range of activities includes eating, dressing, grooming, going to the toilet, bathing, mobility and balance. In addition, domestic and community activities of daily living (often referred to as instrumental ADLs) need to be assessed. These encompass activities such as using a telephone, cooking, housework, taking medications, handling finances, shopping and transportation. The significance of mobility to many of the ADLs and high incidence of falls makes assessing exercise practice and activity status particularly important (Wieland & Hirth 2003). Any impairment in activities of everyday life should be considered in relation to information about the person's environment and social situation.

PSYCHOLOGICAL FUNCTION

This dimension is primarily concerned with cognition (acute and chronic confusion) and mood, although consideration of psychosocial elements in this domain also incorporates social and recreational activity, behaviour patterns, customary routines and life preferences (Dorevitch et al 2004).

Older people with cognitive impairment, even in the absence of dementia, are at increased risk for accidents, delirium, medical and pharmaceutical non-adherence and disability. Therefore, a brief cognitive screen is recommended, especially for those aged 75 years and older (American Geriatrics Society 2008). This should only be performed in those with symptoms or signs of cognitive impairment, whether reported by themselves or others, due to the high percentage of false positives from any test that screens indiscriminately. Such signs include (but are not limited to) memory problems: some people with cognitive impairment retain good memory but have difficulties with word-finding or executive function (such as cooking the family meal). It should be noted that a brief screen is not diagnostic of cognitive impairment, even when in the impaired range, and should be followed up with a more comprehensive cognitive assessment. Commonly used screening tests include the Rowland Universal Dementia Assessment Scale (RUDAS) (particularly for people from a non-English speaking background), the Montreal Cognitive Assessment (MOCA) and the General Practitioner Assessment of Cognition (GPCOG). The Mini-Mental State Examination (MMSE) is still widely used but is now under copyright.

Symptoms of depression below the threshold for a diagnosis of major depression are common in late life and may promote a level of disability that warrants intervention (American Geriatrics Society 2008). Depression is under-diagnosed in the older population but, once recognised, responds well to treatment that includes social and psychological support (Gottfries 2001). A good single question to ask is: 'Do you often feel sad or depressed?'. An affirmative response calls for further evaluation of other depressive symptoms through the use of a standardised instrument.

SOCIAL FUNCTION

Although it has long been recognised that, as the World Health Organization (WHO) definition of health articulates, health is more than an absence of disease and is 'a state of complete physical, mental and social well-being' (WHO 1948), the latter and its role in health status has often been overlooked in the past. Research into inequalities in health has, over time, brought to the forefront the significance of a growing understanding of the 'remarkable sensitivity of health to the social environment', now best known as the social determinants of health (Wilkinson & Marmot 2003). The dimension addressing social assessment consists of several elements, including ethnicity, spirituality and cultural background. Fundamental components of this domain encompass usual living arrangements (type of residence and with whom the person resides), the range and frequency of community and private services received, the availability and adequacy of social support, carer issues (nature of contribution, health literacy, carer burden, adequacy of support and health status), economic wellbeing, living environment (including aspects of safety such as access and home aids/modifications) and whether or not elder abuse or neglect is suspected (American Geriatrics Society 2008, Dorevitch et al 2004).

SOURCES OF ASSESSMENT INFORMATION

The four main sources of assessment information are: older people themselves ('self-report'); others who know the older person well ('informant-report'); observation of the person undertaking various ADLs ('direct observation'); and various other secondary written sources of information (including hospital records, medical reports and investigation results). It is likely that the best comprehensive assessments are those that incorporate information collected from all four sources. Each of the four sources of assessment information is associated with potential limitations and pitfalls.

The accuracy of self-report has generally been shown to be superior to that of informants (Dorevitch et al 2004). However, it may be compromised by various factors including: acute illness; impaired cognition, hearing or communication; limited proficiency with English or other cultural barriers; fear of consequences; or denial as a psychological adaptive mechanism (Dorevitch et al 2004). Even the way the assessor frames the question will impact on the accuracy of the information provided. For example, questions concerning physical function that are framed in terms of 'performance' ('Do you … '), rather than 'capacity' ('Are you able to … ') can result in answers that seemingly reflect a greater level of dependence than might otherwise be elicited.

Unless there is reason to suspect otherwise, the older person should be assumed to be best placed to provide accurate information about their health status, with collateral history sought from other sources if required. While informal or formal community carers may be a useful source of person-related information, particularly concerning physical function, the accuracy of their information may be adversely affected by such factors as a lack of recent or sufficiently frequent observation of the older person's performance or by a conscious or subconscious desire to access additional support (Cohen-Mansfield & Jensen 2007). Permission should be sought from the older person to obtain additional information from other informants such as family, case managers and community or residential aged care providers. Direct observation is really the best source of information about physical function. It is important to recognise that the physical setting in which the observations take place may impact on physical function; what an older person can do in hospital may be quite different from what they can do in their own individualised home environment.

Other sources of information (informant-report, direct observation of physical function or the use of medical records) should ideally be pursued for corroboration of self-reported information—to fill in any gaps in the assessment and to gain important carer and service provider perspectives. However, there are situations where they may have to be relied upon as primary sources. Medical records can contain information gathered from the other three sources, but it is important to keep in mind that there may be significant imprecision or ambiguity in the way this information was initially recorded.

There is a critical association between assessment and care planning, with the quality of any given care plan being largely a function of the accuracy and comprehensiveness of the assessment that informed it. Inaccurate or incomplete assessment information will inevitably lead to the development of suboptimal care plans, which in turn will lead to a less favourable impact upon the health of those most likely to benefit—older people with chronic and complex healthcare needs.

Unless there is reason to suspect otherwise, the older person should be assumed to be best placed to provide accurate information about their health status, with collateral history sought from other sources if required.

HOW TO CONDUCT A COMPREHENSIVE ASSESSMENT

Any framework for assessment should be flexible and able to be adapted to a variety of circumstances and be:
- appropriate to the audience it is intended for
- capable of balancing and incorporating the views of a number of carers, users and agencies, and able to provide a mechanism for bringing different views together, while recognising the diversity and variation within individual circumstances (Dorevitch et al 2004).

Comprehensive assessment can be conducted using standardised, global assessment tools, structured or semi-structured proformas that incorporate domain-specific instruments and checklists where required, or using an unstructured approach based on the professional expertise of the individual assessor.

The format adopted is likely to depend on:
- the assessment setting (acute or subacute hospital ward, outpatient clinic, the older person's home or residential aged care facility)
- the likely assessment workload (a standardised, global assessment tool may take up to two hours to complete, whereas an unstructured,

targeted assessment may take no more than 30 minutes for a suitably trained and experienced health professional)
- who will be involved in the assessment process (one individual assessor or several people contributing to the overall process)
- the level of training and expertise of those undertaking the assessment.

SELECTING THE RIGHT TOOLS FOR ASSESSMENT

The importance of using reliable and valid assessment tools cannot be overstated. The use of tools can facilitate assessment, although, if used inappropriately, can reduce efficiency and undermine the relationship between the assessor and the older person (Osterweil 2003). While a reliance on structured measures alone may not allow for the identification of outstanding needs, the correct tools can provide a solid foundation of information from which to move forward. As Scanlan (2005 p 6) states, 'comprehensive assessment requires both simple screening measures to facilitate identification of problem areas and more detailed evaluation tools to guide the development of targeted interventions'.

Table 12.1, at the end of this chapter, provides a sample of tools widely used for assessment purposes in aged care that can be used in a variety of settings. An example of a tool, with summarised information, has been included for key elements across each domain of comprehensive assessment identified in this chapter. Dimension-specific tools identified have been generally validated for use with older people. The Dementia Outcomes Measurement Suite contains multiple tools to assess most aspects of dementia (www.dementia-assessment.com.au). There are far too many tools available to identify specifically but a useful compendium of assessment tools, including a number of global assessment tools, can be found as a supplement in the Australian publication *Guide for Assessing Older People in Hospital* (Dorevitch et al 2004).

Global assessment tools have not been included in Table 12.1 but a brief word about some of those currently available is warranted. Foreman et al (2004) identified existing, validated, comprehensive assessment tools for assessing people with chronic health conditions and older people with complex care needs for comprehensive review and identified six candidate tools: Camberwell Assessment of Need for the Elderly (CANE—for more information see www.thecane.co.uk) (Orrell & Hancock 2004); Functional Assessment of the Care Environment for Older People (FACE—for more information see www.facecode.com); Handicap Assessment Resource Tool (HART) (Vertesi et al 2000), EASYCare (Philp 2000); Outcomes and Assessment Information Set (OASIS—for more information see www.cms.hhs.gov/OASIS); and InterRAI (and all its components; for more information see www.interrai.org/section/view). While for the purposes and criteria of that review the InterRAI was identified as the strongest, the authors of the review noted that all the short-listed tools 'may be suitable for particular services' (Foreman et al 2004 p 51).

In addition, it is important to note that there are a number of assessment tools that are mandated for use in specific circumstances and may be of interest and value in a range of settings where validated tools are not readily available.

Table 12.1

Sample of tools commonly used for assessment in aged care

ASSESSMENT INSTRUMENT	DESCRIPTION/ADMINISTRATION	INFORMATION/AVAILABILITY
	CLINICAL	
Cumulative Index Rating Scale (CIRS)	Medical assessment tool. Brief but comprehensive tool for assessing physical impairment, overall burden and severity of illness. Can be used across different care settings. Physician administered—relies on clinical judgment.	Copy of tool available in: Linn, B.S., Linn, M.W., Gurel, L., 1968. Cumulative Illness Rating Scale. Journal of the American Geriatrics Society 16 (5), 622–626.
The Centre for Eye Research Australia, Vision Screening Test	Vision test to identify appropriate eye care services and low-vision rehabilitation. Distance visual acuity tested at 6/12, 6/18, 6/60 and 3/60. Near visual acuity measured at N8, N20 and N48. Completed by medical staff using a card with four symbols.	For more information see: http://cera.unimelb.edu.au/publications/reports/vision_screening_for_older_people.pdf
The Clinical Scale to Detect Hearing Loss	Simple test of hearing loss for people aged 55 years and over comprising seven questions to assess sociodemographic and hearing related characteristics via interview.	Copy of questionnaire available in: Reuben, D.B., Walsh, K., Moore, A.A., et al., 1998. Hearing Loss in Community-Dwelling Older Persons: National Prevalence Data and Identification Using Simple Questions. Journal of the American Geriatrics Society 48 (6), 1008–1011.
Mini Nutritional Assessment (MNA)	A nutrition screening and assessment tool that can identify patients aged 65 or older who are malnourished or at risk of malnutrition. For use in any setting, it can be administered in a few minutes and requires no special training.	Further information and forms (pdf and interactive versions) and user guides available in several languages at: www.mna-elderly.com

Tool	Description	Source
The Braden Scale for Predicting Pressure Sore Risk	Allows nurses and other healthcare providers to reliably score a client's level of risk for developing pressure ulcers. The scale is made up of six subscales—three reflect primary factors (sensitivity, activity, mobility) and three reflect factors contributing to diminished tissue tolerance. Administration by nursing staff.	Subject to copyright. Additional information, copy of scale and permission for use can be obtained online at: www.bradenscale.com
The Oral Health Assessment Tool (OHAT)	The OHAT is a modification of the Brief Oral Health Status Examination (BOHSE). It is a tool used for screening purposes only, and does not replace the need for regular examinations by a dentist. The assessment covers the patient's current oral health status, including factors that can contribute to the risk of oral disease and indicate the need for referral.*	Copy of the tool can be viewed and printed from: www.healthcare.uiowa.edu/igec/tools under the oral health category.
The Verbal Descriptor Scale (VDS) / Verbal Rating Scale (VRS)	For pain assessment. A number of scales with five- to seven-word responses to pain that are easy to use. Verbally administered by healthcare workers. Has been found to be the most sensitive and reliable of the various pain scales, with best completion rate for people with cognitive impairment.	Copy of VDS available at: http://www.ndhcri.org/pain/Tools/Verbal_Descriptor_Pain_Scale.pdf For more information on pain assessment see: Pautex, S., Gold, G., 2006. Assessing pain intensity in older adults. Geriatrics Aging 9 (6), 399–402.
Abbey Pain Scale	Brief tool to assess pain in people with dementia. Preliminary validity estimates indicate the tool has merit.	Abbey, J., De Bellis, A., Easterman, A., et al., 2004. The Abbey pain scale: A 1-minute numerical indicator for people with end-stage dementia. International Journal of Palliative Nursing 10 (6), 6–13.

Table 12.1

Sample of tools commonly used for assessment in aged care—cont'd

ASSESSMENT INSTRUMENT	DESCRIPTION/ADMINISTRATION	INFORMATION/AVAILABILITY
	PHYSICAL FUNCTIONING	
Barthel Activities of Daily Living (Modified)	A simple-to-administer tool for assessing self-care and mobility activities of daily living.	Granger, C.V., Albrecht, G.L., Hamilton, B.B., 1979. Outcome of comprehensive medical rehabilitation: Measurement by PULSES Profile and the Barthel Index. Archives of Physical Medicine and Rehabilitation 60, 145–154.
Lawton-Brody Instrumental Activities of Daily Living (IADL)	Intended to be used among older adults. Can be used in community or hospital settings and is most useful for identifying how a person is functioning at the present time, and for identifying improvement or deterioration over time.	Lawton, M.P., Brody, E.M., 1969. Assessment of older people: self-maintaining and instrumental activities of daily living. The Gerontologist 9, 179–186.
Timed Up & Go	Test for quantifying functional mobility that may also be useful in following clinical change over time. The test is quick and requires no special equipment or training.	Potsiadlo, D., Richardson, S., 1991. The Timed Up & Go: A test of basic functional mobility for frail elderly persons. Journal of the American Geriatrics Society 39, 142–148.
Tinetti Performance Oriented Mobility Assessment	A test targeting older people who might be at risk of falling during usual activities of daily living.	Tinetti, M.E., 1986. Performance-oriented assessment of mobility problems in elderly patients. Journal of the American Geriatrics Society 34 (119), 1–26.
	PSYCHOLOGICAL	
Mini-Mental State Examination (MMSE)	A brief screening tool used to assess the severity of cognitive impairment and to document change over time. Can be used in any setting.	Folstein, M.F., Folstein, S.E., McHugh, P.R., 1975. 'Mini-mental State': A practical method for grading the cognitive state of patients for the clinician. Journal of Psychiatric Research 12, 189–198.

The Short Confusion Assessment Method (Short CAM)	The first four items of the complete CAM test (nine items) used to detect delirium in confused older people in an acute hospital setting but reliable and applicable in varied settings. Takes about 10–15 minutes and can be administered by non-psychiatric trained health professionals.	Inouye, S.K., van Dyck, C.H., Alessi, C.A., et al., 1990. Clarifying confusion: The Confusion Assessment Method. Annals of Internal Medicine 113, 941-948.
Geriatric Depression Scale (GDS)	Both 15- and 30-item scales available to identify the presence of depression in older people. Can be used in different settings.	Yesavage, J.A., Brink, T.L., Rose, T.L., et al., 1983. Development and validation of a geriatric depression screening scale: a preliminary report. Journal of Psychiatric Research 17 (1), 37-49. http://www.stanford.edu/%7Eyesavage/GDS.html
Cornell Score for Depression in Dementia (CSDD)	Designed specifically to detect depression in older people with dementia. A 19-item scale that is administered by a clinician, taking about 20 minutes.	Alexopoulos, G.S., Abrams, R.C., Young, R.C., et al., 1988. Cornell Scale For Depression in Dementia. Biological Psychiatry 23, 271-284.
SOCIAL		
Duke Social Support Index	A measure of social support for older people living in the community that can be self-completed or interviewer-administered. A shorter, 11-item version has been adapted by Koenig.	Koenig, H.G., Westlund, R.E., George, L.K., et al., 1993. Abbreviating the Duke Social Support Index for use in chronically ill elderly individuals. Psychosomatics 34, 61-69.
Index of Social Support (ISS)	Nine items and provides separate measures of a person's perceived availability of support and his or her satisfaction with it.	James, O., Davies, A., 1987. Assessing social support and satisfaction in the elderly: Development of a brief assessment instrument, the index of social support. International Journal of Geriatric Psychiatry 2 (4), 227-233.

*For further information see Chalmers J, Johnson V, Tang J H et al 2004 Evidence-based protocol: Oral hygiene care for functionally dependent and cognitively impaired older adults. Journal of Gerontological Nursing 30(11):5-12

For example, the Aged Care Funding Instrument (ACFI) Assessment Pack (see www.health.gov.au/acfi) contains the continence record, includes a '3 day urinary record' and a '7 day bowel record' and behaviour records, in addition to validated tools for cognitive assessment (PAS) and depression (Cornell Scale). Also, the *Guidelines for Medication Management in Residential Aged Care Facilities* provide an example of an assessment of a resident's ability to self-administer medication (Australian Pharmaceuticals Advisory Council 2002). Similarly, the need to provide culturally sensitive assessment and consequent care requires a practical way of evaluating cultural variables and their effects on health and illness behaviours (Rawlings-Anderson 2004), and some resources have been developed with this in mind. For example, Giger and Davidhizar (1995) argue that every person is influenced to some degree by six cultural phenomena: communication, space, social organisation, time, environment control and biological variations. They have developed key questions relevant to each cultural phenomenon to form a framework that assists health professionals to uncover important information that can identify what aspects of the older person's cultural background might impact on the assessment process and consequent care plan.

Many tools in use are not age-specific nor do they cater for cultural differences. Assessment tools are often used to gather information from areas that the tool was not designed to assess. The wise use of tools to aid in gathering information is essential if the results are to be useful in portraying an accurate picture of the strengths and weaknesses of the area being assessed.

The wise use of tools to aid in gathering information is essential if the results are to be useful in portraying an accurate picture of the strengths and weaknesses of the area being assessed.

USE OF DATA FROM ASSESSMENTS

The collection of assessment data must be relevant and take a broad approach to include the present and the past. Often large amounts of information are required to gain a holistic picture of the person and their health status. Past history of medical problems, social indicators and community information, as well as current medical tests and presenting problems, add up to large files. The assessor must not subject data to personal interpretation, as this can lead to making hasty conclusions about the issues found. Only facts must be recorded and not assumptions. Conclusions must be drawn from the data collected and clinical decisions made to form interventions that are recorded on a care plan.

Care plans vary from service to service but the constant factor is the interpretation of the assessment data into specific interventions. This requires a team approach to maximise the benefits of the process of information gathering and to lessen the chances of misinterpretation. Opinions are valid if they are tested and subjective data is recorded as reported.

Evaluation of interventions can be done by repeating the use of a tool after a period of time to measure changes, by observation, by talking to the client, by collecting other results from tests, and by case meetings of the interdisciplinary team. In using any tool as an evaluative index or outcome measure, it is important to remember that not all tools have been designed to have the necessary sensitivity to be responsive to change in health status over time.

ETHICAL RESPONSIBILITIES

All health professionals have a duty of care to do no harm. Gathering information from a client may identify/highlight personal matters that may affect care relationships between family members and divulge legal or distressing topics that the assessor has to record in a sensitive way. Often decisions about care concern family members but the older person may not want them involved, or has issues that they do not want family to know. Written forms of communication are usually not a problem if information is accurate and sensitively recorded, but verbal commentary can be detrimental to the older person. Conversations relayed to other staff can be construed as insensitive. Withholding information is not only unethical but it may also be a legal matter. Often staff forget that not all older people have hearing or cognitive impairments that may impact on their understanding of conversations they overhear. Assessment data are discussed by the team in order to come to a clinical decision about how to improve health, not to critique or judge another.

Summaries of the older person's health problems and admissions should be made available to other health professionals in the community or other establishments in a timely, safe fashion. Such summarised material must include current medication, ongoing requirements for continued treatments, status on discharge and follow-up arrangements. This is essential to prevent repeated questioning of clients for the same information and policies should be put in place to minimise duplication and ensure the flow of information.

RECORD KEEPING

As assessment is an interdisciplinary effort; all data should be kept in a common file accessible to all team members. If data is permitted to be kept by various team members in different places, a holistic approach cannot be developed and the likelihood of duplication of assessment is increased. Medical records or files are kept securely in specified cupboards or filing cabinets according to the policy of the organisation. It is important to consider any legal requirements that may be relevant to keeping and handling personal and health information, particularly in relation to privacy. In Australia the Commonwealth *Privacy Act 1988* provides a definition of personal information and how it may appear in any identification of the person involved. From December 2001 health service providers covered by the Privacy Act have needed to comply with 10 National Privacy Principles that allow for individuals to exercise new rights and choices about how their personal and health information is handled in the private health sector (see the Office of the Privacy Commissioner website at www.privacy.gov.au/health). However, the Privacy Act does not cover an individual's health information that is held by state or territory public hospitals or clinics so it is important to also consider state and territory legislation that may be in place. Other considerations with respect to record keeping may be linked to the healthcare setting specifically. For example, in Australia legal requirements for documentation keeping may vary from state to state but the *Aged Care Act 1997* does stipulate all aged care facilities must keep their records in a securely locked place for three years following discharge or death. State health Acts may stipulate up to 21 years of safekeeping.

USE OF TECHNOLOGY

The development of computerised records and e-health cards is changing the nature of record keeping. It is crucial that information technology has safeguards applied and that people are aware of the safety issues involved. Transfer of a person's information by one computer to another is already being done, for example, from a hospital to a general practitioner. Results from pathology tests are emailed and copies of x-rays can be sent to other healthcare providers. Formal mechanisms to facilitate the efficient, safe transfer of information across care settings should be developed (Dorevitch et al 2004).

PRACTICAL CONSIDERATIONS WHEN CONDUCTING A PERSON-CENTRED COMPREHENSIVE ASSESSMENT

There are certain assumptions that we, as health professionals, inevitably make when we assess older people. We assume they understand why they are being assessed and are willing participants in the process, that they are able to hear us, that they can comprehend what we say, and that they are capable of accurate, intelligible responses. In any given clinical interaction between an older person and a health professional it is generally taken for granted that these preconditions for a successful outcome have been met. This inevitably leads to self-reported information being sought from the older person in the first instance as the preferred approach to conducting a comprehensive assessment. It is also easiest and least time-consuming to question the older person directly, since obtaining information from other sources (particularly if not present at the time of the assessment) adds to the work of the assessor. Embarking on the process of comprehensive assessment without addressing key practical considerations can promote unnecessary negative consequences for both the assessor and the older person being assessed.

FACILITATING PERSON-CENTREDNESS

All older people undergoing comprehensive assessment should be treated with respect and dignity at all times, and their assessment should be carried out in a manner that is consistent with the principles of 'person-centred care'. In general, giving consideration to the following can facilitate person-centredness of assessment (Dorevitch et al 2004, Nay et al 2009, Webster 2004):
- creating the right context by providing a quiet environment, affording privacy and minimal distractions, no feeling of time pressures and the

assessor taking a physical position that does not dominate the older person (e.g. seated facing each other at the same level)

- being aware of cultural differences in questioning and non-verbal communication interpretation, such as Australian Indigenous people
- establishing rapport with the older person at the outset of the assessment by introducing oneself, asking how they would like to be addressed, explaining the purpose of the assessment, asking what they consider the main problem(s) to be and what their goals are (what they would like to see come of the assessment)
- being honest about the purpose of the assessment and the realities of what might be offered
- taking a positive view by acknowledging personal abilities, strengths and resources
- being attentive and open to what the older person is communicating
- being non-judgmental and prepared to listen, making a concerted effort to understand the person's current perspectives, priorities and anxieties
- clarifying what is understood about the conclusions of the assessment and what will come next.

MEDICAL CONSIDERATIONS

If the older person is acutely unwell or physically discomforted, they may find it difficult to meaningfully participate in the assessment process. If impaired cognition is suspected, which may call the accuracy of self-reported information into question, it is advisable to establish this as early in the assessment as possible by asking the patient if they think they have any problem with their memory and administering a simple screening test of cognition such as the Abbreviated Mental Test Score or the Mini-Mental State Examination (MMSE). If an acute confusional state (delirium) is suspected, it may be helpful to administer a tool such as the Confusion Assessment Method (CAM).

Where an older person seems 'flat', is not making eye contact and is giving non-committal responses to questions, consideration should be given as to whether they are depressed. Depression is under-diagnosed in older people and depressed older people can give the appearance of being cognitively impaired (so-called 'pseudo-dementia').

 Depression is under-diagnosed in older people and depressed older people can give the appearance of being cognitively impaired.

COMMUNICATION CONSIDERATIONS

Communicating with older people with hearing or vision impairment or mental health needs can be challenging and requires specific skills and considerations (Heath 2000). The hearing of an older person should be optimised by making sure they are wearing any usual hearing aids and that such aids are operational.

In most cases the assessor should sit directly in front of the older person and speak clearly, slowly and only slightly louder than usual. However, it is important to keep cultural considerations in mind. For example, in Australia cultural protocol in assessing Aboriginal older people would be to sit shoulder to shoulder or on the diagonal, as this is non-confrontational, allows for less direct eye contact to occur and will make the person feel more comfortable (Carrillo et al 1999). A person has functional hearing if they can hear someone speaking at a normal conversational level from one metre away. Particular attention should be given to the environment in which the assessment is taking place.

Where there are concerns about an older person's receptive communication abilities, this can be easily screened by asking them to follow a simple one-stage command (e.g. 'close your eyes') followed by a two-stage command (e.g. 'lift up your hand, then poke out your tongue'). Expressive communication can be tested by asking the patient to repeat a simple phrase (e.g. 'West Register Street is opposite East Register Street') and to name several common objects (e.g. a pen, a watch or a key).

Older people with limited English proficiency have the right to a trained interpreter. Even though there are significant benefits to using trained interpreters, the use of an interpreter during the assessment process can itself present issues that warrant consideration. The relationship between the assessor and the older person becomes a triad when the interpreter is used. Research suggests that the common language as well as the cultural context may result in the person's attention focusing on the interpreter rather than the health professional (Fatahi et al 2005). A lack of time can impact on the quality of the information being communicated, as not only does the transfer of information involve an additional person but culture-related expressions can also take more time to translate because they often need explanation (Fatahi et al 2005). Although the use of trained interpreters can be costly, failure to use interpreters can lead to higher hospitalisation rates, increased testing, misdiagnosis and poor comprehension, which impacts on compliance and satisfaction (Herndon & Joyce 2004). Bilingual staff members can be taught to provide interpretation services when professional interpreters are not feasible (Sevilla & Willis 2004). Family members or friends should not be used as interpreters because they may find it difficult to interpret what is said and unconsciously screen what they hear, giving a summarised interpretation of the information (Herndon & Joyce 2004). This not only decreases the accuracy of the information but it may impact on the assessor–older person relationship. The older person with limited English proficiency may find having a family member present during the assessment comforting, but also be aware that some older people may be unwilling to volunteer sensitive information with a family member or friend in attendance (Herndon & Joyce 2004).

CULTURAL CONSIDERATIONS

The importance of cultural competence in assessment has been brought to attention in recent years. It refers to 'possessing knowledge, awareness and respect for other cultures' (Juckett 2005 p 2269), which is recognised as important to fostering the cultural understanding between health professionals and patients that improves adherence, patient care and clinical outcomes (Carrillo et al 1999). Brown and Varcoe (2006 p 160) argue that 'critical consideration to "difference" is particularly crucial in terms of culture' as underlying assumptions about what culture is and in what ways cultural issues should be addressed have significant implications for the relationships between health professionals and those they care for, and healthcare more broadly. 'Culture, the shared beliefs and attitudes of a group, shapes ideas about what constitutes illness and acceptable treatment' (Juckett 2005 p 2269) and differences within cultural communities also warrant consideration.

For example, in Australia Aboriginal and Torres Strait Islander communities are as diverse as any other community and, as such, there are different traditions and customs, different ways of communicating, different understandings, different sensitive issues and different elders. Cultural guides providing insight for comprehensive assessment highlight the need for flexibility and patience when working with Aboriginal and Torres Strait Islander people (Department of Human Services South Australia 2002). Involving Aboriginal and non-Aboriginal staff in assessment can facilitate a culturally responsive and sensitive process so assistance with the assessment should be sought from a liaison officer or Indigenous health worker as appropriate. The role of elders in communities should be respected.

Cultural and religious beliefs will influence the individual's view of the world and therefore impact significantly on the way they do things in everyday life, their approach to health and healthcare being no exception (Rawlings-Anderson 2004). The cultural distance between the assessor and the older person being assessed is likely to increase the need for more time, particularly when an interpreter is required to overcome language barriers. While assessors may not fully understand the basis of cultural and religious variations, it is possible to use frameworks to help systematically in the comprehensive assessment process (Rawlings-Anderson 2004).

Cultural and religious beliefs will influence the individual's view of the world and therefore impact significantly on the way they do things in everyday life, their approach to health and healthcare being no exception.

To give some appreciation of how important comprehensive assessment is in aged care the following vignette is drawn from an outpatient's clinic.

Vignette

Mr Kostovich presented at the outpatient's department of a busy city hospital accompanied by his 10-year-old grandson. The family decided that someone needed to go with him because he did not speak English and the grandson was the most proficient having been at school in Australia for four years. Through the grandson interpreting it was ascertained that Mr Kostovich had a tummy ache. On examination the medical officer discovered Mr Kostovich had a very distended abdomen and that he required a scan.

This was explained to the grandson who looked very confused as he tried to convey the necessity of this to his grandfather. On arrival at the radiology department the process of explaining what was going to happen with the scan became somehow distorted. Mr Kostovich left the hospital with his grandson without having his scan but returned the next day in more pain.

At no time during the initial visit was another interpreter called who could speak Russian so the importance of the situation was not conveyed clearly and the grandson was too young to appreciate what was happening. The second visit necessitated the interpreter, who explained the situation so treatment could begin.

CONCLUSION

Comprehensive geriatric assessment is important for improving diagnostic accuracy, guiding the selection of interventions to restore or preserve health, recommending an optimal environment for care, predicting health outcomes and monitoring clinical change over time. Regardless of the setting, appropriate communication and interpersonal skills, underpinned by sensitivity to cultural considerations, are essential for successful comprehensive assessment. How person-centredness is facilitated needs to be given consideration throughout the process. The use of appropriate, valid, reliable tools can facilitate assessment, but instruments cannot substitute for good clinical skills and judgment, including the skill of eliciting important items from the person's life history and physical examination. An interdisciplinary approach underpins good person-centred comprehensive assessment.

Reflective questions

1. How do multidisciplinary teams differ from interdisciplinary teams?

2. The new approach to 'social inclusiveness' in government policy may improve the assessment of social function. Will this influence the way you work in aged care?

3. Where does comprehensive assessment data come from?

4. How does the environment impact on comprehensive assessment of older people?

5. The chapter offers some examples of assessment tools but cautions on the reliability and validity issues of some tools. How can you be sure your assessment tools are reliable and valid?

6. Assumptions made from data obtained from assessment must be validated. How can the assessor do this so mistakes are not made?

7. There are many considerations to be aware of when conducting a comprehensive assessment. What role does culture play in obtaining information?

References

American Geriatrics Society, 2008. Geriatrics review syllabus. A core curriculum in geriatric medicine. Sixth edition (GRS6). Chapter Six: Assessment. Online. Available: http://www.geriatricsreviewsyllabus.org/content/agscontent/asses6_m.htm, 18 Apr 2008.

American Geriatrics Society, 2006. Comprehensive geriatric assessment position statement. Annals of Long-Term Care 14 (3), 34–35.

Aminzadeh, F., Byszeqski, A., Dalziel, W., et al., 2005. Effectiveness of outpatient geriatric assessment programs: exploring caregiver needs, goals and outcomes. Journal of Gerontological Nursing 31 (12), 19–25.

Atwal, A., Caldwell, K., 2006. Nurses' perceptions of multidisciplinary team work in acute health-care. International Journal of Nursing Practice 12 (6), 359–365.

Australian Institute of Health and Welfare (AIHW), 2007. Older Australians at a glance, fourth ed. Cat. no. AGE 52. AIHW, Canberra.

Australian Pharmaceuticals Advisory Council, 2002. Guidelines for medication management in aged care facilities. Department of Health and Ageing, Canberra.

Beers, M., Berkow, R., 2000. The Merck manual of geriatrics. Chapter 7. Geriatric Interdisciplinary Teams. Online. Available: http://www.merck.com/mrkshared/ mm_geriatrics/sec1/ch7.jsp, 18 Apr 2008.

Bogardus Jr., S.T., Bradley, E.H., Williams, C.S., et al., 2004. Achieving goals in geriatric assessment: role of caregiver agreement and adherence to recommendations. The Journal of the American Geriatrics Society 52 (1), 99–105.

Browne, A.J., Varcoe, C., 2006. Critical cultural perspectives and health care involving Aboriginal peoples. Contemporary Nurse 22 (2), 155–167.

Carrillo, J., Green, A., Betancourt, J., 1999. Cross-cultural primary care: a patient-based approach. Annals of Internal Medicine 130, 829–834.

Cohen-Mansfield, J., Jensen, B., 2007. Adequacy of spouses as informants regarding older persons' self-care practices and their perceived importance. Families Systems and Health 25 (1), 53–67.

Department of Human Services (South Australia), 2002. Working with Aboriginal People—a cultural guide: for community-based health and home care services in Wakefield, Gawler and mid north areas of rural South Australia. Online. Available: http://in.dhs.sa.gov.au, 21 Apr 2008.

Dorevitch, M., Davis, S., Andrews, G., 2004. Guide for assessing older people in hospital. Published by Metropolitan Health and Aged Care Services Division, Victorian Government Department of Human Services, Melbourne, Victoria on behalf of Australian Health Ministers' Advisory Council.

Edvardsson, D., Winblad, B., Sandman, P.O., 2008. Person-centred care for people with severe Alzheimer's disease – current status and ways forward. The Lancet Neurology 7, 362–367.

Ellis, G., Langhorne, P., 2004. Comprehensive geriatric assessment for older hospital patients. British Medical Bulletin 71 (1), 45–59.

Fatahi, N., Mattsson, B., Hasanppor, J., et al., 2005. Interpreters' experiences of general practitioner-patient encounters. Scandinavian Journal of Primary Health Care 23 (3), 159–163.

Fenton, J., Levnine, M., Mahoney, L., et al., 2006. Bringing geriatricians to the front lines: evaluation of a quality improvement intervention in primary care. The Journal of the American Board of Family Medicine 19 (4), 331–339.

Foreman, P., Thomas, S., Gardner, I., 2004. The review and identification of an existing validated, comprehensive assessment tool: final report. A project undertaken by the Lincoln Centre for Ageing and Community Care Research, Australian Institute for Primary Care at La Trobe University for the Department of Human Services. Online. Available: http://www.health.vic.gov.au/subacute/assess.pdf, 21 Apr 2008.

Giger, J., Davidhizar, R., 1995. Transcultural nursing assessment and interventions, third ed. Mosby, St. Louis.

Gottfries, C.G., 2001. Late life depression. European Archives of Psychiatry and Clinical Neuroscience 251 (Suppl. 2), II57–61.

Harari, D., Martin, F.C., Buttery, A., et al., 2007. The older persons' assessment and liaison team 'OPAL': evaluation of comprehensive geriatric assessment in acute medical inpatients. Age and Ageing 36 (6), 670–675.

Heath, H., 2000. Assessing Older People. Elderly Care 11 (10), 27–28.

Herndon, E., Joyce, L., 2004. Getting the most from language interpreters. Family Practice Management 11 (6), 37–40.

Hickman, L., Newton, P., Halcomb, E., et al., 2007. Best practice interventions to improve the management of older people in acute care settings: a literature review. Journal of Advanced Nursing 60 (2), 113–126.

Juckett, G., 2005. Cross-cultural medicine. American Family Physician 72 (11), 2267–2274.

Jones, A., 2006. Multidisciplinary team working: collaboration and conflict. International Journal of Mental Health 15 (1), 19–28.

Koch, S., Garratt, S., 2001. Assessing older people: a guide for health professionals. Maclennan & Petty, Sydney.

Landefeld, C., 2003. Improving health care for older persons. Annals of Internal Medicine 139 (52), 421–424.

Nay,R., Bird, M., Edvardsson, D., et al., 2009. Person-centred care. In: Nay, R., Garratt, S. (Eds.), Older people: issues and innovations. Churchill Livingston, Sydney.

Orrell, M., Hancock, G., 2004. CANE: Camberwell Assessment of Need for the Elderly. Gaskell, London.

Osterweil, D., 2003. Comprehensive geriatric assessment: lessons in progress. Journal of the American Medical Directors Association 5, 371–374.

Payne, S., Kerr, C., Hawker, S., et al., 2002. The communication of information about older people between health and social care practitioners. Age and Ageing 31 (2), 107–117.

Philp, I., 2000. EASY-Care: A systematic approach to the assessment of older people. Geriatric Medicine 30 (5), 15–19.

Rawlings-Anderson, K., 2004. Assessing the cultural and religious needs of older people. Nursing Older People 16 (8), 28–33.

Ruben, D., Frank, J., Kirsch, S., et al., 1999. A randomised clinical trial of outpatient comprehensive geriatric assessment coupled with an intervention to increase adherence to recommendations. Journal of Geriatrics Society 47 (3), 269–276.

Rubenstein, L.Z., 2004. Comprehensive geriatric assessment: from miracle to reality. The Journals of Gerontology Medical Sciences 59A (5), 473–477.

Scanlan, B.C., 2005. The value of comprehensive geriatric assessment. Care Management Journals 6 (1), 2–8.

Sevilla Mátir, J.F., Willis, D.R., 2004. Using bilingual staff members as interpreters. Family Practice Management 11 (7), 34–36.

Somers, L., Marton, K., Babaccia, J., et al., 2000. Physician, nurse and social worker collaboration in primary health care for chronically ill seniors. Archives if Internal Medicine 160 (12), 1825–1833.

Vertesi, A., Darzins, P., Lowe, S., et al., 2000. Development of the Handicap Assessment and Resource Tool (HART). Canadian Journal of Occupational Therapy 67 (2), 120–127.

Webster, J., 2004. Person-centred assessment with older people. Nursing Older People 16 (3), 22–26.

Wieland, D., Hirth, V., 2003. Comprehensive griatric assessment. Cancer Control 10 (6), 454–462.

Wilkinson, R., Marmot, M., 2003. Social determinants of health: the solid facts, second ed. WHO, Denmark.

Winefield, H., Murrell, T., Clifford, J., et al., 1996. The search for reliable and valid measures of patient-centredness. Psychology and Health 11, 811–824.

Wolfs, C.A., Verhey, F.R., Kessels, A., et al., 2007. GP concordance with advice for treatment following a multidisciplinary psychogeriatric assessment. International Journal of Geriatric Psychiatry 22 (3), 233–240.

World Health Organization, 1948. Preamble to the Constitution of the World Health Organization as adopted by the International Health Conference, New York 19-22 June 1946; signed on 22 July 1946 by the representatives of 61 States (Official Records of the World Health Organization, no. 2, p 100) and entered into force on 7 April 1948.

Zeiss, A., Thompson, D., 2003. Providing interdisciplinary geriatric team care: what does it really take? Clinical Psychology: Science and Practice 10 (1), 115–119.

CHAPTER 13

ALZHEIMER'S DEMENTIA: NEUROPSYCHOLOGY, EARLY DIAGNOSIS AND INTERVENTION

Matthew Summers

Editors' comments

Summers provides a 'state of the art' discussion of where Alzheimer's diagnosis, differentiation and interventions are at. He explains the changes in the brain that result in the expressions of dementia seen by families and staff: 'unexplainable' changes in mood and behaviour, memory losses and so on. This is particularly important because too often families still think that if the person is 'strong' they should be able to manage and overcome the symptoms. Health professionals can make a very difficult time more understandable by ensuring the person with dementia and those around them can make sense of what is occurring. Summers also notes how different interventions may work for some people but not others. In the end Alzheimer's is a terminal condition and the importance of end-of-life planning is illuminated.

INTRODUCTION

Neuropsychology is a subspecialisation of psychology. As such it is concerned with understanding human behaviour, emotions and thoughts. However, the specialisation involves an understanding of the relationship between brain function (*neuro*) and human behaviour, emotions and thought processes (*psychology*).

Neuropsychologists work closely with medical and allied health professionals, providing expert assessments of children and adults with various deficits or changes to brain function that impact on the behaviour, thoughts processes and emotions. Typically, neuropsychologists assess an individual's cognitive abilities, including intellectual, memory, language, visuo-spatial and executive functions. In addition, through observation and interview techniques, the individual's social, emotional and behavioural responses are assessed. The results of such assessment, when combined with knowledge of the relationship between various brain structures and cognition, behaviour and emotion as well as an in-depth understanding of various neuropsychological, neurological, psychiatric and medical diseases, enables neuropsychologists to formulate a diagnosis of disorders such as dementia. Finally, the role of neuropsychologist is often to provide support for rehabilitation and intervention. The neuropsychological assessment can be invaluable in formulating appropriate therapeutic strategies as well as in guiding the treatment approaches used by other health professionals (e.g. medical practitioners, psychologists, social workers, speech pathologists, occupational therapists, nurses and physiotherapists) to maximise the probability of success. For example, a neuropsychological assessment may indicate that the person displays evidence of marked frontal lobe compromise, resulting in impaired judgment, decision making, reasoning ability, attention, impulse control and reactive mood states. For the treatment team such information can be invaluable in guiding the approaches used for intervention as well as informing the underlying cause of disruptive and inappropriate behaviours (e.g. sexually uninhibited behaviour). This pattern of cognitive impairments indicates that traditional psychological and counselling approaches are unlikely to be effective, as 'talking therapies' require a certain level of reasoning, judgment and decision-making capacity, enabling the patient to exert some level of control over their behaviour and to modify the cognitive triggers for that behaviour. Hence, interventions in such cases will be restricted to behavioural modification, environmental modification and pharmacological approaches.

Neuropsychological assessment is frequently required to determine an individual's capacity to make reasoned and informed decisions regarding their care, financial matters, legal affairs and accommodation needs. Often such neuropsychological assessment is sought by guardianship and administration boards to assist in determining an individual's capacity and need for assistance. Such assessments are increasingly required in cases of older adults who have developed or are developing dementia.

Neuropsychological assessment can be critical in determining which part of the brain is affected and appropriate interventions.

DEMENTIA INCIDENCE

Dementia represents a substantial health, social and economic burden in developed countries such as Australia, with estimates of more than 245,000 Australians, or approximately 1.1% of the population, currently living with dementia. Despite difficulties in diagnosis, dementia is the leading cause of disability in adults older than 65 years of age. With the demographic passage of the 'baby boomer' generation, coupled with increased life expectancy, it has been predicted that by 2050 the incidence and frequency of dementia will increase dramatically, with 940,000 Australians (2.8% of the population) living with dementia (Deloitte Access Economics 2011). In 2002–03 a total of $3.85

billion or 4.5% of the Australian health and aged care budget was expended on dementia (Access Economics 2009). It is estimated that by 2060 health spending on dementia will be greater than for any other single health condition, with projected costs of $83 billion or 11% of the Australian health and residential aged care sector expenditure (Access Economics 2009). It has furthermore been estimated that delaying the onset of dementia by just a few months will produce future health savings in the order of billions of dollars by mid-century (Access Economics 2004). Hence, strategies that delay dementia onset and/or increase resistance to ageing-related cognitive decline, would have significant health and economic benefits.

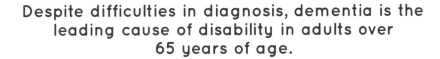

Despite difficulties in diagnosis, dementia is the leading cause of disability in adults over 65 years of age.

WHAT IS DEMENTIA?

Dementia refers to a group of neurodegenerative disorders that produce a condition of cognitive decline and functional impairment. Dementias can be irreversible, static or reversible; however, clinically the term dementia is commonly reserved for the progressive irreversible forms of cognitive and functional decline associated with neurodegeneration of brain tissue.

Traditionally, the progressive irreversible dementias are subgrouped as either cortical or subcortical dementias; however, it is important to note that these subgroups have little diagnostic utility and have limited relevance to directing treatment interventions. Nonetheless, the subdivision of cortical versus subcortical dementias is useful in that it provides a conceptual distinction between the brain structures that are primarily affected in early stages of dementia. Cortical dementias arise from pathological changes in the outer grey matter regions of the cerebral hemispheres, and subcortical dementias result from neuropathological changes in the white matter and deep grey matter regions of the cerebellum and cerebral hemispheres. The distinction between cortical and subcortical dementia is important neuropsychologically, as it reflects a difference in the resulting deficits to cognitive function, emotional and behavioural regulation. Cortical dementias affecting the grey matter regions of the brain typically affect areas of the brain responsible for primary cognitive functions (e.g. learning, memory recall, word knowledge, colour recognition). Consequently, it is this loss of one or more base cognitive functions in cortical dementia that reduces that capacity of the individual to function in their environment, typically seen as impairments to activities of daily living (ADLs). Subcortical dementias predominantly affect the neural pathways connecting the cortical regions together. The cognitive deficits in subcortical dementias reflect a secondary deficit where the base cognitive function is preserved (e.g. learning), but the ability to rapidly combine cognitive functions to produce a coordinated response is impaired. This impediment to coordination across multiple cortical sites is typically seen as slowed processing of information and slowing of reactions to environmental stimuli. Hence, individuals with subcortical deficits retain intact base cognitive functions; their impairment in the real world reflects the speed demands of the environment rather than task complexity. The provision of additional time and reduced environmental demands for rapid responding minimises the severity of cognitive compromise exhibited by people with subcortical compromise, a benefit not seen in those with cortical compromise.

Differences exist between cortical and subcortical dementias. Typically cortical dementias involve the loss of one or more base cognitive functions (e.g. memory), whereas subcortical dementias involve impairment to the ability to coordinate across multiple base cognitive functions.

CORTICAL DEMENTIA

Alzheimer's dementia

Alzheimer's dementia (AD) is the most common form of dementia, accounting for approximately 50% of all cases of dementia in Australia (Access Economics 2009). A definitive diagnosis of AD requires pathological examination of the brain typically at autopsy (but can be by biopsy), identifying the presence of key hallmark pathological features, neurofibrillary tangles and senile/neuritic plaques (McKhann et al 1984, 2011). Tangles and plaques are the pathological markers of neuronal death in the brain and in AD are predominantly present in the temporal, frontal and parietal lobes of the brain (Lezak et al 2012). Further, there is widespread neuronal loss throughout the cortical regions of the frontal, temporal and parietal lobes, resulting in widening of the ventricles of the brain and general shrinkage of brain mass (Lezak et al 2012).

Prior to death, a possible-probable diagnosis of AD is made on the presence of key clinical symptoms of cognitive, behavioural and social impairment. AD is a progressive disease, commencing with mild and relatively circumscribed deficits that gradually worsen to become a severe dementia with widespread and marked impairments to cognitive, social and behavioural functioning. The speed of progression of impairment is variable from individual to individual, with death occurring between two and 20 years post-onset, on average within 10 years post-onset (Alzheimer's Association 2009).

Neuropsychologically, a clinical diagnosis of AD requires the presence of clinically significant impairments to memory as well as to at least one other cognitive domain, typically language, spatial processing or executive functions (McKhann et al 1984, 2011). However, recent research indicates that atypical AD presentations occur in which memory impairment occurs later than impairments to non-memory domains, resulting in a recommended revision to the diagnostic criteria to include a non-amnesic AD diagnosis (McKhann et al 2011). Further, there must be evidence of a slowly emerging decline in function, often confirmed by information sourced by family members or caregivers (McKhann et al 1984, 2011).

Typically, the presentation of AD in the earliest stages is marked by the presence of impairments to memory, most commonly reported being impaired recent memory or memory for recent and/or current events (Lezak et al 2012). This may be accompanied by subtle impairments to a second cognitive domain, such as word-finding difficulties (language), reduced capacity to clearly explain ideas to others (language), becoming lost in unfamiliar locations (spatial) or struggling to cope in unfamiliar environments or with novel tasks (executive). Neuropsychological assessment at this early stage can be essential to differentiate AD from other conditions that can resemble early stage AD, such as depression or delirium.

With disease progression, there is a worsening of the initial deficits seen and a spreading of impairment to incorporate other cognitive functions (Lezak et al 2012).

- Memory functions deteriorate with increasing pathology in the medial temporal lobe structures, resulting in increasingly severe impairments to new learning as well as a progressive loss of access to previously learnt information, such as names of friends and family members.
- Language deficits become increasingly prominent, with increasing pathology in the temporal and parietal lobes of the dominant hemisphere. This leads to the emergence and worsening of various dysphasias, resulting in the person experiencing increasing difficulty understanding what they have been told and deteriorating ability to use language to explain their thinking to others.
- Spatial impairments become increasingly prominent as pathology increases in the parietal lobes of the brain. Initially the AD sufferer may become confused and disoriented in unfamiliar locations, which may worsen and lead to wandering and confusion in most environments except the most familiar (e.g. home).
- Dyspraxias may also emerge with parietal lobe pathology, reflecting a loss of the cognitive representation for use of objects for purposeful action.
- Executive impairments emerge with frontal lobe pathology and can appear at any stage of the development of AD. Executive functions encapsulate a range of higher order cognitive processes including but not restricted to: attention, concentration, capacity to multi-task, planning and organisational capacity, adaptability to changing environments and task demands, reasoning capacity, decision making, impulse control, modulation of behaviour and emotional reactions (Lezak et al 2012). A range of deficits to behaviour, functioning in social situations, emotional control and cognitive processing arise due to executive impairments in AD. These range from difficulty coping with complex tasks, slowing of task completion, emotional changes (irritability, depression, anxiety, affective lability, anger outbursts) and socially inappropriate behaviour (including sexually inappropriate) to at the severe end, an inability to make reasoned and informed decisions regarding self-care, medical, legal, or accommodation issues.

- As the executive deficits worsen, impairments to insight of deficit appear. This lack of awareness can result in increasing difficulties for carers in managing the person with AD because the person believes they have no cognitive problems. With increasing executive compromise there is a dysregulation of emotional responses from executive control resulting in emotional lability. Emotional lability reflects the expression of the raw emotional response to a situation without executive processes (planning, judgment, reasoning) mediating the expression of the emotion in a socially appropriate manner. Due to the dysregulation of emotional response, the person with AD will display rapidly changing emotional reactions ranging from tearfulness, distress and anger, through to happiness and elation.
- Typically, by the advanced stage of dementia, memory impairments have worsened such that the person is no longer capable of maintaining information beyond the immediate experience. As a result, the person is readily distracted from the mood state by the introduction of a new situation or stimulus.
- Characteristically, the emergence of clinically significant impairments to insight, decision making, reasoning and organisational ability triggers the appointment of a guardian or administrator under the relevant state guardianship and administration Act.

There is no known treatment for AD. A number of pharmacological agents are available for early-stage AD and may slow disease progression but do not halt or reverse AD (Machado & Caramelli 2006). Death is the inevitable consequence of AD. Early accurate diagnosis is therefore essential to provide the person and their family with appropriate information and support for future life planning with full involvement of the person with AD.

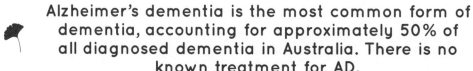

Alzheimer's dementia is the most common form of dementia, accounting for approximately 50% of all diagnosed dementia in Australia. There is no known treatment for AD.

OTHER DEMENTIAS

There is a diverse range of progressive cortical and subcortical dementias other than Alzheimer's dementia; however, these will not be described here in detail so as to remain focused on the most common form of dementia, AD. Cortical dementias such as frontal-temporal lobar degeneration (FTLD) account for approximately 10% of all cases of dementia (Grossman 2002), and dementia with Lewy bodies (DLB), which may also account for up to 20% of all cases of dementia (Lezak et al 2012). Subcortical dementias include dementia due to Parkinson's disease, dementia due to Huntington's disease and dementia due to progressive supranuclear palsy, all of which are relatively uncommon forms of dementia. Dementia can also emerge as a result of repeated vascular insult in the brain, often referred to as vascular dementia. Recent studies indicate that vascular dementia is less common than initially thought, with an autopsy-based study indicating only 12% of all dementia cases being associated with vascular infarct alone, and 42% of all dementia cases constituting a 'mixed' dementia in which vascular infarction was seen in combination with neuropathological markers of AD, Parkinson's disease or DLB (Schneider et al 2007). Additionally, there is a range of multiple rare dementias that include AIDS-related dementia, Jakob-Creutzfeldt dementia, alcohol-related dementia and a range of dementias induced by toxic exposure.

DIAGNOSING DEMENTIA: THE IMPORTANCE OF NEUROPSYCHOLOGICAL ASSESSMENT FOR EARLY DIAGNOSIS AND DIFFERENTIAL DIAGNOSIS

Given the range of different progressive dementias, the similarity between different forms of dementia in the early stages in terms of behavioural and cognitive features and the similarity of symptoms to non-dementing conditions (such as depression and delirium), careful neuropsychological assessment is often the only method by which an accurate early diagnosis can be made. Neuropsychological assessment has excellent reliability and sensitivity in early differential diagnosis of the various forms of progressive dementia (Lezak et al 2012). Further, neuropsychological assessment can inform appropriate intervention based on the unique pattern of cognitive, behavioural and social strengths and weaknesses displayed by the person with dementia throughout the progression of the disease. As AD varies in terms of its exact presentation and rate of progression, neuropsychological assessment can be critical to tailored case management.

Over the past decade there has been increasing interest in identifying those at highest risk of developing dementia. The identification of a prodromal phase to dementia that is accurate and reliable proffers the prospect of providing intervention or treatment *before* dementia emerges. Epidemiological studies from the Mayo Clinic led to the development of a construct referred to as mild cognitive impairment (MCI) (Petersen 2004, Petersen et al 1997, 1999, 2001). MCI describes individuals who display cognitive deficits beyond what is expected for normal ageing but who do not satisfy the diagnostic criteria for dementia (Winblad et al 2004). The initial conceptualisation of MCI was that it was a condition characterised by a subclinical isolated memory impairment in which there was no impairment to ADLs or evidence of dementia (Petersen et al 2001). Various longitudinal studies indicate that people identified with amnestic MCI (aMCI) have an elevated risk of developing AD. However, there is great inconsistency in the estimated risk for AD, with different studies reporting that between 1.85% and 60.5% of those with MCI will develop AD within one year (Morris et al 2001, Solfrizzi et al 2004, Wahlund et al 2003).

Since the initial studies by Petersen et al (1997, 1999, 2001) the classification criteria for MCI have undergone repeated revisions. Current iterations of MCI classification criteria enable the identification of MCI subtypes on the basis of the presence of one or more subclinical cognitive impairments. The pattern of impairments detected on neuropsychological assessment enables the classification of single-domain aMCI, multiple-domain aMCI (aMCI+), single-domain nonamnestic MCI (naMCI) and multiple-domain nonamnestic MCI (naMCI+) (Albert et al 2011, Winblad et al 2004). A meta-analysis of epidemiological studies indicates that the annual conversion rate from each MCI subtype to AD are: 11.7% for aMCI (nine studies; sample size = 646), 12.2% for aMCI+ (eight studies; sample size =446) and 4.1% for naMCI (five studies; sample size = 354) (Mitchell & Shiri-Feshki 2009).

Mild cognitive impairment is conceptually a phase of subclinical cognitive impairment that precedes dementia. Neuropsychological assessment is used to identify subclinical levels of impairment. Research suggests that people with MCI have an increased *risk* of developing dementia.

However, when the epidemiologically derived MCI criteria are applied to diagnosing individuals, there is great inconsistency in diagnostic accuracy. While some people with MCI develop dementia, between 40% and 70% of adults classified with aMCI revert to an unimpaired status or remain stable at follow-up (Ravaglia et al 2006). Recent research suggests that aMCI is a rare and unstable classification (Alladi et al 2006, Saunders & Summers 2010), has low predictive value for developing dementia (Fischer et al 2007, Rasquin et al 2005, Rountree et al 2007) and that cognitive difficulties in areas other than memory can predicate the onset of AD (Storandt et al 2006). As a result of this heterogeneity in outcome, some researchers assert that MCI is a diagnostic nonentity that fails to predict risk of developing dementia (Gauthier & Touchon 2005, Ritchie et al 2001, Tabert et al 2006).

A recent Australian study (the Tasmanian MCI study) examined the capacity for MCI criteria to accurately diagnose risk for dementia in 81 MCI participants and 25 age- and education-matched controls over a two-year period. It was found that 20 months after initial assessment, 12.3% of the MCI participants had developed AD (converted), 25% had improved and no longer displayed MCI (recovered), 41% continued to present with MCI (stable), 15% transitioned to an alternate MCI subtype (unstable), 7% progressed from a single domain MCI subtype (aMCI or naMCI) to a multi-domain MCI subtype (aMCI+) (progressed) and 100% of the controls displayed stable neuropsychological performance from baseline to follow-up (Summers & Saunders 2012). That 25% of the MCI sample reverted to normal levels of function is consistent with previous studies (Comijs et al 2004, Ganguli et al 2004, Larrieu et al 2002, Palmer et al 2002). That such a large proportion of those identified as meeting the epidemiologically derived criteria for MCI reverted to normal levels of function indicates that these epidemiologically derived classification criteria have little utility in the clinical diagnosis of a person's risk of developing dementia. Further analysis of the data in the Tasmanian MCI study found that a combination of measures of visual episodic memory, verbal episodic memory, visual immediate memory span, visual working memory capacity, divided attention and sustained attention and target detection accurately classified outcome at 20 months in 86.3% of cases (Summers & Saunders 2012). Of most importance, this battery of neuropsychological tests accurately identified 100% of the MCI cases that progressed to AD 20 months later (Summers & Saunders 2012).

The results of the Tasmanian MCI study indicate that subclinical impairments across multiple cognitive domains (i.e. aMCI+) predict development of Alzheimer's dementia, whereas single domain subclinical impairments (e.g. aMCI, naMCI) are poor predictors of later development of AD (Summers & Saunders 2012). That multiple-domain MCI represents the best predictor for later AD development is not surprising given that a clinical diagnosis of AD requires the presence of clinically significant impairments in two or more cognitive domains including memory (McKhann et al 2011).

The results of the Tasmanian MCI study indicate that subclinical impairments across multiple cognitive domains (i.e. aMCI+) predict development of Alzheimer's dementia, whereas single-domain subclinical impairments (e.g. aMCI, naMCI) are poor predictors of later development of AD.

NON-PHARMACOLOGICAL TREATMENTS FOR DEMENTIA

Establishment of diagnostic criteria for a prodromal phase of AD, such as MCI, is essential for developing and applying treatments and therapies designed to slow or halt the progression from a prodromal phase to full-blown dementia. While some researchers are focused on identifying diagnostic criteria for MCI with prognostic sensitivity and specificity, other researchers are investigating the capacity of non-pharmacological approaches to slow or halt the progression to dementia.

Several research groups are currently investigating the potential benefit of non-pharmacological intervention approaches in MCI and AD groups. The studies described here do not represent the entire range of studies currently in progress but represent a selection of studies that have a clear non-pharmacological intervention approach.

Accurate and reliable diagnostic criteria for early stage Alzheimer's dementia and prodromal phases of dementia (such as MCI) are essential to ensure that treatments to delay or prevent the development of dementia can be applied at the earliest possible stage.

THE TASMANIAN HEALTHY BRAIN PROJECT

The Tasmanian Healthy Brain Project (THBP) is a world-first study examining the potential beneficial impact that university level education in late adulthood may have on delaying or preventing age-related cognitive decline, MCI and AD (Summers et al 2012). The basic premise behind the THBP is to ascertain whether it is possible to enhance cognitive reserve in older adults and whether this enhancement provides protection against MCI and AD.

Extensive research literature indicates that age-related decline commonly occurs across a range of cognitive functions, most notably information processing speed, attention, concentration and memory performance (Bisiacchi et al 2008, Johnson et al 2009, Salthouse et al 1996). Other studies indicate that ageing is associated with pathological changes to the brain, specifically progressive cortical shrinkage, reduction to grey matter volume in several regions and white matter loss in the prefrontal cortex (Beason-Held et al 2008). However, despite this evidence, there is considerable variability in the degree of cognitive change, as well as the degree and extent of structural pathological changes evident across people of approximately the same age.

The variability in age-related cognitive change and structural brain changes may relate to pre-existing individual differences in information processing capacity or 'cognitive reserve'. The notion of cognitive reserve (CR) stems from repeated observations that the extent of brain pathology or brain damage observed in an individual does not directly relate to the severity of clinical symptoms associated with that damage (Stern 2002, 2009). The CR hypothesis predicts, for example, that older adults with a higher CR will be able to sustain greater insult to the brain before clinical symptoms appear compared with a person with less cognitive reserve. Stern (2002, 2009) distinguished between passive and active components of reserve. The passive component is a product of brain size or number of neurons, thus larger brains can sustain larger amounts of damage before clinical impairments emerge. The active component relates to the ways in which the brain utilises pre-existing cognitive processes to compensate or cope with brain damage, thus two adults with AD can sustain identical patterns of brain damage but the one with greater CR retains a higher level of function than the patient with lower CR. Importantly both genetic predisposition and factors associated with life experiences, such as level of educational and occupational attainment and lifetime patterns of cognitive activity, are seen as contributing to CR (Richards & Sacker 2003).

Previous research indicates that an inverse relationship exists between educational attainment and risk for AD. Longitudinal studies of Catholic clergy indicate that education mediates the risk for AD, such that the higher the level of education the greater the level of neuropathology required before clinical symptoms of AD are evident (Bennett et al 2003). Other studies confirm these findings; individuals with clinical diagnoses of AD have two to three years less formal education than those without a clinical diagnosis (Roe et al 2007). Likewise, a study of Catholic nuns indicated risk for AD increased fourfold in those with low levels of educational attainment and small head circumference, when other factors such as age and genetic risk factors (APOE-ε4 status) were controlled for (Mortimer et al 2003). Both education and occupation have been found to reduce the likelihood that adults with MCI will convert to AD, suggesting that enhanced cognitive reserve may exert a protective effect on adults with preclinical signs of AD (Garibotto et al 2008).

In addition to education and occupation, other factors appear to be important in reducing risk for dementia. In a study of community-based elders it was found that level of social engagement, as measured by size of social networks, mediated the relationship between neuropathology (neurofibrillary tangles and amyloid plaques) and level of cognitive function. That is, participants with higher levels of social engagement displayed higher levels of cognitive function despite increasing neuropathological burden (Bennett et al 2006). Likewise, frequent cognitive activity (playing chess, visiting a library) is associated with reduced risk for AD, with cognitively inactive adults having a 2.6 times greater risk for developing AD (Wilson et al 2007). Therefore, the existing body of research suggests that prior education, occupational history and level of social engagement may mediate the likelihood that a person develops clinically evident AD. The precise nature of this apparent protective relationship is unclear, with some studies suggesting that education and occupation may enhance CR such that an individual can develop significant neuropathology but not display clinically significant cognitive decline. Other studies suggest that education and occupation may mask other factors that may be protective against AD, such as frequency of cognitive activity, socialisation, depressive symptomatology, diet, history of vascular disorder and academic performance.

The THBP commenced in Tasmania in 2011; by mid-2012 in excess of 400 participants had enrolled in the study. The THBP is designed to determine whether late-life university education exerts a protective effect on future risk for MCI and dementia. Participants in the study are 50–79 years of age at the time of enrolling in the study. Each participant is screened for pre-existing health conditions to ensure all are healthy older adults. Of the participant pool 90% will undertake at least 12 months of part-time university study, with each participant being able to engage in additional university-level education should they choose. The remaining 10% of the participant pool will not engage in university-level study and will serve as active controls. Each participant in the study undertakes an annual extensive neuropsychological assessment battery. In addition, measures of psychological health, medical health, social engagement and life satisfaction will also be used on an annual basis. This extensive assessment protocol will enable the contribution of pre-existing CR in determining if CR increases following education intervention and whether CR is related to eventual outcome for the participants in the study.

As the THBP is in the initial phases, there are few results available. However, preliminary results are available on a subset of 99 participants (80 experimental, 19 control) who have completed baseline testing and the first annual assessment. These results indicate that both groups displayed an increase in CR; however, the magnitude of the increase in CR is significantly higher in the experimental than the control group. The increase in the control group most likely represents a practice effect observed commonly in test-retest trials. The greater increase in CR in the experimental group compared with the control group suggests that the increase in CR in the experimental group is significantly greater than that seen due to practice effects (Summers et al 2012). However, these remain preliminary results on a subset of the complete sample in the study; further results will become available over the ensuing five years.

Variability between individuals in their response to non-pharmacological interventions may reflect inter-individual differences in cognitive reserve or the influence of prior life experience (education, occupation, etc.) on the level of cognitive performance displayed by an individual.

THE ACTIVE STUDY

The ACTIVE study is a large-scale study in the United States examining the potential benefit of cognitive training in healthy older adults (Willis et al 2006). The ACTIVE study is a randomised controlled trial of 2832 adults aged on average 73 years who were living independently in the community. The study design involved three different treatment groups and a non-intervention control group. Treatment options were reasoning training, memory training or processing speed training. For each treatment option there were 10 treatment sessions, each session lasting 60–75 minutes in duration (Willis et al 2006). Participants were also provided with booster sessions at 11 and 35 months following initial training. The results of the study indicate that participants in all three treatment groups displayed an increase in objectively assessed cognitive functions evident immediately following the treatment protocol (Willis et al 2006). Further, the improvement in function was maintained in all three treatment groups when they were reassessed five years later (Willis et al 2006).

The ACTIVE study demonstrated that in community-residing older adults the provision of cognitive training increased the cognitive ability of these adults for up to five years following the cognitive training.

THE ACE STUDY

A recent study undertaken at the University of Tasmania is the *Active Cognitive Enhancement* study (ACE study). The ACE study is a multi-domain cognitive training program targeting age-related cognitive decline in healthy older adults residing in the community (Summers et al 2010). The ACE study employs a waitlist treatment crossover design in which half of the participants undertake the intervention, while the remainder act as a control group and undertake the treatment protocol after the first group has completed the treatment. The treatment program consists of two-hour weekly group training sessions for a period of 10 weeks. Each treatment group is led by a treatment facilitator through activities targeting visual and verbal memory, attention, concentration, information processing speed and problem solving. Initial results from 117 participants who had completed the ACE training program indicated that significant improvements were observed on objective measures of visual learning, visual memory, attention, working memory and executive functions (Summers et al 2010). Recently reported results of the three-, six- and 12-month follow-up testing of 315 participants (253 experimental, 62 controls) indicated that performance enhancement following the ACE intervention varied according to premorbid cognitive level. Specifically, participants who displayed the highest improvement in objective memory performance were those who were older males, less educated and with lower premorbid intellectual capacity (Wolf et al 2012). These results suggest that cognitive training programs may have differential effects, with greatest effects seen in those with premorbid lower cognitive function and lower levels of education, whereas for those with higher levels of education or intellectual ability there is little benefit from cognitive training (Wolf et al 2012).

> The ACE study demonstrated that in community residing older adults the provision of cognitive training increased cognitive functions in adults with lower levels of education, but had minimal effect on those adults with higher levels of prior education. These results suggest that the potential benefit of cognitive training in older adults may be mediated by an individual's level of cognitive reserve.

COGNITIVE TRAINING IN MILD COGNITIVE IMPAIRMENT

Recently a group of researchers in Melbourne have examined the ability for memory training strategies targeting prospective memory to improve memory performance in adults with aMCI (Kinsella et al 2009, 2012). Prospective memory refers to memory for future events and intentions, differentiating it from episodic memory, which refers to memory for past events and information—the basis for the classification of aMCI. In the initial study, Kinsella et al (2009) report randomly assigning a sample of 54 participants with aMCI to treatment and waitlist treatment groups. The treatment program involved a five-week program of five weekly 90-minute sessions. Treatment sessions involved information on memory processes as well as training in the use of various memory strategies including external memory aids (Kinsella et al 2009). The results of the study indicate that the treatment group displayed improved prospective memory performance at follow-up assessments conducted two weeks and four months following completion of the treatment protocol

(Kinsella et al 2009). Despite this improvement on objective measures of prospective memory, there was no improvement detected on subjective measures of memory (Kinsella et al 2009).

Recently, Kinsella et al (2012) reported the results of a larger scale treatment program for prospective memory in MCI participants, the LaTCH Memory Group Program. In a randomised controlled trial of 220 adults diagnosed as either aMCI or healthy older controls, participants were allocated to early or late treatment groups. Treatment involved the use of memory groups to provide information on the use of compensatory memory strategies. The results of the study indicate that both the aMCI and healthy controls displayed a significant increase in subjective measures of memory function, such as satisfaction with memory ability (Kinsella et al 2012). However, in contrast to the 2009 study, there was no evidence of a significant change to performance on objective measures of episodic memory in either group. This indicates that the intervention did not improve episodic memory performance, the defining feature of aMCI (Kinsella et al 2012).

 A key advantage to non-pharmacological treatments is the absence of adverse physiological side effects that are common in pharmacological approaches.

THE IMPORTANCE OF EARLY DIAGNOSIS OF DEMENTIA

TREATMENT OPTIONS

A diagnosis of dementia is required in order to access medications under the Pharmaceuticals Benefit Scheme (PBS). There are two broad groups of medication available for symptom relief in Alzheimer's dementia: cholinergic treatments and memantine. Cholinergic treatments typically involve using anticholinesterase inhibitors, which inhibit the activity of the synaptic enzyme anticholinesterase, resulting in increased availability of the neurotransmitter acetylcholine in the synapse. Memantine blocks another neurotransmitter, glutamate, resulting in a reduction in the level of calcium moving into neurons reducing the rate of neuronal damage (Crouch 2009).

Anticholinesterase inhibitors are available for use with early-stage AD and are subsidised under the PBS for confirmed diagnoses of early stage AD. Further, if there is evidence of improved cognitive function in the first six months of treatment, the person is then able to access further PBS-subsidised supplies of medication. Memantine is only approved for use in people with moderately severe to severe AD and is subsidised under the PBS for those people who meet specific criteria for disease severity (Le Couteur et al 2011).

It is important to note that existing medications do not alter the pathology of AD but can be used only to improve symptoms. A review of 13 randomised, placebo-controlled, double-blind trials of anticholinesterase inhibitors indicated that those with mild, moderate or severe AD treated for six to 12 months show an improvement in cognitive function of 2.7 points on the ADAS-Cog (Birks 2006). However, these treatment effects are not large, nor are there studies of treatment efficacy beyond 12 months. Further, improvement in symptoms was only seen in 7% of those treated, with 17% improving without medication and 76% worsening even when taking anticholinesterase inhibitors (Birks 2006). Finally, up to 50% of trial participants ceased taking anticholinesterase inhibitors due to adverse side effects (Birks 2006). Memantine, when given to patients with moderate to severe AD for six months, resulted in a 3% increase on a cognitive test score but only a 1% increase when used in mild–moderate AD (McShane et al 2009). Reports indicate that up to 12% of patients cease using memantine due to adverse side effects (McShane et al 2009).

It is imperative to note that at best medications such as anticholinesterase inhibitors and memantine offer temporary symptom relief. Further, this symptom relief is observed in a minority of people, with the majority displaying progressive cognitive decline despite receiving the medication. These drugs do not treat dementia, with AD remaining a terminal disease.

QUALITY-OF-LIFE ISSUES

Early diagnosis of AD is vital in ensuring quality of life for the person. Accurate early diagnosis empowers the person with dementia to participate in the process of decision making for future care planning before disease progression robs them of insight and the capacity to make reasoned and informed decisions. Such empowerment is seen in those with other forms of terminal illness (e.g. cancer). Knowledge that one has a terminal illness enables the person to grieve for the forthcoming loss and to be actively involved in making decisions regarding future care and end-of-life planning. A clear early diagnosis can assist the person with dementia to make decisions regarding accommodation needs as well as identifying critical points during the development and progression of dementia, such as when a power of attorney may be required or when a legally appointed administrator/guardian may be appointed. For the caregiver/family, prior knowledge of the wishes of the sufferer can reduce the emotional burden felt when decision points for transitions in level of care are reached. End-of-life planning for the individual with dementia can be facilitated by a suitably experienced neuropsychologist or health professional and should be considered to be a form of palliative care for the person with dementia.

CONCLUSION

Progressive dementias such as AD are terminal illnesses. Despite decades of research the underlying cause of AD remains unknown, although the pathological processes involved in the neurodegeneration of Alzheimer's disease are well described. In the absence of knowledge of the underlying cause of dementia, effective treatments that treat or cure dementia remain unknown. Existing pharmacological therapies at best slow disease progression, but dementia remains insidiously progressive and ultimately terminal.

Consequently, accurate early diagnosis is essential to maximise quality of life for the person with dementia and to empower them in end-of-life planning. Non-pharmacological therapies offer some hope in delaying the time of onset of dementia and may assist in preventing dementia in some, although further research is required to determine treatment efficacy.

Neuropsychological assessments provide accurate early diagnosis of the various subtypes of dementia as well as the capacity to differentially diagnose dementia from other non-dementing conditions in the older person such as delirium and depression. Neuropsychologists are able to provide compassionate and informed diagnoses to people with dementia and can be critical in assisting the individual with end-of-life planning.

Reflective questions

1. Early diagnosis can lead to a positive experience of end-of-life planning, with the person with dementia actively involved in the decision making and planning. However, some will express a desire for active euthanasia. What are the ethical and legal issues that arise when a patient with an early diagnosis of dementia expresses a plan for 'assisted suicide'?

2. With the rapidly ageing population of Australia, how well placed is the healthcare system to provide appropriate care and support for dementia?

3. In your profession, consider the potential benefit of early diagnosis of dementia in terms of care and management.

4. If you reconsider dementia as a terminal illness, how does your professional practice change when working with people with dementia and their carers/families?

References

Access Economics, 2004. Delaying the onset of Alzheimer's disease: projections and issues. Report for Alzheimer's Australia 1–15.

Access Economics, 2009. Keeping dementia front of mind: incidence and prevalence 2009-2050. Final Report for Alzheimer's Australia 1–109.

Albert, M.S., DeKosky, S.T., Dickson, D., et al., 2011. The diagnosis of mild cognitive impairment due to Alzheimer's disease: recommendations from the National Institute on Aging-Alzheimer's Association workgroups on diagnostic guidelines for Alzheimer's disease. Alzheimer's & Dementia 7, 270–279.

Alladi, S., Arnold, R., Mitchell, J., et al., 2006. Mild cognitive impairment: applicability of research criteria in a memory clinic and characterisation of cognitive profile. Psychological Medicine 36, 507–515.

Alzheimer's Association, 2009. 2009 Alzheimer's disease facts and figures. Alzheimer's & Dementia 5, 234–270.

Beason-Held, L.L., Kraut, M.A., Resnick, S.M., 2008. I. Longitudinal changes in aging brain function. Neurobiology of Aging 29, 483–496.

Bennett, D.A., Schneider, J.A., Tang, Y.X., et al., 2006. The effect of social networks on the relation between Alzheimer's disease pathology and level of cognitive function in old people: A longitudinal cohort study. Lancet Neurology 5, 406–412.

Bennett, D.A., Wilson, R.S., Schneider, J.A., et al., 2003. Education modifies the relation of AD pathology to level of cognitive function in older persons. Neurology 60, 1909–1915.

Birks, J., 2006. Cholinesterase inhibitors for Alzheimer's disease. Cochrane Database Syst Rev Jan 25: CD005593.

Bisiacchi, P.S., Borella, E., Bergamaschi, S., et al., 2008. Interplay between memory and executive functions in normal and pathological aging. Journal of Clinical and Experimental Neuropsychology 30, 723–733.

Comijs, H.C., Dik, M.G., Deeg, D.J.H., et al., 2004. The course of cognitive decline in older persons: results from the Longitudinal Aging Study Amsterdam. Dementia and Geriatric Cognitive Disorders 17, 136–142.

Crouch, A.M., 2009. Treating dementia. Australian Prescriber 32, 9–12.

Deloitte Access Economics, 2011. Dementia across Australia: 2011-2015, report prepared by Deloitte Access Economics. 15.

Fischer, P., Jungwirth, S., Zehetmayer, S., et al., 2007. Conversion from subtypes of mild cognitive impairment to Alzheimer dementia. Neurology 68, 288–291.

Ganguli, M., Dodge, H.H., Shen, C.Y., et al., 2004. Mild cognitive impairment, amnestic type: an epidemiologic study. Neurology 63, 115–121.

Garibotto, V., Borroni, B., Kalbe, E., et al., 2008. Education and occupation as proxies for reserve in aMCI converters and AD: FDG-PET evidence. Neurology 71, 1342–1349.

Gauthier, S., Touchon, J., 2005. Mild cognitive impairment is not a clinical entity and should not be treated. Archives of Neurology 62, 1164–1166.

Grossman, M., 2002. Frontotemporal dementia: a review. Journal of the International Neuropsychological Society 8, 566–583.

Johnson, D.K., Storandt, M., Morris, J.C., et al., 2009. Longitudinal study of the transition from healthy aging to Alzheimer disease. Archives of Neurology 66, 1254–1259.

Kinsella, G.J., Ames, D., Storey, E., et al., 2012. Knowledge-transfer following cognitive intervention for amnestic mild cognitive impairment. Alzheimer's & Dementia 8, 235.

Kinsella, G.J., Mullaly, E., Rand, E., et al., 2009. Early intervention for mild cognitive impairment: a randomised controlled trial. Journal of Neurology, Neurosurgery & Psychiatry 80, 730–736.

Larrieu, A., Letenneur, L., Orgogozo, J.M., et al., 2002. Incidence and outcome of mild cognitive impairment in a population based prospective cohort. Neurology 59, 1594–1599.

Le Couteur, D.G., Robinson, M., Leverton, A., et al., 2011. Adherence, persistence and continuation with cholinesterase inhibitors in Alzheimer's disease. Australasian Journal on Ageing: doi: 10.1111/j.741-6612.2011.00564.x.

Lezak, M.D., Howieson, D.B., Bigler, E.D., et al., 2012. Neuropsychological assessment, fifth ed. Oxford University Press, Oxford.

Machado, J.C., Caramelli, P., 2006. Treatment of dementia: anything new? Current Opinion in Psychiatry 19, 575–580.

McKhann, G.M., Drachman, D., Folstein, M., et al., 1984. Clinical diagnosis of Alzheimer's disease: report of the NINCDS-ADRDA work group under the auspices of Department of Health and Human Services Task Force on Alzheimer's disease. Neurology 34, 939–944.

McKhann, G.M., Knopman, D.S., Chertkow, H., et al., 2011. The diagnosis of dementia due to Alzheimer's disease: recommendations from the National Institute on Aging-Alzheimer's Association workgroups on diagnostic guidelines for Alzheimer's disease. Alzheimer's & Dementia 7, 263–269.

McShane, R., Areosa, S.A., Minakaran, N., 2009. Memantine for dementia. Cochrane Database Syst Rev 21 Jan.

Mitchell, A.J., Shiri-Feshki, M., 2009. Rate of progression of mild cognitive impairment to dementia—meta-analysis of 41 robust inception cohort studies. Acta Psychiatrica Scandinavica 119, 252–265.

Morris, J.C., Storandt, M., Miller, J.P., et al., 2001. Mild cognitive impairment represents early-stage Alzheimer disease. Archives of Neurology 58, 397–405.

Mortimer, J.A., Snowdon, D.A., Markesbery, W.R., 2003. Head circumference, education and risk of dementia: findings from the Nun study. Journal of Clinical and Experimental Neuropsychology 25, 671–679.

Palmer, K., Wang, H.X., Bäckman, L., et al., 2002. Differential evolution of cognitive impairment in nondemented older persons: results from the Kungsholmen project. American Journal of Psychiatry 159, 436–442.

Petersen, R.C., 2004. Mild cognitive impairment as a diagnostic entity. Journal of Internal Medicine 256, 183–194.

Petersen, R.C., Doody, R., Kurz, A., et al., 2001. Current concepts in mild cognitive impairment. Archives of Neurology 58, 1985–1992.

Petersen, R.C., Smith, G.E., Waring, S.C., et al., 1997. Aging, memory and mild cognitive impairment. International Psychogeriatrics 9, 65–69.

Petersen, R.C., Smith, G.E., Waring, S.C., et al., 1999. Mild cognitive impairment: clinical characterization and outcome. Archives of Neurology 56, 303–308.

Rasquin, S.M.C., Lodder, J., Visser, P.J., et al., 2005. Predictive accuracy of MCI subtypes for Alzheimer's disease and vascular dementia in subjects with mild cognitive impairment: a 2-year follow-up study. Dementia and Geriatric Cognitive Disorders 19, 113–118.

Ravaglia, G., Forti, P., Maioli, F., et al., 2006. Conversion of mild cognitive impairment to dementia: predictive role of mild cognitive impairment subtypes and vascular risk factors. Dementia and Geriatric Cognitive Disorders 21, 51–58.

Richards, M., Sacker, A., 2003. Lifetime antecedents of cognitive reserve. Journal of Clinical and Experimental Neuropsychology 25, 614–624.

Ritchie, K., Artero, S., Touchon, J., 2001. Classification criteria for mild cognitive impairment: a population-based validation study. Neurology 56, 37–42.

Roe, C.M., Xiong, C.J., Miller, J.P., et al., 2007. Education and Alzheimer disease without dementia: support for the cognitive reserve hypothesis. Neurology 68, 223–228.

Rountree, S.D., Waring, S.C., Chan, W.C., et al., 2007. Importance of subtle amnestic and nonamnestic deficits in mild cognitive impairment: prognosis and conversion to dementia. Dementia and Geriatric Cognitive Disorders 24, 476–482.

Salthouse, T.A., Fristoe, B.N., Rhee, S.H., 1996. How localized are age-related effects on neuropsychological measures? Neuropsychology 10, 272–285.

Saunders, N.L.J., Summers, M.J., 2010. Attention and working memory deficits in mild cognitive impairment. Journal of Clinical and Experimental Neuropsychology 32, 350–357.

Schneider, J.A.M.D., Arvanitakis, Z.M.D., Bang, W.M.S., et al., 2007. Mixed brain pathologies account for most dementia cases in community-dwelling older persons. Neurology 69, 2197–2204.

Solfrizzi, V., Panza, F., Colacicco, A.M., et al., 2004. Vascular risk factors, incidence of MCI and rates of progression to dementia. Neurology 63, 1882–1891.

Stern, Y., 2002. What is cognitive reserve? Theory and research application of the reserve concept. Journal of the International Neuropsychological Society 8, 448–460.

Stern, Y., 2009. Cognitive reserve. Neuropsychologia 47, 2015–2128.

Storandt, M., Grant, E.A., Miller, J.P., et al., 2006. Longitudinal course and neuropathologic outcomes in original vs revised MCI and in pre-MCI. Neurology 67, 467–473.

Summers, J.J., Wolf, A., Elder, S., et al., 2010. Cognitive training in older adults. Alzheimer's & Dementia 6, S163–S164.

Summers, M.J., Saunders, N.L.J., 2012. Neuropsychological measures predict decline to Alzheimer's dementia from mild cognitive impairment. Neuropsychology 26, 498–508.

Summers, M.J., Valenzuela, M.J., Summers, J.J., et al., 2012. The Tasmanian Healthy Brain Study (THBS): does late-life education prevent age-related decline and dementia? Alzheimer's & Dementia 8, 147.

Tabert, M.H., Manly, J.J., Liu, X.H., et al., 2006. Neuropsychological prediction of conversion to Alzheimer disease in patients with mild cognitive impairment. Archives of General Psychiatry 63, 916–924.

Wahlund, L.-O., Pihlstrand, E., Jonhagen, M.E., 2003. Mild cognitive impairment: experience from a memory clinic. Acta Neurologica Scandinavica 107, 21–24.

Willis, S.L., Tennstedt, S.L., Marsiske, M., et al., 2006. Long-term effects of cognitive training on everyday functional outcomes in older adults. Journal of the American Medical Association 296, 2805–2814.

Wilson, R.S., Scherr, P.A., Schneider, J.A., et al., 2007. Relation of cognitive activity to risk of developing Alzheimer disease. Neurology 69, 1911–1920.

Winblad, B., Palmer, K., Kivipelto, M., et al., 2004. Mild cognitive impairment – beyond controversies, towards a consensus: report of the International Working Group on Mild Cognitive Impairment. Journal of Internal Medicine 256, 240–246.

Wolf, A., Gomez, R., Summers, M.J., et al., 2012. Verbal memory performance in healthy older adults: predicting inter-individual differences in cognitive training outcomes. Alzheimer's & Dementia 8, 385.

CHAPTER 14

DEPRESSION AND SUICIDE IN OLDER PEOPLE

Christine Neville and Gerard Byrne

Editors' comments

The significance of depression in older people cannot be overstated; normally we would argue too many drugs are prescribed to older people but in the case of depression it is the opposite. A frail, quiet person can be seen as the 'perfect patient' when in fact they are experiencing a major depression that has been ignored because the person is not disruptive. Antidepressants could in such cases prevent suicide and certainly improve quality of life. Links between depression and dementia are highlighted as is the tendency of older people to deny their depression because it was stigmatised by their parents and cohort.

INTRODUCTION

Depression and suicide are two closely linked and pertinent clinical issues in older people. Depression is the leading mental illness to affect older people and it is the major risk factor for suicide. In Australia and many other developed countries, older men have a higher rate of completed suicide than any other age and gender group. This chapter examines recent developments in managing depression and suicide in older people and discusses some of the more controversial aspects of this topic.

DEPRESSION

EPIDEMIOLOGY

Although there are quite a number of different types of depression recognised in nosologies such as the American Psychiatric Association's (2013) *Diagnostic and Statistical Manual of Mental Disorders*, 5th edition (DSM-5), the archetypal depressive illness is the one referred to as 'major depression'. It is this type of clinically significant depression that will be emphasised in this chapter. However, it is worth noting that chronic low-grade depression is referred to as dysthymia; depressive reactions to adverse life events that do not meet diagnostic criteria for major depression are referred to as 'adjustment disorders with depressed mood'. However, it is critical to appreciate that major depression remains major depression, regardless of whether it has occurred in the context of an adverse life event.

The prevalence of major depression in older people is the subject of some dispute (O'Connor 2006). In particular, there is a debate about whether its prevalence actually declines with age as indicated by large-scale epidemiological studies. Many of these studies systematically excluded people who were not living at home at the time of the survey. So older people living in hostels, nursing homes and hospitals were generally not counted. We know that the prevalence of depression in these settings is much higher than in the general community, so it is likely that population studies that are based on household surveys have systematically underestimated the number of older people with depression. In addition, the survey instruments commonly used to generate diagnoses of depression, such as the Diagnostic Interview Schedule (DIS) or the Composite International Diagnostic Interview (CIDI), usually exclude symptoms that might be due to general medical conditions. This is not such a problem in young and middle-aged populations but in older people may have the effect of under-counting symptoms of depression, as older people have a much higher prevalence of general medical problems.

The 2007 Australian National Survey of Mental Health and Wellbeing (Slade et al 2009) found that 1.9% of men and 2.9% of women aged 65 years and over living in the community met diagnostic criteria for major depressive disorder within the previous 12 months. However, this survey did not include older people in residential aged care settings and it is now well established that between 5% and 25% of older people living in aged nursing homes have a major depression (Seitz et al 2010). The prevalence of depression in older people receiving domiciliary nursing care and in older hospital inpatients is reported to be even higher. In an American study (Steffens et al 2000) that surveyed community and institutionalised older people in Cache County, Utah, the point prevalence of major depression was 2.7% in men and 4.4% in women, and the estimated lifetime prevalence of depression was 9.6% in men and 20.4% in women.

RISK FACTORS

Risk factors for developing a depressive disorder include the following:
- family history of mood disorder (particularly for early-onset depression)
- personality factors (particularly trait neuroticism)
- history of childhood physical, emotional or sexual abuse
- recent bereavement or other loss events
- stroke and acute myocardial infarction

- prescribed medications (e.g. steroids, interferon, gonadotropin-releasing hormone (GnRH) agonists, reserpine, propranolol, alpha methyldopa, levodopa and some chemotherapy agents).

CLINICAL FEATURES

Depression in older people may present in several different ways and it is important to appreciate that many depressed older people will deny feeling depressed, even when asked directly. A diagnosis of depression is made by a trained clinician on the basis of the symptoms and signs exhibited by the person and in the absence of alternative explanations for those symptoms and signs. An appropriate work-up for a first episode of depression in an older person includes detailed history-taking from the person, mental state examination, physical examination, laboratory tests and, where relevant, a brain scan. In many cases it is also appropriate to obtain further history from an informant, such as a family member or a friend. This is particularly important if the older person is thought to have cognitive impairment.

Many depressed older people will deny feeling depressed, even when asked directly.

By definition, major depression is characterised by either depressed or irritable mood, or by a loss of interest and pleasure in usual activities, or by both. In addition, older people may have a number of other symptoms that involve their thought content, neurovegetative function or behaviour. Thought content symptoms include thoughts of guilt or hopelessness and thoughts of suicide. Neurovegetative symptoms include abnormalities of sleep, appetite and energy. Behavioural symptoms include psychomotor agitation or retardation. Crying tends to be uncommon in major depression, although displays of exaggerated distress in relation to the vicissitudes of life or exaggerated sadness in relation to real or perceived evils of the world, are common. Some older depressed people adopt a type of importuning behaviour that might lead the clinician to the incorrect conclusion that they have serious personality difficulties. Some older people experience and report the distress associated with their depression in the form of somatic symptoms such as headache, dizziness, chest pain or shortness of breath. It is not uncommon for older depressed people to display socially sanctioned smiling when engaged in interviews with health workers. Such superficial smiling has given rise to the term 'smiling depression'.

Some people experience a single episode of depression and make a complete recovery, whereas others experience a remitting and relapsing course. In later life it is useful to divide depression according to the age of onset of the first episode. Most depression has its onset in young and middle-aged people and such individuals often go on to experience further episodes in later life. However, some people experience their first episode of depression in later life. This late-onset depression is often a harbinger of cognitive decline and later dementia or occurs in the context of a general medical problem, or one of the other vicissitudes of later life.

Late-onset depression is often a harbinger of cognitive decline and later dementia.

COMORBIDITY

Major depressive episodes in older people are commonly associated with other comorbid disorders, the more common of which are the following:

- anxiety disorders, particularly generalised anxiety disorder (GAD)
- mild cognitive impairment and dementia
- alcohol abuse and dependence
- sedative or analgesic abuse and dependence
- general medical conditions including heart attack, stroke and cancer.

DIFFERENTIAL DIAGNOSIS

It is important to avoid the tendency to reduce most human misery to the notion of 'depression' and, in so doing, to fail to appreciate that there are many things that may superficially resemble depression but require a different interpretation and response.

Avoid the tendency to reduce most human misery to the notion of 'depression'.

In older people it is particularly important to distinguish depression from grief and demoralisation (Clarke & Kissane 2002). Grief is a normal human response to loss and is a very common experience among older people (Byrne & Raphael 1997). Symptoms of grief include crying, thoughts about the deceased, insomnia, a sense of presence of the deceased, hallucinations of the deceased and thoughts of death. Although the manifestations of grief vary considerably between cultures, grief tends to come in waves—the so-called 'pangs' of grief—and generally settles spontaneously with the passage of time and without treatment. Grief may be pathologically severe or prolonged in cases where the death was traumatic or unexpected, or in cases where the attachment was ambivalent. Grief counselling may be warranted in such cases. In Western culture, at least, grief is associated with considerable tearfulness, whereas depression is often associated with an inability to cry. One implication of this is that it is important to allow people to grieve in their own culturally appropriate way, and to avoid medicalising a common, normal phenomenon. However, in a minority of cases grief is complicated by depression and this depression requires treatment in the usual manner. Depression complicating grief may be associated with pervasive anhedonia or the development of suicidal intent.

Demoralisation is a common consequence of adversity, particularly where this is prolonged. Many older people with chronic medical conditions or chronic disability following acute medical conditions such as a heart attack or stroke develop demoralisation. This is not the same as depression. Treatment of demoralisation requires a different approach (see Clarke & Kissane 2002).

It is also important to distinguish depression from delirium, dementia and sedative drug-induced states. Delirium is a clinical chameleon and often mimics depression. Dementia is frequently complicated by depression and is often preceded by depression. Drug-induced sedation in older people often leads to psychomotor slowing that can be confused with depression.

It is also important to distinguish depression from delirium, dementia and sedative drug-induced states.

Emotionalism (pathological crying or laughing) associated with stroke and other manifestations of cerebrovascular disease, including subcortical vascular damage, can sometimes be mistaken for depression. Assessment in the context of stroke can be challenging and often calls for expert opinion. Curiously, both emotionalism and depression respond to treatment with antidepressant medication.

Parkinson's disease is often associated with a paucity of movement (bradykinesia) and with a reduction in facial expression. These clinical features can easily be mistaken for depression. However, Parkinson's disease is also commonly associated with depression.

OTHER ASSESSMENT ISSUES

Given the high rate of suicide associated with depression it is essential that all older people with depression have a risk assessment undertaken by a well-trained health worker. This is discussed in detail in the second half of this chapter. Some older people with depression stop eating and drinking and this can be dangerous, particularly if they live in a socially isolated situation or if they live in a harsh climate.

About 10% of people with severe depression develop psychotic symptoms including delusions and hallucinations. Often these psychotic symptoms are mood-congruent and take on depressive themes. Common themes include those of guilt, poverty and hypochondriasis.

PSYCHOLOGICAL TREATMENTS

The main evidence-based psychological treatments used in depression are cognitive behaviour therapy (CBT) and interpersonal psychotherapy (IPT). A number of other psychological treatment approaches, including problem-solving therapy (PST) and acceptance and commitment therapy (ACT), are associated with increasing levels of empirical evidence. Although most clinical trials of CBT and IPT have been conducted in young and middle-aged people, there is a growing body of evidence that suggests that these treatments are also effective in older people (Laidlaw et al 2003). In the oldest of the old it is necessary to modify the application of the standard techniques used in these treatments. For instance, it is often necessary to increase the number of sessions and decrease the homework requirements. Sensory impairment (vision and hearing) and cognitive impairment are both significant challenges to psychological treatment. Although CBT and IPT have traditionally been administered by clinical psychologists or psychiatrists, they can be administered by trained therapists from any disciplinary background.

A recent systematic review has suggested that behaviour therapy might be as effective as CBT in treating depression (Ekers et al 2008). If this is confirmed, it is likely to be very important for managing depression in older people. Pleasant events, scheduling physical activity, exposure techniques and other behaviour therapy interventions are often easier to implement in older people than formal CBT.

 A recent systematic review has suggested that behaviour therapy might be as effective as cognitive behaviour therapy in treating depression.

DRUG TREATMENTS

A variety of antidepressant medications are now available to treat depression. The use of antidepressant medication is usually essential for treating severe depression and is often needed for treating moderate depression. In most people the combination of antidepressant medication and a psychological treatment works better than either alone. In many cases of mild depression and some cases of moderate depression psychological treatments may be used alone.

The 'number needed to treat' for most modern antidepressants lies between three and five. In other words, one person with depression will respond to pharmacological treatment for every three to five people treated. That does not mean that only one in three to five people will get better, but it does mean that only one in three to five gets better due to the antidepressant. The usual response rate in antidepressant trials is about 60%, of which about 35% is due to the placebo effect and about 25% is due to the effect of the drug.

What this means is that it is often necessary to trial more than one antidepressant before finding one that works in a particular person. Often it is prudent to use an antidepressant that has worked previously in the person or in a first-degree relative.

Although early clinical trials suggested that antidepressant medications worked in major depression occurring in the context of Alzheimer's disease, more recent evidence (Banerjee et al 2011) suggests that this is not the case. Fortunately, major depression occurring in the context of other general medical problems, such as heart attack and stroke, does respond to treatment and such treatment is also associated with a better outcome from the general medical condition.

In older people, the usual initial doses of antidepressants are reduced and doses are increased more slowly than in young or middle-aged people. Certain adverse effects are more common in older people, including postural hypotension (low blood pressure on standing) and hyponatraemia (low serum sodium).

Older antidepressants

The original antidepressants are still in use, particularly in older people, and so will be discussed briefly here. The tricyclic antidepressants (TCAs), so named because of their characteristic three-ring chemical structure, were introduced in the 1950s and proved to be highly effective. Examples include amitriptyline, imipramine and clomipramine. However, nortriptyline is considered to have the best adverse effect profile and is the preferred tricyclic antidepressant today. The TCAs are thought to work by blocking the reuptake of both noradrenaline and serotonin at central nervous system (CNS) synapses. By this mechanism, they increase the availability of these two neurotransmitters and lead to down-regulation of noradrenergic and serotonergic receptors. All tricyclic antidepressants have significant side effects, which limit their use and increase the risk of death by overdose. The main side effects are dry mouth, blurred vision, postural hypotension, constipation, urinary hesitancy (especially in older males), sedation and weight gain.

 All tricyclic antidepressants have significant side effects, which limit their use and increase the risk of death by overdose.

Around the same time, the monoamine oxidase inhibitors (MAOIs) were introduced. Examples include phenelzine and tranylcypromine. These drugs irreversibly block the monoamine oxidase A and B enzymes and increase levels of the monoamine neurotransmitters serotonin, noradrenaline and dopamine. The person must be on a special tyramine-free diet to avoid dangerously high blood pressure. The MAOIs also have a similar side effect profile to the TCAs. They are no longer commonly used. In the 1980s a new MAOI was produced, moclobemide. This drug is a selective, reversible inhibitor of monoamine oxidase A and does not require a tyramine-free diet.

A drug called mianserin was also introduced in the 1980s. This drug has a four-ring structure and so is referred to as a tetracyclic. It is less toxic than the TCAs and old-style MAOIs, although does cause postural hypotension and sedation at higher doses. It is now only rarely used in older people.

Newer antidepressants

In the late 1980s and early 1990s a series of antidepressant drugs belonging to a new class were introduced. These are called the selective serotonin reuptake inhibitors (SSRIs), the name reflecting their mode of action. These drugs increase the availability of the neurotransmitter serotonin at central synapses. The first drug in this class was fluoxetine and its original trade name was Prozac. Fluoxetine was immediately popular, particularly among women, because it was not sedating and did not cause weight gain (in fact weight loss was common). It was soon used widely in older people because of its safer side effect profile. Although it did cause nausea, insomnia and agitation, it did not cause postural hypotension or any of the anticholinergic side effects of the

TCAs (blurred vision, dry mouth, constipation and urinary hesitancy). Subsequently, another five SSRIs were marketed. In addition to fluoxetine, we now have sertraline, citalopram, escitalopram, fluvoxamine and paroxetine. Of these five SSRI antidepressants, sertraline is most suitable for use in older people. Citalopram and escitalopram are also commonly used in older people, although their dose should be limited to avoid rare cardiac adverse effects. Fluvoxamine also has a place in older people with agitated depression because it is somewhat sedating, although it does have drug-drug interactions. Paroxetine should be rarely used in older people because it has more anticholinergic side effects than the other SSRIs.

Since the advent of the SSRI antidepressants, several newer drugs have been marketed. These newer drugs have more complicated methods of action. Venlafaxine and desvenlafaxine are serotonin and noradrenaline reuptake inhibitors (SNRIs), mirtazapine and duloxetine have complex modes of action, and reboxetine is a selective noradrenaline reuptake inhibitor. A novel antidepressant that works on both the serotonergic and melatonergic systems, agomelatine, has recently been marketed. Although these drugs are used as first-line agents in certain situations, they are more often reserved for people who have not responded to an SSRI.

The major limitations in using antidepressant medications, other than relatively modest efficacy, are adverse effects and adherence. Many people experience adverse effects, even with the modern drugs that have improved tolerability profiles. With the SSRI medications, people commonly experience nausea and insomnia. Initial agitation is also not uncommon. In older people, these drugs sometimes cause hyponatraemia (low serum sodium concentration), which often mimics worsening depression and may sometimes be life-threatening.

 In older people, these drugs sometimes cause hyponatraemia (low serum sodium concentration), which often mimics worsening depression and may sometimes be life-threatening.

Fortunately, the modern antidepressant medications are generally safe in overdose, unless combined with other drugs. Unlike the case in adolescents, there is no evidence of an increased risk of suicide in the first few days or weeks of treatment with modern antidepressant drugs in older people. Antidepressant drugs are not habit-forming or addictive, although some people may experience mild withdrawal symptoms, particularly if a substantial regular dose is suddenly ceased. It is not usually necessary to use more than one antidepressant at a time, and there is little scientific evidence in support of this practice.

Other treatments

Antipsychotic drugs are used in combination with antidepressants in older people with psychotic depression. The antipsychotic drug most commonly used in older people is risperidone, usually in low dose. Mood stabilisers such as lithium, valproate and carbamazepine, which are commonly used to treat bipolar disorder, are sometimes also used to augment the effect of antidepressants in the treatment of severe depression or in the prevention of relapses of depression in people in remission. Although lithium is an excellent mood stabiliser, it is excreted exclusively via the kidneys and significant renal impairment may make lithium treatment dangerous. Older people in warmer climates might also be prone to dehydration, which adds to the risk of lithium. If lithium is used, regular blood tests to check the serum lithium level need to be arranged. Carbamazepine has a tendency to interact with other drugs, making valproate the most useful mood stabiliser in older people with renal impairment.

Antipsychotic drugs are used in combination with antidepressants in older people with psychotic depression.

Electroconvulsive therapy (ECT) is a treatment for severe, life-threatening depression or depression that has not responded to conventional treatments. The person is given a short general anaesthetic and then an electric current is applied to their scalp, usually to the non-dominant hemisphere. The electric current induces a grand mal seizure that is highly modified by the general anaesthetic. The precise mode of action of ECT is unknown, although it may work by causing the liberation of monoamine neurotransmitters in the brain. ECT is particularly useful in older people who are unable to tolerate, or who do not respond to, treatment with antidepressant medication.

In people with depression as part of seasonal affective disorder (SAD), bright light has been used successfully as a method of resetting the circadian rhythm (including the sleep–wake cycle) and has contributed to the resolution of depression. Most of this work has been done in colder climates and in young and middle-aged people. The effects of bright light seem to be short-lived. Aerobic exercise and weight training have both been demonstrated, in randomised controlled trials, to be effective treatments for people living in the community with mild to moderate depression without melancholic, psychotic or suicidal features. In contemporary practice, psychiatrists often recommend daily morning exercise outside in an attempt to boost the effect of conventional drug and psychological treatment for depression.

Thyroid hormone, psychostimulants such as dexamphetamine and methylphenidate, and complementary therapies such as St John's wort (*Hypericum perforatum*) have been used in case series and small clinical trials. Although some of the findings are promising, there is insufficient evidence to recommend their use to treat depression outside of specialised mood disorder units.

Transcranial magnetic resonance (TMR) is an experimental treatment for depression. TMR involves using a powerful electromagnetic coil to induce a small electric current in the brain. No anaesthetic is required. To date, evidence of efficacy has been mixed, and no clinical trials have demonstrated superiority to ECT. Vagal stimulation is an experimental treatment carried out by implanting a pacemaker (that is similar to a cardiac pacemaker) with leads that stimulate the vagus nerve. Case series suggest that this might be a useful treatment for some people with depression. Deep brain stimulation (DBS) using an implantable electrode has been used to treat severe, unremitting depression.

PREVENTION

The evidence base for preventing depression in older people is meagre (Byrne 1995). However, potential preventive interventions might include timely intervention in pathological grief, control of chronic pain, secondary prevention of cerebrovascular disease and relapse prevention using a combination of antidepressant medication and a psychological treatment (Reynolds et al 1999). Attention to risk factors earlier in life, including reducing the prevalence of childhood abuse and neglect, is likely to reduce the prevalence of both depression and anxiety throughout the lifecycle. It may also be important to deal with risk factors for cerebrovascular disease, including smoking, hypertension, hypercholesterolaemia, diabetes and physical inactivity.

PROGNOSIS

Although many older people who experience an episode of depression for the first time in later life respond well to treatment, some require extended treatment for many years. Around 30% of people with major depression experience chronic depression lasting at least two years (Murphy & Byrne 2012) and socioeconomic disadvantage is a risk factor for persistent depression (Almeida et al 2012a). A small number of depressed people do not get better despite intensive treatment. These people require ongoing care and support. Others exhibit a remitting and relapsing course. It is important to appreciate that depression is often a chronic condition, more like diabetes than influenza, that requires multimodal treatment on a continuing basis.

 Depression is often a chronic condition that requires multimodal treatment on a continuing basis.

SUICIDE

Suicide in older people is generally a subject not taken seriously by older people themselves, lay people and health professionals alike. These tolerant attitudes of such a tragic event may develop when a pessimistic view of old age is held. That is, old age is seen as a time of life characterised by losses (e.g. the loss of a spouse, friends, physical and mental health or meaningful employment) and being seen as a burden on society. If an older person has nothing to live for and they are near the end of their life, why bother intervening if they want to die? Of course the answer is not simple and the intention of this section is not to debate the value of older people to society, but rather to examine the issue of suicide in older people.

Old age is a known predictor of completed suicide. Suicide in older people is a complex, real and significant issue and when it is encountered by health professionals they need to be able to implement effective care. Knowledge of the spectrum of suicidal behaviours, epidemiology, methods, risk factors, management and suicide prevention in older people, as well as being cognisant of controversial issues such as medically assisted suicide, is fundamental to providing such care.

> ## Old age is a known predictor of completed suicide.

THE SPECTRUM OF SUICIDAL BEHAVIOURS

Suicidal behaviour in older people can range from thoughts of hopelessness or suicidal ideation and indirect self-destructive behaviour through to deliberate self-harm and completed suicide (Harwood 2002). Thoughts of hopelessness or suicidal ideation such as saying 'I would be better off dead' are relatively common in older people, but when pressed there is rarely an actual wish to die. More serious suicidal thoughts are usually associated with depression, physical disability, pain, sensory impairments, institutionalisation and being single. Passive, indirect self-destructive behaviours, such as refusing nourishment (with the intent of starvation) and noncompliance with medical treatments, do not necessarily have a suicidal intent, but the likelihood of dying is increased and this occurs commonly in women and the institutionalised very old. Deliberate self-harm is different from suicidal thoughts and indirect self-destructive behaviour because there is a definite and more immediate response.

EPIDEMIOLOGY

In Australia suicide rates in older people have declined substantially since the 1980s, a trend mirrored by many other developed countries (Australian Institute for Suicide Research and Prevention 2003, Kreisfeld et al 2004). Older males commit suicide at a higher rate than older females. In Australia in 2010, males over the age of 65 years had a suicide rate of 20.9 per 100,000, whereas in 1995 it was 22.7 per 100,000. Males aged over 75 years have always had a higher suicide prevalence rate than their younger counterparts; for example, in 2010, the prevalence rate per 100,000 for males aged 65–74 years was 14.5, whereas for males aged 75 years or older it was 24.6. In contrast, the suicide rates for females aged 65 years and older in Australia in 2010 was 4.6 per 100,000, which is not a great change from the 5.6 per 100,000 recorded in 1995, and there were no significant variations between the age groupings for females (Australian Bureau of Statistics 2012).

RISK FACTORS

Many of the well-identified risk factors that are associated with suicide in older people are listed below, with no single factor being totally causal (Blazer 2003, Conwell et al 2002, Draper 1996, Nowers 1993):

- being single, divorced or widowed
- lack of a confidant
- family discord
- interpersonal problems
- social isolation
- poor sleep quality
- low socioeconomic status
- physical illness (e.g. cancer [particularly the first year after diagnosis], stroke, multiple sclerosis or epilepsy)
- development of a disability
- pain
- grief, especially recent spouse bereavement
- depressive disorder
- early dementia
- prior suicide attempts
- alcohol abuse
- sedative or hypnotic abuse
- personality disorder (particularly with anxiety and anankastic traits)
- preparations for imminent death
- verbal statements (e.g. 'I want to die' or 'Life is not worth living').

Detection of risk factors in older people may differ from younger people in a number of ways, such as fewer warnings or explicit cues, particularly if the older person is socially isolated. In cases of social isolation, any risks may be unnoticed or not raised because fewer people are aware of, or interested in, the older person's wellbeing. Older people have a higher prevalence of hopelessness, comorbid depression and painful medical conditions, as well as less contact with mental health services than younger people (Levy et al 2011, Minayo & Cavalcante 2010). It has been suggested that the determination of older people to end their life is greater than for younger people, with 80% committing suicide on the first attempt (de Leo et al 2001b). Older people are also generally frailer physically and more susceptible to the effects of potentially lethal attempts.

METHODS

Males of all ages adopt more violent and lethal methods for suicide than females and this fact is thought to account for the higher rate of completed suicide in males. Hanging, shooting and carbon monoxide poisoning (car exhaust fumes) are the most common methods for older males within Australia. Older females prefer drug overdose, with paracetamol, analgesics and antidepressants being the three most frequent drug classes, followed by hanging and carbon monoxide poisoning (de Leo et al 2001b).

MANAGEMENT

As with many controversial issues that confront health workers, the individual needs to examine their own beliefs about suicide so that this does not interfere with their ability to care for an older person in a life-threatening situation. After this reflective exercise, what is required are well-developed interview skills and assessment practices because of the frequently complex presentation of older people. Many older people cannot or are reluctant to disclose how they are feeling. Some of the reasons for this may be the shame related to having a mental health problem and the fear of the consequences of bringing up such issues; for example, if it is felt that they are not coping at home then pressure may be brought on for them to move to a residential aged care facility (Conwell 2001). Classically, an older person will describe psychological symptoms in terms of more socially acceptable physical symptoms and somatic complaints. These situations can be further clouded with the presence of painful, acute and chronic medical conditions that are more prevalent with increasing age. If the treatment of the medical conditions becomes the primary focus, the symptoms of depression may go undetected or be perceived as 'understandable' when these are masked by physical symptoms.

If treating the medical conditions becomes the primary focus, the symptoms of depression may go undetected or be perceived as 'understandable' when masked by physical symptoms.

An individualised and thorough interview should take place, with the health worker not being reluctant to directly ask the older person if they are suicidal (Crawford et al 2011). A risk assessment is helpful at this stage and gaining information from close family, friends and neighbours may be appropriate to improve the accuracy of the assessment. There are some tools, such as the Scale for Suicide Ideation (Beck et al 1979) that may assist in this process. When a person is assessed as suicidal there are suicide intervention protocols available for use (e.g. see Brown et al 2001, Szanto et al 2002) or there may be locally developed ones for individual services. Depending on the level of assessed suicidality, such protocols generally include determining the suicide plan and access to means, removing the means, and constant supervision in a safe environment, such as a hospital's acute psychiatric unit. Admission to hospital could be under involuntary status by use of a mental health Act. When inpatient care is over, intensive follow-up is still required because the immediate post-discharge period is also a time for high suicide risk, even with older people who seem to be quite 'mentally well'. Despite these actions from identifying risks through to active intervention, there will be some older people who still manage to commit suicide; health workers need to be aware that suicide can be unpredictable and it is sometimes only with hindsight that the indicators can be identified.

TREATING SUICIDAL BEHAVIOUR

When suicidal ideation is linked with depressive illness, antidepressants and ECT can be effective treatments. Psychological therapies, such as problem-solving therapy, psycho-education, CBT and mindfulness-based cognitive therapy may be efficacious in reducing suicidal ideation and attempts (Sakinofsky 2007). Additionally, although specific scientific data may not be available, health workers cannot discount the therapeutic value of interpersonal contact made during frequent, routine clinical visits, particularly for older people who are socially isolated.

SUICIDE PREVENTION IN OLDER PEOPLE

Leading the way in suicide prevention strategies that have shown a reduction in suicide rates was the introduction of the *National Suicide Prevention Strategy* by the Australian Government in 1999 (de Leo et al 2001a). From this formalised national approach, more specific strategies have developed at local levels of health service delivery.

Screening, diagnosis and treatment of depression and suicide behavior are important preventative interventions for older people. Health practitioners in primary care settings have a pivotal role in this prevention strategy (Almeida et al 2012b). Evidence has shown that 50% of potential suicide victims had an appointment with their general medical practitioner within one month prior to their death, although the appointment may not have been specifically about suicidal ideation (Harwood et al 2000). Many suicidal deaths involve prescription medications, so attention to prescribing procedures such as restricting the overprescribing of certain medications and more use of non-pharmacological treatments are simple but important preventative strategies that can be implemented.

Targeting high-risk groups such as recently bereaved males, the socially isolated, older people with depression or chronic physical illnesses and older people who are engaged in deliberate self-harm behaviours has also proven to be an effective strategy. Healthcare workers can play an important role in providing more comprehensive care to high-risk individuals by developing skills in risk assessment and having better communication processes for information exchange between the different healthcare personnel.

Targeting high-risk groups such as recently bereaved males, the socially isolated, older people with depression or chronic physical illnesses and older people who are engaged in deliberate self-harm behaviours has proven to be an effective strategy.

ASSISTED SUICIDE

Assisted suicide, which involves a healthcare worker providing the means by which a competent person can end their life after they have explicitly requested assistance in hastening their death (Hendin 1998), is a controversial issue in Australia, as evidenced in the mid-1990s when it was legal for a short time in the Northern Territory. The legal/illegal status of assisted suicide is reflected in other parts of the world as well (Prokopetz & Lehmann 2012). The people at the centre of this debate usually have a terminal illness or a degenerative disease where there is no cure or hope for improvement and the prognosis for their quality of life is extremely poor. The role of healthcare workers may not be providing the means, but it may be dealing with the revelation that the older person is contemplating suicide. As stated at the beginning of this section about suicide in older people, the answers are not simple. As with any complex issue, healthcare workers have to be very clear in their own mind about their beliefs and values and how these impact on the care they provide. Due consideration must also be given to the legal and ethical issues involved with assisted suicide.

CONCLUSION

This chapter has explored issues surrounding depression and suicide in older people. After detailing epidemiology, risk factors and clinical features, how to undertake a comprehensive assessment was presented. The prevalence of depression and suicide in older people attests to the need for active and timely intervention by health practitioners. The use of a range of psychosocial, pharmacological and non-pharmacological interventions has made successes possible for what often presents as a hopeless and intractable situation.

Vignette

Joe is a 75-year-old retired motor mechanic and former rally car driver. He is married with two sons. At the time of his referral to the Older Persons Mental Health Service (OPMHS) he was residing in a nursing home receiving high-level care. He had been diagnosed with dementia of the Alzheimer's type on a background of recurrent major depressive disorder with psychotic features. Prior to admission to the nursing home, Joe had received treatment elsewhere with antidepressant medication and a short course of ECT. He initially improved to some extent, but this was not maintained and he was noted to have significant cognitive impairment. Joe scored 23 out of 30 on the Mini-Mental State Examination (MMSE). A CT brain scan showed generalised atrophy and a SPECT brain scan showed reduced tracer uptake in both temporal lobes. The cognition enhancer galantamine was added to his ongoing treatment with the antidepressant venlafaxine. He was assessed by the Aged Care Assessment Team (ACAT) as eligible for dementia-specific high-level care.

At that time Joe was noted to have little spontaneous speech, poor sleep, reduced oral intake and urinary incontinence. He was also wandering and somewhat resistive to care. Following this assessment, Joe was admitted to the nursing home, where he stayed for just under a year. However, his wife and the director of care at the nursing home became concerned that Joe might be depressed and referred him to the OPMHS. When seen by the OPMHS community outreach team in the nursing home he was noted to have low mood, poor appetite, weight loss of 35 kg over one year, lack of speech, isolative behaviour, somnolence and poor memory. He was admitted to hospital for further assessment and treatment. He was difficult to assess because he was essentially mute and lying in the fetal position in bed. He was not eating and drinking and had double incontinence. He scored 20 out of 30 on the MMSE. He had a repeat CT brain scan, which showed atrophy and deep white matter ischaemic changes. An electroencephalogram (EEG) was normal.

He scored 24 out of 30 on the GDS. His dose of the antidepressant venlafaxine was increased and the antipsychotic medication risperidone was added, but he did not improve.

Approval for a longer course of ECT was obtained from the Mental Health Review Tribunal and he was given 14 right unilateral ECT treatments with excellent response. He gained weight and was bright, cheerful and optimistic. He fully recovered from his major depression and his post-ECT MMSE score rose to 28/30. He regained the capacity to undertake all of his own activities of daily living. He was commenced on weekly maintenance ECT and discharged home. Maintenance ECT was continued for one year at increasing intervals and he was subsequently maintained on venlafaxine. He has now been living happily at home with his wife for more than two years and has taken an overseas trip without difficulty. He is restoring an old Porsche in his shed and enjoying his normal social life. There is no sign of clinically significant cognitive impairment. The final diagnosis was major depressive disorder, severe, with pseudo-dementia.

Reflective questions

1. If depression is the major risk factor for suicide in older people, how can we prevent this from occurring in the community?

2. Obtaining data from the person presenting with depressive signs can be made difficult if cognitive impairment is present. Is information from family and friends reliable in determining diagnosis?

3. Older people living in residential care usually have multiple comorbidity problems. How does this influence a depressive state?

4. What other treatment modalities are available for depression apart from medication?

5. Understanding the past often reveals clues to the present mental health status of people. How can you improve the reported social history of your clients?

References

Almeida, O.P., Pirkis, J., Kerse, N., et al., 2012a. Socioeconomic disadvantage increases risk of prevalent and persistent depression in later life. Journal of Affective Disorders 138 (3), 322–331.

Almeida, O.P., Pirkis, J., Kerse, N., et al., 2012b. A randomized trial to reduce the prevalence of depression and self-harm behavior in older primary care patients. Annals of Family Medicine 10, 347–356.

American Psychiatric Association, 2013. Diagnostic and statistical manual of mental disorders, fifth ed. American Psychiatric Publishing, Arlington VA.

Australian Bureau of Statistics, 2012. Causes of death, Australia, 2010. ABS, Canberra.

Australian Institute for Suicide Research and Prevention, 2003. International suicide rates—recent trends and implications for Australia. Australian Government Department of Health and Ageing, Canberra.

Banerjee, S., Hellier, J., Dewey, M., et al., 2011. Sertraline or mirtazapine for depression in dementia (HTA-SADD): a randomised, multi-centre, double-blind, placebo-controlled trial. The Lancet 378 (9789), 403–411.

Beck, A.T., Kovacs, M., Weissman, A., 1979. Assessment of suicidal intention: the scale for suicidal ideation. Journal of Consulting and Clinical Psychology 47 (2), 343–352.

Blazer, D.G., 2003. Depression in late life: review and commentary. Journal of Gerontology 58 (3), 249–265.

Brown, G.K., Bruce, M.L., Pearson, J.L., 2001. PROSPECT Study Group: high risk management guidelines for elderly suicidal patients in primary care settings. International Journal of Geriatric Psychiatry 16 (6), 593–601.

Byrne, G.J.A., 1995. Opportunities for preventive intervention for mental disorders in the elderly. In: Raphael, B., Burrows, G. (Eds.), Handbook of preventive psychiatry. Elsevier, Amsterdam, pp. 185–202.

Byrne, G.J.A., Raphael, B., 1997. The psychological symptoms of conjugal bereavement in elderly men over the first 13 months. International Journal of Geriatric Psychiatry 12, 241–251.

Clarke, D.M., Kissane, D.W., 2002. Demoralization: its phenomenology and importance. Australian and New Zealand Journal of Psychiatry 36 (6), 733–742.

Conwell, Y., 2001. Suicide in later life: a review and recommendations for prevention. Suicide and Life-threatening Behaviour 31 (Suppl), 32–47.

Conwell, Y., Duberstein, P.R., Caine, E.D., 2002. Risk factors for suicide in later life. Biological Psychiatry 52 (3), 193–204.

Crawford, M.J., Thana, L., Methuen, C., et al., 2011. Impact of screening for risk of suicide: randomized controlled trial. British Journal of Psychiatry 198, 379–384.

de Leo, D., Hickey, P.A., Neulinger, K., et al., 2001a. Ageing and suicide. Commonwealth Department of Health and Aged Care, Canberra.

de Leo, D., Padoani, W., Scocco, P., et al., 2001b. Attempted and completed suicide in older subjects: Results for the WHO/EURO multicentre study of suicidal behaviour. International Journal of Geriatric Psychiatry 16, 300–310.

Draper, B., 1996. Attempted suicide in old age. International Journal of Geriatric Psychiatry 11, 577–587.

Ekers, D., Richards, D., Gilbody, S., 2008. A meta-analysis of randomized trials of behavioural treatment of depression. Psychological Medicine 38, 611–623.

Harwood, D., 2002. Suicide in older persons. In: Jacoby, R., Oppenheimer, C. (Eds.), Psychiatry in the elderly. Oxford University Press, Oxford.

Harwood, D.M.J., Hawton, K., Hope, T., 2000. Suicide in older people: mode of death, demographic factors, and medical contact before death in one hundred and ninety-five cases. International Journal of Geriatric Psychiatry 15, 736–743.

Hendin, H., 1998. Suicide by death: doctors, patients, and assisted suicide. Norton, New York.

Kreisfeld, R., Newson, R., Harrison, J., 2004. Injury Deaths, Australia, 2002. Cat. No. INJCAT 65. AIHW, Adelaide.

Laidlaw, K., Thompson, L.W., Dick-Siskin, L., et al., 2003. Cognitive behaviour therapy with older people. John Wiley, Chichester.

Levy, T.B., Barak, Y., Sigler, M., et al., 2011. Suicide attempts and burden of physical illness among depressed elderly inpatients. Archives of Gerontology and Geriatrics 52, 115–117.

Minayo, M.C., Cavalcante, F.G., 2010. Suicide in elderly people: a literature review. Rev Saúde Pública 44, 750–757.

Murphy, J.A., Byrne, G.J., 2012. Prevalence and correlates of the proposed DSM-5 diagnosis of chronic depressive disorder. Journal of Affective Disorders, 139 (2), 172–180.

Nowers, M., 1993. Deliberate self-harm in the elderly: a survey of one London borough. International Journal of Geriatric Psychiatry 8, 609–614.

O'Connor, D.W., 2006. Do older Australians truly have low rates of anxiety and depression? A critique of the 1997 National Survey of Mental Health and Wellbeing. Australian and New Zealand Journal of Psychiatry 40, 623–631.

Prokopetz, J.J.Z., Lehmann, L.S., 2012. Redefining physicians' role in assisted dying. New England Journal of Medicine 367, 97–99.

Reynolds III, C.F., Frank, E., Perel, J.M., et al., 1999. Nortriptyline and interpersonal psychotherapy as maintenance therapies for recurrent major depression. A randomized controlled trial in patients older than 59 years. Journal of the American Medical Association 281, 39–45.

Sakinofsky, I., 2007. Treating suicidality in depressive illness. Part 2: Does treatment cure or cause suicidality? The Canadian Journal of Psychiatry 52 (1), 85S–101S.

Seitz, D., Purandare, N., Conn, D., 2010. Prevalence of psychiatric disorders among older adults in long-term care homes: a systematic review. International Psychogeriatrics 22 (7), 1025–1039.

Slade, T., Johnston, A., Browne, M.A.O., et al., 2009. 2007 National Survey of Mental Health and Wellbeing: Methods and key findings. Australian and New Zealand Journal of Psychiatry, 43 (7), 594–605.

Steffens, D.C., Skoog, I., Norton, M.C., et al., 2000. Prevalence of depression and its treatment in an elderly population: the Cache County study. Archives of General Psychiatry 57 (6), 601–607.

Szanto, K., Gildengers, A., Mulsant, B., et al., 2002. Identification of suicide ideation and prevention of suicidal behaviour in the elderly. Drugs & Aging 19 (1), 11–24.

CHAPTER 15

PERSISTENT PAIN IN OLDER PEOPLE

Stephen J Gibson, Samuel Scherer, Benny Katz and Rhonda Nay

Editors' comments

Pain for most people is unwelcome and can result in numerous adverse outcomes including depression, disability, social isolation, confusion, irritability and anxiety. Older people experience more chronic pain, acute-on-chronic pain and other types of pain at the same time—such as neuropathic and nocioceptive—because of the comorbidities associated with older age. However, recognition, assessment, treatment and documentation of pain is far from optimal. There are various reasons for this and the authors of this chapter, after outlining the epidemiology of pain, discuss the varying pain experiences, issues with under-recognition and provide valuable information in relation to assessment tools and treatments.

INTRODUCTION

Pain is recognised as being a complex and inherently personal experience with sensory-discriminative (e.g. location, intensity, quality of sensation), affective-motivational (unpleasantness, anxiety, actions to withdraw–avoid further harm) and cognitive-interpretive dimensions (meaning of pain symptoms, context, beliefs). Pain may be considered as being either acute (short-term, resolves with the cessation of noxious stimulation or recovery from injury/disease) or chronic, persistent pain. Chronic pain should not be regarded as a simple perpetuation of an acute pain episode. Rather, modern conceptualisations of pain emphasise a biopsychosocial perspective in which biological, psychological, behavioural and social factors all play a relevant role in shaping the experience (Turk & Flor 1999). Common factors associated with chronic pain include: interference and disability, mood disturbance, problems with sleep, effects of disuse, poor quality of life, a high and ongoing consumption of medications and other treatments as well as adverse side effects and iatrogenesis resulting from past treatment attempts to cure pain. As pain persists beyond the usual time of healing, the original injury or pathological cause often becomes less important than the ongoing pain and suffering. In other words, the pain becomes the major problem needing timely treatment. Indeed, there is now growing recognition of chronic pain as a disease entity in its own right (Niv & Devor 2004, Siddall & Cousins 2004). Considerable progress has been made in understanding the basic pathophysiology of pain processing and the role of selected psychological and social factors that impact on the perceptual experience. The development of new, and more targeted, pharmacological and non-pharmacological treatment strategies for managing pain has also been forthcoming over recent years as our fundamental knowledge about pain has improved. Nonetheless, the assessment and management of bothersome pain can be a particularly challenging prospect, and in none more so than those of advanced age.

 Modern conceptualisations of pain emphasise a biopsychosocial perspective in which biological, psychological, behavioural and social factors all play a relevant role in shaping the experience.

EPIDEMIOLOGY OF PAIN IN OLDER PEOPLE

Older people are more likely to suffer painful degenerative disease, require hospitalisation or undergo medical interventions, many of which will be painful. Epidemiologic studies of pain prevalence in the community setting show that acute pain remains approximately similar across different age cohorts at 5% of the population (Helme & Gibson 2001). In contrast, persistent pain (defined as pain on most days persisting beyond three months) shows an age-related increase in prevalence until at least the seventh decade of life and then a slight decline into very advanced age (Blyth et al 2001, Helme & Gibson 2001, Jones & Macfarlane 2005). Prevalence rates of persistent pain vary widely between different studies, nonetheless, a consensus view might suggest that about 18% of young adults suffer from persistent, bothersome pain rising to a peak of 30–65% in those aged 55–65 years and then declining somewhat to about 25–55% of the population in those aged 85 years or older living in the community (Blyth et al 2001, Gibson 2007, Helme & Gibson 2001, Jones & Macfarlane 2005). Several studies also show an exceptionally high prevalence of pain (up to 80%) in people living in residential aged care facilities (Helme & Gibson 2001, Takai et al 2010).

PAIN PREVALENCE IN PEOPLE WITH DEMENTIA

Advancing age is associated with a high prevalence of chronic pain and of dementia. Although not causally related the two conditions are likely to co-exist in many older people. This is of special importance for those in residential care facilities. The presence of dementia can affect the perception of pain as well as the emotional and behavioural impacts. The aetiology and stage of dementia may be important considerations, as studies show differential impacts at mild levels of cognitive impairment versus more moderate and severe dementia. For instance, several studies have shown a similar pain experience and prevalence in those with mild cognitive impairment (Cole et al 2006, Shega et al 2010). By contrast, both the frequency and severity of identified pain was reduced in those with severe dementia and the magnitude of this difference is large (with 61% of cognitively intact residents identified with pain versus 31% of those with dementia) (Proctor & Hirdes 2001). This observed decrease in pain prevalence occurs when using either self-report rating scales as well as proxy-rated observational pain scales (Gibson & Lussier 2012, Scherder et al 2009). Given the similar findings with both self-report and observational assessments, it appears that the reduced pain prevalence in those with dementia is not simply due to a loss of verbal skills but rather reflects the increased difficulty in identifying pain or some genuine reduction in pain processing with advancing dementia. The exact reasons for reduced pain are still being investigated but include impaired communication skills (verbal and behavioural), the possibility of less comorbid disease or some alteration in pain processing related to degenerative neurophysiological changes that accompany many dementing illnesses. Despite the demonstrations of less pain in those with dementia, these findings do not suggest that pain is less bothersome when it is actually reported. On the contrary, it is likely that any complaint of pain (verbal or via behavioural markers) made in the presence of marked cognitive impairment requires even greater attention and a more proactive approach to assessment and treatment.

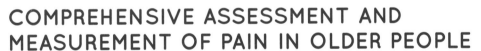

Pain in people with dementia is more difficult to diagnose and is undertreated.

COMPREHENSIVE ASSESSMENT AND MEASUREMENT OF PAIN IN OLDER PEOPLE

Whether pain is acute or chronic, it is important to develop a picture of all factors that may contribute to the pain, including the role of physical pathologies, documentation of aggravating and relieving factors, prior history and consideration of relevant medical issues as well as the prospect of remedial or curative actions. With chronic pain, a comprehensive approach is also required, including evaluating physical functioning (disability, interference with daily activities), psychosocial function (mood, interpersonal relationships, sleep, cognitive function), beliefs/attitudes to pain (fear of harm, ability to cope, meaning of symptoms) and general quality of life. Identifying those factors that might interfere with pain reporting and treatment options (i.e. hearing impairment, cognitive impairment, renal impairment) is also advised. Each of these aspects of a comprehensive assessment are important components in designing a tailored pain management program to meet the specific needs of older people and are important indicators of the efficacy of an integrated treatment approach (Herr 2005).

Medical assessment, contributing to an accurate multidimensional diagnostic formulation, is integral to effectively manage pain in older people and is informed by the expertise of both geriatric and pain medicine.

The key components of assessing chronic pain in older people include:
- pain history
- concurrent medical conditions, past medical history and current medications
- physical examination
- mental state examination and mood state
- diagnostic investigations.

A person's self-report, through a structured history that ascertains onset, location, intensity, periodicity, quality, aggravating and relieving factors, and impact of pain, should be the standard first step in pain assessment whenever possible (American Geriatrics Society (AGS) 2009, Herr 2005). The older person should be given every opportunity to provide this history. Even in the presence of communicative or cognitive impairment important information can often be obtained given adequate time. The person taking the history should be a skilled communication partner and necessary time, proximity, lighting and sensory-assistive devices should be used. The pain history should also encompass information about past pain-directed investigations and treatments as well as their tolerability and effectiveness.

The older person should be given every opportunity to provide this history notwithstanding the presence of communicative or cognitive impairment.

While the medical assessment and diagnosis of pain in younger people often progresses in a relatively linear or single-pointed trajectory, the process in many older people tends to becomes interwoven with the fact that they often have pathology in several bodily systems (e.g. musculoskeletal, vascular, neurological) that may contribute to the pain through a variety of mechanisms. Therefore pain in a single location could be contributed to by more than one disease process (e.g. foot pain due to both arthritis and neuropathy); pain in multiple locations could have either a single underlying pathological cause or a set of entirely different causes.

If not directly contributing to the underlying cause of their pain, concurrent illnesses may also be associated with other symptoms, impairments and disabilities (e.g. insomnia, weakness, falls) that can exacerbate or be relevant to the clinical presentation, cause and management of the pain (Leong et al 2007). In addition, it is important to evaluate all medications that the person is already taking, especially in the context of renal or hepatic disease, alertness, cognitive impairment, balance problems and general frailty, since the available pharmacological pain treatment options may become much fewer.

The physical examination should include specific focus on the site(s) of reported pain for any evidence of diagnostic clues such as inflammation or other local changes as well as the mapping out of the area of pain (Hadjistavropoulos 2005), particularly in relation to patterns of neuroanatomical distribution. Generally the focus is on the musculoskeletal system (e.g. evidence of spinal or large or small joint deformity and restriction in range of movement) or neurological systems (e.g. evidence of weakness or sensory changes such as allodynia, hyperalgesia or hyperpathia) (AGS 2009), and it is important to assess such pain on movement not just when sitting or lying.

Informed by the results of the history and examination, the health professional should consider the formulation including the likely diagnoses and contributions to the person's pain. If there has been a recent increase or change in pain report, the possibility that there is a new condition requiring specific treatment (e.g. a recent bone fracture, renal calculus) should be pursued with appropriate diagnostic investigations. Other significant changes in the person's condition such as unexplained weight loss, fever or neurological signs may also indicate the need for further investigation. Metastatic disease should be considered in any person with a past history of malignancy. Last but not least, the health professional should not overlook opportunities for effective treatment through diagnosing a modifiable underlying disease process (e.g. joint arthroplasty for osteoarthritis, ischaemic pain responsive to stenting a blocked artery or rheumatoid arthritis responsive to disease-modifying medication) (Australian Pain Society 2005). When considering whether to undertake any new investigations it is important to recognise the high occurrence of incidental pathology (e.g. radiographic osteoarthritis in the absence of symptoms) and that abnormal findings may often be unrelated to the pain symptoms (Carragee 2005). The history and physical examination should guide the acquisition of additional diagnostic studies/tests and the need for such tests should be considered with care. Radiological imaging may reassure the person that the pain is not due to serious pathology, enabling a focus on a rehabilitative approach. Correlation of symptoms with abnormal investigation findings is often challenging in older people, but this should not preclude a focus on symptom management and rehabilitation when the underlying cause of pain cannot be identified or treated (Weiner et al 2004). A summary of a comprehensive assessment approach to persistent pain in older people is provided in Table 15.1

Health professionals should not overlook opportunities for effective treatment through diagnosing a modifiable underlying disease process.

PSYCHOMETRIC APPROACHES TO A COMPREHENSIVE ASSESSMENT OF PAIN

The successful identification and treatment of a bothersome, persistent pain problem relies on a comprehensive assessment of all of those factors that contribute to the person's pain, suffering and disability, yet systematic research efforts have only just started to focus on the reliability and validity of common pain assessment tools when used in older populations. The need for a

Table 15.1

Summary of a comprehensive assessment approach to persistent pain in older people

| ISSUE OF INTEREST DOMAIN | CLINICAL AND PSYCHOMETRIC ASSESSMENTS OF PAIN IN OLDER PEOPLE | | |
| | APPROACH TO ASCERTAINMENT OF INFORMATION | | |
	Clinical history	Clinical examination	Psychometric measures
Onset and duration of history of pain	Circumstances of onset of pain history (e.g. compensable issues) and chronicity (months, years, decades) may help define diagnosis and prognosis		
Pain intensity and/or unpleasantness	Listen carefully as the person describes their pain; facilitate dialogue to elaborate details of severity and quality of the pain	Observe for emotional valence during pain report and evidence of pain behaviours both at rest and during examination	**Verbal** Verbal descriptor scales Numeric ratings (i.e. 0–10) Coloured Analogue Scales Faces Pain scales Pain thermometer **Multidimensional scales** Brief Pain Inventory Multidimensional Pain Inventory McGill Pain Questionnaire Geriatric Pain Scale **Non-verbal** PAINAD PACSLAC Abbey Pain Scale DOLOPLUS-2 NOPAIN

Location and local findings	Ask about precise location; consider likelihood of deep somatic versus superficial somatic pain versus visceral pain	Map out sites; consider anatomical (including neuroanatomical) patterns; observe for local inflammation or skin changes; test for allodynia/hyperalgaesia	Body map
Pain periodicity and exacerbating and relieving factors	Define the person's pain experience as they go through their typical 24-hour cycle	Observe for pain behaviours and their interpersonal-communicative and physical-protective context	**Verbal** Brief Pain Inventory
Pain impact on physical function	Ask whether pain interferes with personal and domestic/instrumental activities of daily living and whether help is given/available/needed	Examine range of movement of joints and back; look for pain evoked by movement; evaluate upper and lower limb function—is walking range and standing time limited?	**Verbal** Brief Pain Inventory Geriatric Pain Scale Multidimensional Pain Inventory—section 3 Rolland Morris Sickness Impact Profile Oswestry SF-36

Table 15.1

Summary of a comprehensive assessment approach to persistent pain in older people—cont'd

CLINICAL AND PSYCHOMETRIC ASSESSMENTS OF PAIN IN OLDER PEOPLE			
ISSUE OF INTEREST DOMAIN	APPROACH TO ASCERTAINMENT OF INFORMATION		
	Clinical history	Clinical examination	Psychometric measures
Pain impact on psychosocial function	Ask about, anxiety, depression, interpersonal relationships and medication-related cognitive changes	Evaluate alertness mood; affective reactivity; and cognitive function	**Verbal** The Geriatric Depression Scale Zung Depression Scale Spielberger State-Trait Anxiety Inventory Spielberger Anger Inventory Profile of Mood States Questionnaire Depression-Anxiety and Stress Scale **Non-verbal** Neuropsychiatric Inventory Cohen Mansfield Inventory
Past history	Both general past history and conditions that could be directly related to the pain should be reviewed (e.g. history of osteoporosis or shingles)	Look for evidence of potentially relevant morbidity such as kyphosis, surgical scars or hemiparesis associated with unilateral sensory loss	

Comorbidity and burden of pathology	Does the person have a single clear-cut pain and health problem such as OA hip, or is the diagnosis or formulation more complex with multiple disease processes contributing to pain and other symptoms, impairments and disabilities?	Evaluate overall level of resilience or frailty. Is pain the main limiting issue or do one or more other conditions (e.g. cardiac, respiratory, neurodegenerative) impose greater or cumulative disabilities?	**Verbal and non-verbal** Cumulative illness rating Charlston Index
Sleep	Ask about sleep disturbance and the degree to which this is related to pain; evaluate pattern of insomnia—sleep habits, onset, offset, duration, and daytime somnolence		**Verbal** Pittsburgh Sleep Quality Index Sleep Questionnaire
Beliefs and attitudes to pain	Ask about meaning of symptoms such as fear of progressive condition, harm/damage, loss of independence, catastrophic thinking		**Verbal** Coping Strategies Questionnaire Survey of Pain Attitudes Pain Attitudes Questionnaire Pain Self Efficacy Questionnaire Cognitive Risk Profile
Quality of life	Ask about the person's goals and what he or she would be enabled to do if the pain could be managed		**Verbal** Brief Pain Inventory SF-36 AQual EuroQual

Verbal: Patient able to provide self-report.
Non-verbal: Patient not able to provide self-report.

multifaceted, comprehensive assessment is well recognised and should include: pain intensity; quality and variations over time and situation; the extent of psychological disturbance; utilisation of coping strategies, beliefs and attitudes towards pain; functional impairment in activities of daily life; and the social impacts of chronic pain.

Measurement of pain

Self-report measures of pain have become the de facto gold standard for pain assessment and are recognised as being the only valid method to truly convey a latent, subjective state that is really only known to the individual who suffers. Numerous unidimensional and multidimensional self-report measures of pain have been developed and, in general, tools with demonstrated merit in younger adult populations are also thought to be useful with older adults. Several different types of self-report scales exist, including verbal descriptors (i.e. none, mild, moderate, strong severe), numeric ratings (i.e. 0–10), visual analogue scales in which current pain intensity is marked on a 10 cm line between extremes of 'no pain' and 'worst possible pain', complex qualitative word lists (i.e. MPQ) and more graphic representations, such as the pain thermometer, coloured analogue scale or FACES pain scale (i.e. Baker Wong). Several studies to directly compare different self-report pain measurement tools suggest that the verbal descriptor scales are most preferred by older people and have the strongest evidence of utility, reliability and validity (Herr 2005, Mendoza et al 2004, Wynne et al 2000). Other acceptable measures include numeric rating scales (i.e. 0–10, Wood et al 2010), box rating scales, pictorial pain scales (i.e. pain thermometer, faces scales), the multidimensional McGill pain questionnaire and Brief Pain Inventory (Gagliese & Katz 2003, Herr et al 2004, Pautex et al 2005). There is less uniform support for visual analogue scales and several authors raise concerns when using this measure with older adults (Gagliese & Katz 2003, Herr et al 2004). However, it is important to note that there is no one best measure of pain and a failure to complete one type of scale does not preclude success with other pain assessment tools (Ferrell 1995).

In clinical practice it may be best to select tools that are consistent with the personal preference of the individual when it is known, or to try several different types of scales before giving up on using self-report tools.

PAIN ASSESSMENT IN PEOPLE WITH DEMENTIA

Given that self-report has become the de facto gold standard for pain assessment, whenever possible, this should remain as the preferred option in people with dementia. People with mild to moderate cognitive impairment often remain capable of valid self-report (Ferrell et al 1995), especially in relation to current pain severity or pain 'right now' (Herr 2005). Clinicians should focus on simple and direct questions such as 'How bad is your pain now?' rather than questions requiring higher cognitive skills: 'How is your pain compared with last week?'. There are several self-report pain assessment tools that are valid and reliable in cognitively impaired people, including verbal descriptor scales, numeric rating scales, pain thermometers and facial pain scales (Herr et al 2004, 2007, Pautex et al 2005). Moreover, self-report scales have been shown to be more reliable than the alternative of using opinions of surrogate reporters regarding a person's pain experience (Horgas & Tsai 1998, Weiner et al 1999).

Pesonen et al (2009) compared the utility of various unidimensional pain tools across participants with various stages of dementia, such as a verbal rating scale, red wedge scale, visual analogue scale and FACES scale. The verbal rating scale (no pain, slight pain, moderate pain, severe pain) was successfully completed by a higher proportion of participants across all severity of dementia, although more than half the participants with moderate to severe dementia (MMSE 11–16) were still able to complete the other rating scales. In severe stages of dementia (MMSE ≤10) only the verbal rating scale had a successful completion rate of greater than 50%.

With the progression of dementia the ability to comprehend and verbally report painful experiences is increasingly compromised and ultimately becomes impossible. This raises serious challenges for pain assessment, and people with severe dementia are at significant risk of having their pain under-recognised and under-assessed (Morrison & Siu 2000, Teno et al 2003). There are now more than 25 observer-rated behavioural pain assessment tools developed for specific use in those with dementia. Most instruments grade the presence of various behaviours (facial grimace or wince, negative vocalisation, changes in body language, rubbing, guarding, restlessness, altered breathing or physiologic signs) that are thought to be indicative of pain. Each observer-rated scale has typically undergone some limited validation testing on a small sample of older adults and has demonstrated inter-rater reliability, although large methodologically rigorous studies are still needed to better establish the utility of these instruments (Hadjistavropoulos et al 2007). Recommended examples include the PAINAD, PACSLAC, ABBEY and DOLOPLUS-2 behaviour rating scales (Australian Pain Society 2005, Hadjistavropoulos et al 2007, Herr et al 2006). These scales represent a welcome addition to the battery of available pain assessment tools and provide an important first step to improving the quality of pain management in this highly dependent and vulnerable group.

MEASUREMENT OF PSYCHOSOCIAL IMPACTS OF PAIN

The longer that bothersome pain persists, the greater the probability that the older person will become depressed, socially withdrawn, irritable and somatically preoccupied. Anger, frustration, loss of ability to cope and increased anxiety also occur as the person tries and fails with a variety of medical and non-medical therapies (Gibson et al 1994). As a result, the measurement of mood disturbance and social impacts are now considered as an integral component of any comprehensive clinical evaluation and should be incorporated as a routine part of the assessment plan.

A number of standardised tools have demonstrated reliability and validity for use in older adults. The Geriatric Depression Scale, Zung Depression Scale, Spielberger State-Trait Anxiety Inventory, and the Depression, Anxiety and Stress scale are widely used and appropriate for older adult populations and particularly in those with chronic pain (Gibson 1997, Woods et al 2010). The initial assessment may also include evaluation of other common psychological associations and mediators of pain including: anger (e.g. Spielberger Anger Inventory); cognitive and behavioural coping strategy use (i.e. Coping Strategies Questionnaire); beliefs and attitudes; stoicism (Survey of Pain Attitudes, Pain Attitudes Questionnaire) (Jensen et al 1986, Yong et al 2003); sleep (Menefee et al 2000); spousal bereavement; and suicide risk (Gibson & Chambers 2003). Developing a better understanding of the person's social situation, beliefs, attitudes and current coping strategies in relation to their pain provides an important starting point towards individualising the eventual management plan. However, the comprehensive contextual information gained from such an assessment must be weighed against the increased respondent burden on the older person with bothersome pain.

Understanding the person's social situation, beliefs, attitudes and current coping strategies in relation to their pain provides an important starting point towards individualising the eventual management plan.

MEASUREMENT OF ACTIVITY, DISABILITY AND PAIN-RELATED INTERFERENCE WITH DAILY ACTIVITIES

Chronic pain has a major impact on function and is likely to interfere with many of the activities of daily life (Williamson & Schulz 1992). A number of options exist for measuring activity levels or disability, ranging from objective measures of uptime/movement and direct observation of activity task performance, through to self-report psychometric questionnaires of activities of daily living and activity dairies. The psychometric scales typically used to measure function in geriatric populations (i.e. Barthel Index, Katz ADL scale, Cape, Lawton & Brody, FIM) may be useful to monitor the personal and instrumental activities of daily living in older people with chronic pain, although they tend to lack sensitivity and fail to measure the more discretionary activities that are most commonly affected by chronic pain (i.e. leisure and pastimes, home maintenance, social interactions, gardening and more strenuous activities). One must also exercise some care with the interpretation of activity measures, whether they be self-report or observational, because activity restriction can also occur as a consequence of a change in social circumstances, medical factors or other concurrent disease states rather than as a consequence of pain (Gibson et al 1994). Moreover, regardless of whether measures are via self-report or objective markers, activity performance is highly dependent upon motivational factors and the context in which measurement is undertaken. As a result, studies of chronic pain populations have tended to focus on measures of perceived pain-related interference in activity/disability rather than documenting the actual levels of activity performance.

Validated measures of pain interference include the Brief Pain Inventory interference scales, the SF-36, Pain Disability Index, Oswestry Disability Questionnaire, and the Roland Morris Questionnaire. These instruments are multidimensional and typically monitor several domains of activity performance including ambulation, sleep/rest, mobility, self-care, social interaction, communication, work, emotional behaviours, leisure activities and pastimes. The evidence for reliability and validity in older chronic pain populations is somewhat lacking, but all of these tools have been used in geriatric populations with good effect. It has been noted that older people with chronic pain often respond more dramatically with respect to improvements in function than in pain intensity following an efficacious treatment plan (Cook 1998, Ferrell 2003) and that functional outcomes are often considered as the most important outcome for older people (Ersek et al 2003, Theiler et al 2002, Weiner et al 2003). For this reason, the measurement of disability and perceived interference should become an essential component of any routine comprehensive pain assessment.

A COMPREHENSIVE APPROACH TO TREATING CHRONIC PAIN IN OLDER PEOPLE

While there is a very high prevalence of pain among older adults living in the community, many individuals are able to manage their pain with little or no help. This is particularly true in cases of short-term, mild aches and pains, where symptomatic relief may be all that is required. This type of pain will not be considered further in this chapter. In other cases, the pain may persist, although many older adults can still self-manage and remain high-functioning. For some, all that may be required is assistance from a primary care clinician to gain symptomatic relief at times when pain is particularly problematic. Specialist help may be required if the pain persists and is bothersome or fails to respond to more conventional treatment strategies. Careful diagnosis of the pain (nociceptive, neuropathic and exacerbating factors), adoption of more advanced treatment methods (including the potential to modify disease components, such as arthroplasty in those with ongoing pain from osteoarthritis) and greater attention to the negative impacts of pain is typically required. Finally, there is a relatively small proportion of people with chronic pain for whom pain becomes all-consuming and affects all aspects of life. The complexity of the chronic pain problem and the lack of response to standard treatments necessitate a different, more comprehensive, multidisciplinary approach to evaluation and management.

Multiple factors contribute to the lack of adequate treatment of pain. Broadly speaking they may be grouped into factors relating to the individual, those involving health professionals or medical factors.

Individual factors include:
- inability to report pain due to cognitive or communication impairment
- reluctance to report pain
- accepting pain as an inevitable part of ageing
- fear of the meaning of pain
- not wanting to bother busy staff
- reluctance to take treatment due to stoicism or fear of side effects.

Health professional factors include:
- inadequate skills to undertake and document pain assessment
- not allocating enough time to identify and assess pain
- not believing the person about pain
- reluctance to administer treatment, such as opioids
- role ambiguity regarding responsibility for managing pain.

Medical factors include:
- concurrent medical/psychiatric conditions limiting investigation and/or treatment
- intolerance of treatment
- refractory pain states such as neuropathic pain.

While pain cannot be eradicated in all cases we do have the ability to achieve better outcomes. Some people will not voluntarily report pain. They may need to be specifically asked about the presence of pain, functional limitations caused by pain, and observed during activities likely to aggravate pain. The individual must be given adequate time to describe their symptoms. They should not feel rushed or that the assessor is not interested in their problem. Once pain has been identified, the next step must be negotiated with the individual. Some people are able to cope well and may consider further evaluation or treatment more of a burden than the pain.

While pain cannot be eradicated in all cases we do have the ability to achieve better outcomes.

If pain is identified to be a problem, then a decision needs to be made as to the balance between diagnostic evaluation and symptomatic management. In general, investigation should be limited to situations where the result has the potential to alter management or for the purpose of excluding serious pathology. A negative x-ray or scan may help reassure the individual, enabling the focus to shift to pain management. Unnecessary investigations can have a detrimental effect, moving the focus to the search for a cure.

Uncertainty or role ambiguity about the management of pain may create a barrier to effective management, particularly when the care plan is simultaneously provided by professionals from different healthcare disciplines. Professionals from one discipline should not assume that pain is the responsibility of another discipline, for example, a nurse believing that pain management is the responsibility of the doctor. There are situations where simple measures such as information, a hot pack or repositioning are more effective than potent analgesic medications. Conventional approaches to pain management using either pharmacological or non-pharmacological approaches, or a combination of the two, often provide adequate relief even when pain eradication is not achieved. This is best handled in a coordinated multidisciplinary fashion, covering physical, psychological and medical aspects of the pain. Good communication is the key to a successful outcome.

Vignette

Mr Peters was described by staff as 'a grumpy old man' with cognitive impairment. He was refusing to participate with rehabilitation following repair of a fractured neck of femur. He was 'verbally aggressive' to staff and refusing to eat or take his medications. Taking a person-centred approach meant sitting down and really listening to his story. He was convinced that the medications were making him aggressive and he was embarrassed by his behaviour. He felt dizzy and nauseated upon standing and that was why he would not take his medications or attend rehabilitation. He believed that the medications were making him worse. He felt a terrible burden on his wife and felt quite useless. Interventions included: appreciation of his description of his pain; reviewing his medications, reviewing the analgesic and stopping a benzodiazepine (which did cause aggression) and starting an antidepressant after diagnosis of depression; and introducing some of his favoured foods. He and his wife were encouraged to talk about what he could do on return home to 'be useful'. Within days Mr Peters was getting out of bed and setting goals for how far he would walk each day. He returned home within three weeks feeling in control of his pain. Initially staff were only focused on *their* goals of rehabilitation for his fractured hip and not listening to what was important to him. Taking a holistic and interdisciplinary approach to assessing his pain and using an analgesic regimen that was acceptable to him resulted in the cessation of 'behaviours' and a successful outcome.

 Do not label or assume 'dementia' explains everything—assess and treat for pain.

MEDICAL MANAGEMENT OF CHRONIC PAIN IN OLDER PEOPLE

The preferred approach to managing pain is to treat the underlying cause, for example, corticosteroids for polymylagia rheumatica or joint replacement surgery for osteoarthritis. A symptom-based approach may be required in the interim or if cure is not feasible. Pharmacological therapies form the mainstay of the Western medical approach, although they are often more effective when combined with non-pharmacological approaches. A summary of pharmacological approaches to pain management in older people in provided in Table 15.2.

There is a wide range of pharmacological treatment options and different modes of drug delivery. Many of the medications have been in use for a long time and have not undergone the rigorous evaluation now required prior to the marketing of a new agent. Many of the drug trials specifically exclude people with comorbid medical conditions or other issues that may confound the evaluation of efficacy. This often results in the exclusion of frail and older

Table 15.2

Summary of pharmacological approaches to pain management in older people

	MEDICATION USE IN OLDER PEOPLE	
MEDICATION	INDICATIONS	COMMENTS
Paracetamol (also known as acetaminophen)	• First-line treatment for common pain conditions • May have opioid-sparing effects in severe pain	• Dose adjustment not usually required except for small stature, alcoholics, poor nutritional status or advanced liver disease • Widely available and inexpensive • Risk of inadvertent overdose because of multiple brand names
Aspirin	• May be used for acute pain, but not widely used as a single agent for persistent pain • May be used in combination analgesics	• Gastrointestinal adverse effects of aspirin limit its use in the elderly • Low-dose aspirin is frequently prescribed as an antiplatelet agent, to reduce cardiovascular events. The dose for this indication does not confer analgesia • Gastrointestinal (GI) sparing effect of selective COX-2 inhibitors are counterbalanced by concurrent low-dose aspirin therapy
Non-steroidal anti-inflammatory drugs (NSAIDs)	• Widely used, specific indication for inflammatory arthropathies	• Preferred by people because of convenience of dosing compared with paracetamol • Increased risk of adverse effects in the elderly, especially GI bleeds, renal and cardiovascular • Should only be used in the lowest effective dose for the shortest duration • Topical NSAIDs are widely used, and may offer pain relief with lower risk of systemic adverse effects than oral NSAIDs
Tramadol	• Acute and chronic pain. Evidence of efficacy for neuropathic pain	• Short- and slow-release preparations • Lower maximum dose in older people is 300 mg per day • Less respiratory depression, constipation and potential for dependency than with other opioids • Caution regarding serotonin syndrome when coadministered with antidepressants

Drug	Indication	Notes
Codeine	• Acute and chronic pain, usually in combined with paracetamol, ibuprofen or aspirin	• Common side effects include constipation, nausea and drowsiness • Dose often limited by side effects or the agent it is combined with, especially paracetamol • May be an ineffective analgesic in individuals unable to transform codeine into active metabolite (morphine), up to 10% of Caucasians • More suitable for short-term use for acute than for chronic pain
Strong oral opioids including oxycodone and morphine	• Severe acute, chronic and cancer pains	• Short-acting and sustained-release oral preparations • Usually start at lower doses in elderly, 25–50% of the usual starting dose, adjusted according to response • Oxycodone has more predicable blood levels than morphine and possibly fewer cognitive effects in older people • Opioid side effects including nausea, constipation, cognitive effects and respiratory depression • Trend for increasing use in chronic non-cancer pain • Oxycodone-naloxone combined tablet causes less opioid-induced constipation
Transdermal patches—buprenorphine and fentanyl	• Severe cancer and non-malignant pain	• Not appropriate for acute pain because of slow onset of action • Patients should generally be stabilised on shorter acting analgesics before transfer to an opioid patch • Slow onset of action • Avoid direct application of heat to the patch • Slow offset after patches removed • Fentanyl patches should not be initiated in opioid-naïve people • Opioid-related GI side effects may be less severe with patches
Tricyclic antidepressants (e.g. amitriptyline and nortriptyline)	• Naturopathic pain (e.g. painful peripheral neuropathy or post-herpetic neuralgia)	• Good evidence of efficacy but generally not well tolerated in older people • Start at lowest possible dose (e.g. 10 mg nocte) and titrate slowly • Analgesic effect occurs at a lower dose than antidepressant effect • Side effects include drowsiness, confusion, postural hypotension, falls, dry mouth, constipation and urinary retention • Inexpensive

Table 15.2

Summary of pharmacological approaches to pain management in older people—cont'd

MEDICATION	INDICATIONS	COMMENTS
	MEDICATION USE IN OLDER PEOPLE	
Newer antidepressants such as selective serotonin reuptake inhibitors (SSRIs) (e.g. sertaline citalopram, duloxetine and venlafaxine)	• No evidence to support the use of SSRIs for pain indications • Evidence of efficacy in neuropathic pain	• Start in low dose, titrate slowly • Check current regulations prior to prescribing • In Australia, duloxetine is approved for diabetic peripheral neuropathy, but does not attract a PBS/RPBS subsidy for this indication
Anticonvulsants carbemazepine	• Drug of choice for trigeminal neuralgia	• Little evidence to support its widespread use for neuropathic pain apart from trigeminal neuralgia • Common side effects include drowsiness, confusion, dizziness, ataxia; start with low dose
Gabapentin and pregabalin	• Painful diabetic neuropathy and post-herpetic neuralgia • Various other chronic pain states	• Better tolerated than tricyclic antidepressants but still must be used with caution • Start with low dose and titrate slowly • May take some weeks to achieve therapeutic doses with gabapentin • Expensive; refer to current regulations before prescribing
Valproate	• Neuropathic pain	• Often tried when other anticonvulsants are not tolerated or unaffordable, although its use in pain is not supported by evidence
Lignocaine patches (also known as Lidocaine)	• Post-herpetic neuralgia and other neuropathic pains	• Not currently marketed in Australia • Evidence of efficacy with fewer side effects than systemic therapies

people from drug trials, yet this is the population most likely to use the medications (Van Spall et al 2007). Therefore, many of the commonly used treatments in older people do not have an evidence base to support their use in this population. Where a medication has been found to be efficacious in a younger person it is likely to be efficacious in an older person, but in general, older people do not tolerate medications as well. The issue is not one of efficacy, so much as tolerability. In some cases this can be managed by commencing a medication at a lower dose and titrating the dose slowly according to the response. This deals with altered drug sensitivity and drug handling in older people. For example, the initial dose of an opioid analgesic is often quarter to half of the starting dose in younger people. The response to the analgesic must be monitored, and adjusted according to response.

Older people are more likely to have other health problems in addition to their pain. These issues may influence the selection and dose of medications. This can be highlighted using NSAIDs as an example. NSAIDs are one of the most commonly prescribed drug classes in older people and the leading cause of adverse drug effects requiring hospitalisation (Pirmohamed et al 2004). The risks associated with NSAID use rise exponentially with age. The most important adverse effects include gastrointestinal toxicity (dyspepsia, peptic ulcer disease and bleeding) acute renal failure, hypertension and cardiovascular events (myocardial infarction and stroke). This is further compounded by drug-drug interactions. For instance, the risk of renal impairment with an NSAID is increased by the coadministration of an angiotensin-converting enzyme inhibitor (ACE inhibitor). Some individuals find that a topical application of NSAIDs provides adequate pain relief, and can use this approach at much lower risk than with systemic therapy. Some people may find the side effects of treatment more troublesome than the pain, such as dyspepsia with NSAIDs and opioid–induced constipation.

Paracetamol, also known as acetaminophen, is one of the most widely used medications in the world. It is often commenced by people before seeking professional advice. Most pain guidelines have paracetamol as the starting point (AGS 2009, WHO 1990).

Special care is required when using paracetamol. Its wide availability without prescription under different brand names may result in a person with unrelieved pain seeking another analgesic unaware that it also contains paracetamol, resulting in an inadvertent paracetamol overdose. Paracetamol toxicity is the major cause of preventable liver failure (Larson et al 2005). This raises the issue of the recommended maximum dose of paracetamol for older people. Generally no maximum dose reduction is required (i.e. up to 4000 mg over a 24-hour period is typically safe); however, the maximum recommended dose should be reduced in people of small stature, poor nutritional intake, liver dysfunction or in alcoholics. People should be warned against exceeding the maximum recommended dose for pain exacerbations. If pain is inadequately controlled, the timing of dosing of paracetamol should be reviewed, as it has a short half life. If this does not achieve the desired result then the coadministration of another analgesic should be considered. These include NSAIDs, tramadol and opioid analgesics.

The risk of serious adverse effects may be worth taking, but this needs to be an individualised decision. The dose and duration of treatment of NSAIDs should be kept to a minimum. The newer anti-inflammatory agents, cyclo-oxygenase 2 selective anti-inflammatory inhibitors (COX 2 inhibitors), have not completely eradicated the safety concerns of the conventional NSAIDs as was initially hoped. In particular, any benefit in reducing gastric bleeding and ulceration may be lost when COX-2 inhibitors are coadministered with low-dose aspirin required for prophylaxis of cardiovascular or cerebrovascular disease (Silverstein et al 2000).

The risk of serious adverse effects may be worth taking, but this needs to be an individualised decision.

Codeine is frequently used in combination with paracetamol, using different doses for moderate or severe pain such as Panadeine and Panadeine Forte. Codeine is an opioid analgesic used for mild to moderate pain. It has a ceiling effect, and further dose increases do not confer greater analgesia but increase the risk of paracetamol toxicity when used in combination preparations. The analgesic effects of codeine are dependent on its biotransformation to morphine in the liver. Genetic factors and several commonly prescribed medications may affect this pathway rendering codeine an ineffective analgesic, while other people who are ultrarapid metabolisers may develop toxicity even with low doses of codeine. Common side effects include constipation, drowsiness and cognitive changes (Analgesic Expert Group: Therapeutic Guidelines 2007).

Tramadol is often used in the post-operative setting because it causes less constipation, respiratory depression and abuse potential than other opioid analgesics. It is also available in sustained-release preparations for chronic pain. Side effects are more common in older people and the maximum daily dose should be reduced to 300 mg for older people. It should be used with caution in people with a history of epilepsy, and should not be used in combination with tricyclic or SSRI antidepressants because it may precipitate a serotonin syndrome. The serotonin syndrome is a medical emergency. Features include agitation, confusion, myoclonus, coma, tachycardia, sweating and fever.

Tramadol should be used with caution in people with a history of epilepsy, and should not be used in combination with tricyclic or selective serotonin reuptake inhibitor antidepressants.

Opioid analgesia was traditionally reserved for people with severe acute pain and cancer-related pain. In recent times there has been increasing trend to use opioid analgesic for managing persistent non-malignant pain. There is some evidence of efficacy of opioids used over short periods for persistent pain, but evidence of efficacy for long-term use is lacking (Kalso et al 2004). The prescription of opioids for persistent non-malignant pain should involve a process of explanation and informed consent, and should be regarded as a therapeutic trial, ideally with measured and predetermined goals over an agreed timeframe. Failure to achieve benefit should result in cessation of opioid treatment. There are a large number of opioid analgesics to choose from, varying in chemical structure, duration of effect, route of delivery and side effect profile. The selection is based on individual factors and preference. Opioid patches are not suitable for acute pain. Persistent pain states are best managed with sustained-release preparations, either oral or transdermal, with a short-acting agent for breakthrough pain. Fentanyl patches are too potent to be initiated in individuals who are not already stabilised on opioid analgesics. There is no evidence that one opioid or route of delivery is superior to the others. Selection is based on tolerability and individual preference. Nausea, drowsiness and confusion tend to be transient, whereas the tendency to constipation persists and prophylactic laxative treatment should always be considered when the opioids are commenced. A combination oxycodone-naloxone tablet is available to reduce opioid-induced constipation, but aperients are still often required in older people. Transdermal preparations may cause fewer side effects than oral preparations. A person on long-term opioid analgesia may be able to resume driving once on a stable dose and with no ongoing side effects that impair driving ability.

Pain related to disease or damage of the somatosensory system ('neuropathic' pain) is often very distressing and difficult to treat. Evidence-based guidelines have been published to help guide clinicians (Finnerup et al 2010). Standard analgesics should be tried, but if the pain remains bothersome then adjuvant analgesia should be tried. Adjuvant agents are not strictly analgesics. Their main indication is for other purposes, but in certain circumstances, such as neuropathic pain, they may have analgesic effects. The most common causes of neuropathic pain in older people include peripheral neuropathies and postherpetic neuralgia. Multiple studies have demonstrated that adjuvant analgesics are of benefit. In general terms, three or four people with neuropathic pain would need to be treated with an adjuvant analgesic for one more person to have a successful outcome beyond that reported in those treated with placebo. In these trials, a successful outcome is usually defined as a 50% reduction in pain, not total pain eradication. The dose of these medications, and probably efficacy, is limited by drug side effects.

The tricyclic antidepressants (e.g. amitriptyline and nortriptyline) are efficacious adjuvant agents for neuropathic pain but are not particularly well tolerated in older people. Common side effects include sedation, falls and anticholinergic side effects such as dry mouth, blurred vision, constipation, postural hypotension and urinary retention, especially in men. The newer selective SSRIs are better tolerated but have not been shown to be effective adjuvant analgesics. Duloxetine, a selective serotonin and noradrenalin reuptake inhibitor (SNRI), has been shown to be of benefit in painful diabetic neuropathy and fibromyalgia. Venlafaxine is in the same drug class.

Anticonvulsants are frequently used for neuropathic pain. Carbemazepine is the drug of choice for trigeminal neuralgia and is often used for other naturopathic conditions despite lack of evidence of efficacy. There is a large body of evidence to support the use of gabapentin and pregabalin for the common neuropathic pain states. Side effects include sedation, confusion, dizziness and ataxia. The starting dose should be reduced for older people. Although demonstrated to be effective, not all of these medications are approved or subsidised in Australia for pain indications. The doctor should take this into consideration before prescribing.

A comprehensive review of all pharmacological therapies is beyond the scope of this chapter. The key point is that a wide range of analgesic and adjuvant medications are available. The choice of agent should be based on the nature of the pain, other concurrent conditions the older person may have, availability and individual preference. Side effects can be minimised by starting with a low dose and titrating slowly according to the response. Total pain eradication may not be feasible.

A wide range of analgesic and adjuvant medications are available, but total pain eradication may not be feasible.

Over more recent times complementary and alternate therapies have become widely used by older people with bothersome pain. Complementary therapies encompass a broad range of biological and traditional holistic treatments. Some treatments have been subject to critical appraisal using randomised controlled trials, often with conflicting results. For instance, the Rotta preparation of glucosamine was found to be superior to placebo for pain and function in osteoarthritis, whereas other non–Rotta preparations have failed to show similar benefits (Towheed et al 2006, 2009). Some herbal remedies have demonstrated similar efficacy to NSAIDs (Gagnier et al 2006). Most clinical trials support the safety of complementary and alternate therapies, although adverse interactions of dietary supplements and herbal therapies with prescription medications may be of concern. More detailed information about various complementary and alternate modalities is available on the National Centre for Complementary and Alternate Medicines website (www.nccam.nih.gov).

MEDICAL MANAGEMENT OF PAIN IN PEOPLE WITH DEMENTIA

There is growing evidence to suggest that people with Alzheimer's disease (AD) are routinely prescribed and administered fewer analgesics than cognitively intact peers, even after controlling for the presence of painful disease (Farrell et al 1996, Farrell et al 1997). Only 33% of people with AD received appropriate analgesic medication compared with 64% of adults without dementia (Scherder & Bouma 1997). This was true for NSAIDs as well as other classes of analgesics (opiates, acetaminophen), even though the need for pain relief was judged equivalent according to the treating clinician. Others have confirmed this undertreatment (Horgas & Tsai 1998), particularly with reference to persistent pain (Pickering et al 2006). Consistent with an earlier study (Feldt et al 1998), Morrison and Siu (2000) found that people with dementia recovering from hip fracture surgery received only one-third of the amount of morphine sulphate equivalents administered to cognitively intact adults and that 76% of people with AD had no standing order for postoperative analgesia. Nonetheless, all of these studies are focused on usage rates of analgesics rather than whether such treatments are effective.

There have been very few randomised controlled trials of treatment efficacy in people with dementia, yet such research is essential in order to help guide clinical practice. A randomised study using a step-wise pain treatment protocol (including successive serial administration of non-pharmacological and pharmacological approaches) demonstrated a 25% improvement in discomfort scores of people with severe dementia in the treatment group but a 20% increase in discomfort in the non-treatment control group over a four-week period (Kovach et al 2006). This effect was improved if treatment options were extended to include more potent analgesic treatments (Kovach et al 2012). Husebo et al (2011) also demonstrated a 40% improvement in observer-rated behavioural pain scores following a step-wise analgesic protocol in people with severe dementia after eight weeks but no change in the control group. Moreover, the provision of appropriate analgesic treatment resulted in a significant 17% reduction in agitation and aggression scores, which is comparable to the treatment effect size of administering a neuroleptic agent, such as resperidone. This hallmark finding is of considerable importance and highlights the potential widespread benefits of treating unrelieved pain in people with dementia.

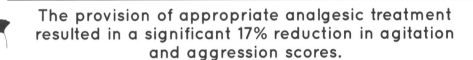

The provision of appropriate analgesic treatment resulted in a significant 17% reduction in agitation and aggression scores.

PSYCHOLOGICAL APPROACHES TO PAIN MANAGEMENT

As pain is a sensory and emotional experience and given that psychological factors play an important role in most persistent pain states, attempts to manage pain symptoms using only pharmacological treatments is likely to fail. Two major psychological models have been most frequently used to treat persistent pain:

- cognitive therapy, which seeks to alter the belief structures, attitudes and thoughts of the person in order to modify the experience of pain and suffering
- behavioural operant conditioning, which seeks to reinforce healthy behaviours and ignore or extinguish maladaptive pain behaviours (e.g. inactivity, excessive medication use).

Table 15.3 describes psychological therapies for managing persistent pain in older adults.

A principle that is fundamental to all types of cognitive therapy is the notion that one's beliefs, appraisals and the meanings attributed to a situation will, in a large part, determine the emotional and behavioural responses to it. People with persistent pain often exhibit maladaptive, distorted or dysfunctional beliefs that contribute to greater levels of pain and greater pain impact. The basic

Table 15.3

Psychological therapies for managing persistent pain in older adults

COMPONENTS OF THERAPY	DESCRIPTION AND EXAMPLES
Education	Discuss expectations of therapy Agree on common treatment goals (control versus cure) Discuss the role of emotional state on pain perception Challenge the view that pain is indicative of serious pathology The response to pain can be changed even if the pain signal cannot
Restructure bad thoughts/ reconceptualisation	Teach the individual to identify negative or distorted thoughts (e.g. *I can't stand the pain, it overwhelms me, there is nothing that I can do to relieve my pain*) Replace with more adaptive thoughts (*I can deal with this pain, I have done it before and I can do it again, if I plan my activities I can usually avoid increasing my pain*)
Relaxation/ biofeedback	Methods of relaxation include: • pre-recorded calming relaxation tapes • deep, controlled breathing exercises, often with a calming message to oneself on each outward breath • progressive muscle relaxation involving the voluntary tightening and systematic relaxation of individual muscles Biofeedback guided by machine feedback of physiological signs (temperature, muscle tension and galvanic skin resistance)
Coping skills	Attention distraction (watch TV, play a game, read) Reinterpretation of pain sensations (think of warmth or tickling) Positive self-coping statements (*I can deal with this, I have managed before, it will pass soon*) Prayer (*I pray to God and I know my faith will help*) Increased activity (*I move, I start an enjoyable activity*) Guided imagery (*I imagine that I am sitting on a warm beach, I can hear the calming waves break on to the beach, I can smell the salt air and feel the wind through my hair*)

Table 15.3

Psychological therapies for managing persistent pain in older adults—cont'd

COMPONENTS OF THERAPY	DESCRIPTION AND EXAMPLES
Problem solving	Adaptive problem solving, identification of the true problem, considering alternative modes of action, benefits and risks of alternatives , assessment of success, reformulation of new strategies, pace activity and break tasks into smaller, more manageable fragments
Behaviour reactivation/ operant conditioning	Reward for engaging in healthy behaviour Encourage gradual increase in meaningful activities according to pre-set goals and ignore maladaptive or disruptive pain-associated behaviours
Other skills that may be applicable to certain residents	Improved communication skills, social interaction, stress management, sleep hygiene, anger management, conflict resolution, marital counselling, cognitive therapy for depression, anxiety or fear-avoidance

Adapted with permission from the Australian Pain Society 2005.

aims of cognitive treatment are to educate the person regarding the strong interrelationship between thoughts, emotions and the consequent levels of pain and suffering. A reconceptualisation of such thoughts and providing alternative and more effective coping strategies (e.g. positive self-coping statements, reinterpreting sensations) constitute the main treatment approach. The person is encouraged to take an active role in this process and to accept responsibility for the pain and its impact, rather than being regarded as a passive victim. Typically, a multidimensional model of pain is presented and is contrasted with the sensory/physiologic model in which all pain is seen as equating to tissue damage. This leads to a better understanding of the importance of psychological states, such as fear, anxiety, depression and helplessness, in worsening the pain experience. It also helps to demonstrate the ability of the individual to change the cognitive and emotional components of pain even if the sensory aspects remain unchanged. Cognitive methods are seldom given in isolation and may incorporate relaxation therapy, biofeedback, guided imagery exercises and stress-reduction techniques.

Pain behaviours such as limping, using a walking aid, groaning, inactivity and medication use can be either operant or respondent in nature. Respondent behaviour refers to the responses elicited directly by a painful input, while operant behaviour is that which becomes reinforced by various social, environmental and other non-pain influences. The main goal of behaviour therapy is to reduce operant pain behaviours by offering rewards for healthy choices and for meeting preset behavioural goals related to exercise and reactivation. An explicit contract is usually made with the person to achieve realistic goals for increased activity, a reduction in excessive medication use and increased social interaction. Analgesic medication is usually administered on a time-contingent schedule (using around-the-clock analgesia rather than as required) and in conjunction with staff, friends and relatives, positive reinforcement is given for successfully achieving preset goals and all other maladaptive behaviour is ignored. Aspects of both cognitive and behavioural treatments have been combined into a cognitive behavioural approach that has gradually evolved into the mainstay of psychological therapy for managing persistent pain.

It is important to recognise that cognitive behaviour therapy is more than just a collection of cognitive and behavioural coping methods. To be effective, therapy must be given in a structured and systematic fashion (Kerns et al 2001, Turk & Meichenbaum 2000, Turner & Keefe 1999). The important principles include some initial sessions devoted to a full discussion about the historical, physical, psychosocial and treatment aspects of the pain problem. Educational information on pain and its consequences is provided as well as an explanation of cognitive behavioural approaches and likely treatment gains. This is followed by a reconceptualisation of maladaptive thoughts, new skills acquisition with cognitive and behavioural rehearsal as well as later sessions on the maintenance of treatment gains and how to prevent and cope with future flare-ups and setbacks (Kerns et al 2001, Turk & Meichenbaum 2000, Turner & Keefe 1999). Moreover, there is a systematic structure within each individual treatment session comprising a review of material presented in previous sessions, training and education in a new concept or skill and consolidation and practice of the new skill. Without this type of formal educational structure, many of the described techniques are likely to be less effective (Kerns et al 2001, Turk & Meichenbaum 2000, Turner & Keefe 1999).

Numerous cohort studies have demonstrated the benefits of cognitive-behavioural therapy for the management of chronic pain disorders in older adults (e.g. Sorkin et al 1990, Middaugh et al 1988, see Gibson et al 1996 for review). Significant reductions in pain severity, levels of self-rated disability, depression, anxiety and mood disturbance as well as reduced utilisation of healthcare resources has been reported. Increased coping skills, engagement in social activity and an overall improvement in quality of life are also said to result. There have also been some randomised controlled trials demonstrating the efficacy of cognitive behaviour therapy when administered to older adults living in the community (Ersek et al 2003, Keefe et al 1990, Puder 1988) and one trial conducted in a nursing home setting (Cook 1998). A cognitive behavioural program given to residents over 10 weekly group sessions was shown to be efficacious in reducing pain and pain-related disability when compared with an attention/social support control group. The treatment effects were maintained at four months follow-up. The program involved two sessions of education and reconceptualisation of pain, five sessions dealing with behavioural and cognitive coping skills (including progressive relaxation, imagery and attention diversion) and finally, three sessions of skills consolidation and problem-solving techniques. Note that several participants had cognitive impairment.

Despite strong scientific evidence in support of cognitive behavioural approaches for pain management in older people (Ersek et al 2003, Keefe et al 1990, Puder 1988), including those from a residential care setting (Cook 1998), this type of therapy is rarely used for older people with bothersome pain.

PHYSICAL THERAPIES

There is a wide range of non-pharmacological strategies that involve physical therapies. Exercise is often the first choice of physical therapy for older adults with chronic pain and can provide pain relief through disease modification as well as delivering beneficial effects on physical functioning and mood. When correctly administered, physical exercise programs have negligible adverse risk.

Two types of strengthening exercises, isotonic and isometric, are applicable to older people and are particularly suitable for those with chronic musculoskeletal pain (the most common type of persistent in this population). Isotonic and isometric exercise is much better suited than aerobic exercise in older people with pain because of the typical diminished capacity in functional performance. Evidence strongly supports the use of strengthening exercises, especially isotonic exercises, for improved pain management. Isotonic exercises have been shown to reduce the intensity of pain in older people with musculoskeletal disorders by about 30 per cent (Fransen et al 2002, 2003). They also improve the mood of older people with depression (Huang et al 2003, Singh et al 1997), including people with high levels of comorbidity (Singh et al 2001). These results are comparable to aerobic exercise, although it may be more difficult to ensure compliance with strengthening programs in this population (Penninx et al 2002).

Frail older people can also achieve very substantial increases in strength and associated improvements in functional capacity with isotonic exercises (Binder et al 2002, Fiatarone et al 1990, 1994, Timonen et al 2002). Isotonic exercises involve resisted contractions of major muscle groups through a prescribed joint range. This requires effort if high levels of resistance are used. However, low numbers of repetitions mean that a program targeting a circumscribed number of major muscle groups can be performed within a short time, making direct supervision feasible. The major effect of isotonic exercises is to increase the maximum force that a muscle can generate although aerobic-type exercises; they are also more efficacious in increasing muscle action endurance. Isotonic exercises usually consist of a few repetitions of muscle contraction against a high level of resistance. Ideally, three or four repetitions of movements against resistance of 70–80% of the weight that can be lifted in a single repetition should be used for isotonic exercises in order to ensure the maximal increase in muscle power. Isometric exercises require static contractions of major muscle groups without joint movement and are usually performed within the mid-range of the muscle. Isometric exercises have significantly less impact on pain reports (Sullivan et al 2001) than isotonic exercises but are well tolerated by older people just beginning an exercise program. Aerobic exercise programs can have a role in pain treatment, but their strenuous nature and risk of adverse reactions in older people can be problematic and they appear no more effective at pain relief than strengthening-type (isometric and isotonic) exercise programs.

PHYSICAL MODALITIES

The application of physical modalities, such as superficial heat/ cold, vibration and transcutaneous electrical nerve stimulation (TENS), are designed to reduce pain intensity. Using physical modalities with older adults who cannot give accurate feedback about the sensations produced carries the risk of tissue damage and/or additional pain. Further, the modalities described in this section all involve stimulation of cutaneous and subcutaneous tissues and may, therefore, exacerbate pain if applied to sensitive skin. It is important to remember that skin sensitivity (i.e. hyperalgesia) can increase dramatically in association with painful conditions such as diabetic neuropathy or post-herpetic neuralgia and this needs to be taken into account when considering such superficial physical treatment modalities. Most physical modalities for pain relief have relatively brief periods of efficacy and are not practical for managing more persistent pain, although repeated applications may be warranted for a limited time during acute pain episodes or exacerbation of persistent pain states.

Superficial heat

The application of superficial heat has strong anecdotal support for managing acute and persistent musculoskeletal pain (Chou et al 2007). While superficial heat may be well tolerated, any associated reduction in pain is usually transient. Moreover, all methods that increase skin temperature carry some risk of superficial burns. Therefore, older adults must have intact thermal sensation and adequate communicative and cognitive abilities to be able to provide accurate feedback on the degree of warmth experienced when the superficial heat is applied. Research suggests that superficial heat should not be applied within 48 hours of pain developing as it may increase swelling and hyperalgesia (increased tenderness) (Metules 2007). Heat packs can be a helpful preventive treatment when activities are likely to provoke incident-related pain or when there is likely to be an exercise-induced exacerbation of musculoskeletal pain.

Superficial cold

The application of a cold pack to a site of injury or disease has been shown to assist with the management of acute pain states and may have some role with treating an exacerbation of an inflammatory persistent pain condition (Meeusen & Leivens 1986). However, the duration of relief associated with superficial cooling does not support its use as a regular pain-relieving technique. Its frequent application requires active and ongoing management with little expectation of improvements in the chronic pain experiences of older people (Brosseau et al 2003, Robinson et al 2002). Prolonged cooling of the skin also has the potential to cause tissue damage and is not well tolerated by most people. The brief local reductions in pain perception associated with prolonged or intense cooling are less apparent in older people than in younger people (Washington et al 2000) and so superficial cold therapies are not recommended as a chronic pain relieving modality in older adults.

Vibration

Vibration is considered as a potentially useful treatment strategy for managing pain, based on the implications of the gate control theory of pain in which activation of large nerve fibres (touch) can inhibit small nerve (pain) fibre function. However, there is a paucity of empirical evidence to support the use of vibration in managing clinical pain states. Under experimental conditions, vibration produces small reductions in pain ratings, but these are reversed within seconds of the vibration ceasing (Ward et al 1996). The delivery of vibration requires dedicated equipment and is not recommended as a pain relieving modality in aged populations.

Transcutaneous electrical nerve stimulation

TENS involves the application of a low-frequency current ($\approx$2 to 100 Hz) via electrodes that are taped or self-adhere to the skin, and this technique has demonstrated efficacy for pain relief in a variety of clinical conditions common in older adults, including osteoarthritis and post-herpetic neuralgia. A battery-operated TENS unit is portable, fits into a pocket or clips onto a belt, and does not interfere with usual functional activities. TENS electrodes should not be positioned where they may interfere with cardiac pacemakers, nor over the carotid sinuses. TENS can relieve pain for minutes or even hours when used for one hour daily (Cheing et al 2003) and may be applied for many hours consecutively if pain persists throughout the day and night. The capacity of TENS to be used for long periods with minimal supervision makes this technique a viable option for pain management of aged care residents. While providing guarded support for TENS, meta-analytic reviews have noted substantial methodological shortcomings in many studies (Carroll et al 2001, Milne et al 2001, Osiri et al 2000). Nonetheless, the simplicity and intrinsic safety of TENS suggests that a trial of the technique is warranted in most older people with bothersome pain to assess its efficacy, provided that the individual has adequate cognitive capacity to understand the purpose of the unusual sensations being experienced. In order to have a therapeutic effect, it is recommended that TENS be used to produce a strong but comfortable tingling sensation that exceeds the perception threshold, although optimal TENS parameters for pain relief are yet to be determined. Excessive levels are uncomfortable and can be painful. Stimulation parameters should be determined by trial and error, balancing efficacy (assessed with serial pain measures) and tolerance of the evoked sensations. Low-frequency (2–5 Hz, 'acupuncture-like TENS') and high-frequency TENS (80–100 Hz) have provided comparable levels of analgesia (Carroll et al 2001). Electrode adhesives can occasionally cause skin reactions, but these are typically minor and can easily be treated.

> ## There are many non-pharmacological approaches to pain management that are often successful and rarely used in older people.

In summary, there is an extensive range of pharmacological, non-pharmacological and complementary-alternative therapies that are widely used for managing persistent pain, with varying degrees of scientific evidence to support their use. The individual suffering with persistent pain is only interested in whether the therapy is effective, accessible, affordable and safe. It is therefore reasonable to trial a range of different treatment options to find the best outcome for the person with bothersome, persistent pain.

MULTIDISCIPLINARY APPROACHES TO PAIN MANAGEMENT

There are a small number of people who remain distressed by pain despite standard treatment approaches. These individuals should be considered for referral to a multidisciplinary pain management clinic, or a pain specialist who has access to other health disciplines.

The first multidisciplinary pain management clinic was established in Seattle in the 1960s by Dr John Bonica. The model has been adopted in thousands of sites worldwide and subsequent research has revealed that this is the preferred approach for people with pain refractory to standard approaches. In the past many pain clinics did not admit older people or did not have the resources to deal with their special needs. Concern that older people do not gain the same benefit as younger cohorts became a barrier to accessing these services. Helme et al (1996) established the first multidisciplinary pain management clinic catering exclusively for older people in Melbourne, Australia in 1986, and then a second clinic the following year. There are now a number of multidisciplinary pain management clinics specialising in older adults in Victoria and several clinics overseas have now adopted this general model. These clinics represent a hybrid of the practices of pain medicine and geriatric medicine, with a strong emphasis on a multidisciplinary approach being a common theme of both disciplines.

Most of the multidisciplinary pain clinics in Victoria have operated with specialist clinicians in geriatric medicine, and at times one other medical specialty, together with nursing and four other allied health specialties, including clinical psychology, physiotherapy, occupational therapy and pharmacy. All clinicians are trained in aged care and have expertise in evaluating people with dementia and other concurrent illnesses. Access to other healthcare disciplines and medical specialists is readily available upon referral, but these do not constitute part of the core staffing of most clinics as they do not attend the interdisciplinary team meetings.

There is now good evidence in support of the efficacy of multidisciplinary pain management clinics in treating bothersome persistent pain in older adults (Gibson et al 1996 for review, Ersek et al 2003). The question is no longer whether older people gain as much benefit from a pain clinic as younger cohorts but whether the benefit older people obtain is worthwhile. The answer to this question is affirmative. However, clinics that do not modify their programs to suit the abilities and requirements of older people cannot expect to achieve the equivalent level of benefit (Katz et al 2005).

One may question why multidisciplinary pain management clinics for older people have proven to be more effective than standard care. This is possibly related to four factors:

- All staff have expertise in aged care as well as pain management.
- The structure of the clinic allows more time to be spent on assessment, management, education of the person and family, and monitoring adherence to the management plan. Unlike a primary care setting the clinic does not become distracted by other problems unrelated to the pain. The person continues to attend the pain clinic but may be referred elsewhere for the unrelated problem.
- Education forms an important part of pain management—all members of the team impart the same message.
- Probably the single most important factor is the multidisciplinary approach.

CONCLUSION

Pain is common in older people wherever they live. Pain is under-recognised and undertreated in older people, especially those with dementia. Self-report of pain is considered the gold standard assessment and despite the loss of verbal skills many people with dementia can still report pain.

Although the need for better assessment tools is urgent, there are a number of valid and reliable tools available. It is important to assess pain during functioning and not just in a chair/ bed. It is also necessary to recognise and assess the different causes and types of pain and previous medication before commencing new ones. Non-pharmacological interventions are also available and there is some evidence of their effectiveness. Interdisciplinary care assessment and treatment is more likely to achieve a positive outcome.

Complete elimination of persistent pain is unusual, even with the resources available in a pain management clinic. Misperceptions must be dealt with, for example: that the pain means that ongoing damage is occurring; that activity is detrimental; or a reluctance to use analgesics unless the pain is severe. Realistic goals must be negotiated at the outset. A mismatch between the person's expectations and that of the staff will lead to an unsuccessful outcome. An important step is to move the goal of treatment away from the pain intensity alone, for instance, improved function such as walking distance before being stopped by pain, reduced medication side effects, improved mood and better sleep are more likely to be achieved. People who have undergone a successful pain management program often comment that they still have pain but that it no longer worries them.

Reflective questions

1. Opioid patches are the first line of treatment for very severe acute pain—true or false? Why?

2. Many staff refuse to give opioids to older people as they fear addiction or that they are hastening death and do not want to give 'the last dose'—how would you respond to these concerns?

3. People with dementia often cannot verbalise pain—what strategies could be used to assess pain in these situations?

References

American Geriatrics Society, 2009. Panel on Pharmacological Management of Persistent Pain in Older Persons. Pharmacological management of persistent pain in older persons. Journal of the American Geriatrics Society 57 (8), 1331–1346.

Analgesic Expert Group, 2007. Therapeutic guidelines: analgesic. Version 5. Therapeutic Guidelines Limited, Melbourne.

Australian Pain Society, 2005. Pain in residential aged care facilities: management strategies. APS, Sydney.

Binder, E.F., Schechtman, K.B., Ehsani, A.A., et al., 2002. Effects of exercise training on frailty in community-dwelling older adults: results of a randomized, controlled trial. Journal of the American Geriatrics Society 50 (12), 1921–1928.

Blyth, F.M., March, L.M., Brnabic, A.J., et al., 2001. Chronic pain in Australia: a prevalence study. Pain 89 (2–3), 127–134.

Brosseau, L., Yonge, K., Robinson, V., et al., 2003. Thermotherapy for treatment of osteoarthritis. Cochrane Database Systematic Reviews (4), CD004522.

Carragee, E.J., 2005. Clinical practice. Persistent low back pain. New England Journal of Medicine 352 (18), 1891–1898.

Carroll, D., Moore, R.A., McQuay, H.J., et al., 2001. Transcutaneous electrical nerve stimulation (TENS) for chronic pain. Cochrane Database Systematic Reviews (3), CD003222.

Cheing, G.L., Tsui, A.Y., Lo, S.K., et al., 2003. Optimal stimulation duration of TENS in the management of osteoarthritic knee pain. Journal of Rehabilitation Medicine 35 (2), 62–68.

Chou, R., Huffman, L.H.; American Pain Society; American College of Physicians, 2007. Nonpharmacologic therapies for acute and chronic low back pain: a review of the evidence for an American Pain Society/American College of Physicians clinical practice guideline. Annals of Internal Medicine 47 (7), 492–504.

Cole, L., Farrell, M.J., Tress, B., et al., 2006. Pain sensitivity and fMRI pain related brain activity in persons with Alzheimer's disease. Brain 129, 2957–2965.

Cook, A.J., 1998. Cognitive-behavioral pain management for elderly nursing home residents. Journals of Gerontology B Psychological Sciences Social Sciences 53 (1), P51–59.

Ersek, M., Turner, J.A., McCurry, S.M., et al., 2003. Efficacy of a self-management group intervention for elderly persons with chronic pain. Clinical Journal of Pain 19, 156–167.

Farrell, M.J., Katz, B., Helme, R.D., 1996. The impact of dementia on the pain experience. Pain 67 (1), 7–15.

Feldt, K.S., Ryden, M.B., Miles, S., 1998. Treatment of pain in cognitively impaired compared with cognitively intact older patients with hip-fracture. J Am Geriatr Soc 46 (9), 1079–1085.

Ferrell, B.A., 1995. Pain evaluation and management in the nursing home. Annals of Internal Medicine 123, 681–687.

Ferrell, B.A., 2003. Acute and chronic pain. In: Cassell, C.K. (Ed.), Geriatric medicine: an evidence-based approach. SpringerVerlag, New York.

Ferrell, B.A., Ferrell, B.R., Rivera, L., 1995. Pain in cognitively impaired nursing home patients. Journal of Pain and Symptom Management 10 (8), 591–598.

Fiatarone, M.A., Marks, E.C., Ryan, N.D., et al., 1990. High-intensity strength training in nonagenarians. Effects on skeletal muscle. Journal of American Medical Association 263 (22), 3029–3034.

Fiatarone, M.A., O'Neill, E.F., Ryan, N.D., et al., 1994. Exercise training and nutritional supplementation for physical frailty in very elderly people. New England Journal of Medicine 330 (25), 1769–1775.

Finnerup, N.B., Sindrup, S.H., Jensen, T.S., 2010. The evidence for pharmacological treatment of neuropathic pain. Pain 150 (3), 573–581.

Flor, H., Turk, D., 2011. Chronic pain: an integrated biobehavioral approach. IASP Press, Seattle.

Fransen, M., McConnell, S., Bell, M., 2002. Therapeutic exercise for people with osteoarthritis of the hip or knee. A systematic review. Journal of Rheumatology 29 (8), 1737–1745.

Fransen, M., McConnell, S., Bell, M., 2003. Exercise for osteoarthritis of the hip or knee. Cochrane Database Systematic Review (3), CD004286.

Gagliese, L., Katz, J., 2003. Age differences in postoperative pain are scale dependent: a comparison of measures of pain intensity and quality in younger and older surgical patients. Pain 103, 11–20.

Gagnier, J.J., vanTulder, M., Berman, B., et al., 2006. Herbal medicine for low back pain. Cochrane Database Systematic Review.

Gibson, S.J., 1997. Measurement of mood states in elderly adults. Journals of Gerontology B Psychological Sciences Social Sciences 52B, P167–P174.

Gibson, S.J., 2007. The IASP Global Year Against Pain in Older Persons: highlighting the current status and future perspectives in geriatric pain. Expert Reviews in Neurotherapeutics, 7 (6), 627–635.

Gibson, S.J., Chambers, C., 2003. Pain across the life span: a developmental perspective. In: Hadjistavropoulos, T., Craig, K.D. (Eds.), Pain: psychological perspectives. Lawrence Erlbaum, Mahwah, NJ, pp. 113–154.

Gibson, S.J., Farrell, M.J., Katz, B., et al., 1996. Multidisciplinary management of chronic nonmalignant pain in older adults. In: Ferrell, B.A., Ferrell, B.R. (Eds.), Pain in the elderly. IASP Press, Seattle, WA, pp. 91–101.

Gibson, S.J., Katz, B., Corran, T.M., et al., 1994. Pain in older persons. Disability and Rehabilitation 16 (3), 127–139.

Gibson, S.J., Lussier, D., 2012. Prevalence and relevance of pain in older persons. Pain.

Hadjistavropoulos, T., 2005. Pain assessment in older persons with verbal communication skills. In: Gibson, S.J., Weiner, D.K. (Eds.), Pain in older persons, progress in pain research and management, vol. 35. IASP Press, Seattle, pp. 135–151.

Hadjistavropoulos, T., Herr, K., Turk, D.C., et al., 2007. An interdisciplinary expert consensus statement on assessment of pain in older persons. Clinical Journal of Pain 23 (Suppl 1), S1–S43.

Helme, R.D., Gibson, S.J., 2001. The epidemiology of pain in elderly people. Clinics in Geriatric Medicine 17 (3), 417–432.

Helme, R.D., Katz, B., Gibson, S.J., et al., 1996. Multidisciplinary pain clinics for older people. Do they have a role? Clinics in Geriatric Medicine 12 (3), 563–582.

Herr, K., 2005. Assessing pain in older persons with severe limitations in ability to communicate. In: Gibson, S.J., Weiner, D.K. (Eds.), Pain in older persons, progress in pain research and management, vol. 35. IASP Press, Seattle, pp. 111–133.

Herr, K., Coyne, P.J., Key, T., et al., 2006. American Society for Pain Management Nursing. Pain assessment in the nonverbal patient: position statement with clinical practice recommendations. Pain Management Nursing 7 (2), 44–52.

Herr, K., Spratt, K., Mobily, P., Richardson, G., 2004. Pain intensity assessment in older adults: Use of experimental pain to compare psychometric properties and usability of selected pain scales with younger adults. Clinical Journal of Pain 20, 207–219.

Herr, K., Spratt, K.F., Garand, L., et al., 2007. Evaluation of the Iowa pain thermometer and other selected pain intensity scales in younger and older adult cohorts using controlled clinical pain: a preliminary study. Pain Med 8 (7), 585–600.

Horgas, A.L., Tsai, P.F., 1998. Analgesic drug prescription and use in cognitively impaired nursing home residents. Nursing Research 47 (4), 235–242.

Huang, M.H., Lin, Y.S., Yang, R.C., Lee, C.L., 2003. A comparison of various therapeutic exercises on the functional status of patients with knee osteoarthritis. Seminars in Arthritis and Rheumatology 32 (6), 398–406.

Husebo, B.S., Ballard, C., Sandvik, R., et al., 2011. Efficacy of treating pain to reduce behavioural disturbances in residents of nursing homes with dementia: cluster randomised clinical trial. BMJ 15 (343), d4065.

Jensen, M.P., Karoly, P., Braver, S., 1986. The measurement of clinical pain intensity: a comparison of six methods. Pain 27 (1), 117–126.

Jones, G.T., Macfarlane, G.A., 2005. Epidemiology of pain in older persons. In: Gibson, S.J., Weiner, D.K. (Eds.), Pain in older persons. IASP press, Seattle, WA, pp. 3–24.

Kalso, E., Edwards, J., Moore, R.A., et al., 2004. Opioids in chronic non-cancer pain: systematic review of efficacy and safety. Pain 112, 372–380.

Katz, B., Scherer, S. Gibson, S.J., 2005. Multidisciplinary pain management in older persons. In: Gibson, S.J. Wiener, D.K. (Eds.), Pain in older adults. IASP publications, Seattle, WA, pp. 309–328.

Keefe, F.J., Caldwell, D.S., Williams, D.A., et al., 1990. Pain coping skills training in the management of osteoarthritis knee pain: a comparative study. Behavior Therapy 21, 49–62.

Kerns, R.D., Otis, J.D., Marcus, K.S., 2001. Cognitive-behavioral therapy for chronic pain in the elderly. Clinics in Geriatric Medicine 17, 503–523.

Kovach, C.R., Logan, B.R., Noonan, P.E., et al., 2006. Effects of the Serial Trial Intervention on discomfort and behavior of nursing home residents with dementia. American Journal of Alzheimer's Disease & Other Dementias 21 (3), 147–155.

Kovach, C.R., Simpson, M.R., Joosse, L., et al., 2012. Comparison of the effectiveness of two protocols for treating nursing home residents with advanced dementia. research in gerontological Nursing 17, 1–13.

Larson, A.M., Polson, J., Fontana, R.J., et al., 2005. Acute liver failure study group. Acetaminophen-induced acute liver failure: results of a United States multicentre, prospective study. Hepatology 42, 1364–1372.

Leong, I.Y., Farrell, M.J., Helme, R.D., et al., 2007. The relationship between medical comorbidity and self-rated pain, mood disturbance, and function in older people with chronic pain. The Journal of Gerontology: Biological Sciences and Medical Sciences 62 (5), 550–555.

Meeusen, R., Lievens, P., 1986. The use of cryotherapy in sports injuries. Sports Medicine 3 (6), 398–414.

Mendoza, T.R., Chen, C., Brugger, A., et al., 2004. The utility and validity of the Modified Brief Pain inventory in a multiple-dose postoperative analgesic trial. Clinical Journal of Pain 20 (5), 357–362.

Menefee, L.A., Cohen, M.J., Anderson, W.R., et al., 2000. Sleep disturbance and nonmalignant chronic pain: a comprehensive review of the literature. Pain Medicine 1, 2–32.

Metules, T.J., 2007. Hands-on help. Hot and cold packs. RN 70 (1), 45–48.

Middaugh, S.J., Levin, R.B., Kee, W.G., et al., 1988. Chronic pain: its treatment in geriatric and younger patients. Archives Physical Medicine and Rehabilitation 69, 1021–1026.

Milne, S., Welch, V., Brosseau, L., et al., 2001. Transcutaneous electrical nerve stimulation (TENS) for chronic low back pain. Cochrane Database Systematic Reviews (2), CD003008.

Morrison, R.S., Siu, A.L., 2000. A comparison of pain: its treatment in advanced dementia and cognitively intact patients with hip fracture. Journal of Pain and Symptom Management 19, 240–248.

Niv, D., Devor, M., 2004. Chronic pain as a disease in its own right. Pain Practice 4 (3), 179–181.

Osiri, M., Welch, V., Brosseau, L., et al., 2000. Transcutaneous electrical nerve stimulation for knee osteoarthritis. Cochrane Database Systematic Reviews (4), CD002823.

Pautex, S., Herrmann, F., Le Lous, P., et al., 2005. Feasibility and reliability of four pain self-assessment scales and correlation with an observational rating scale in hospitalized elderly demented patients. The Journal of Gerontology: Biological Sciences and Medical Sciences 60, 524–529.

Penninx, B.W., Rejeski, W.J., Pandya, J., et al., 2002. Exercise and depressive symptoms: a comparison of aerobic and resistance exercise effects on emotional and physical function in older persons with high and low depressive symptomatology. Journals of Gerontology B Psychological Sciences Social Sciences 57 (2), P124–132.

Pesonen, A., Kauppila, T., Tarkkila, P., et al., 2009. Evaluation of easily applicable pain measurement tools for the assessment of pain in demented patients. Acta Anaesthesiol Scand. 53 (5), 657–664.

Pickering, G., Jourdan, D., Dubray, C., 2006. Acute versus chronic pain treatment in Alzheimer's disease. Eur J Pain 10 (4), 379–384.

Pirmohamed, M., James, S., Meakin, S., et al., 2004. Adverse drug reactions as cause of admission to hospital: prospective analysis of 18 820 patients. BMJ 329, 15–19.

Proctor, W.R., Hirdes, J.P., 2001. Pain and cognitive status among nursing home residents in Canada. Pain Research & Management 6 (3), 119–125.

Puder, R.S., 1988. Age analysis of cognitive-behavioural group therapy for chronic pain outpatients. Psychology and Aging 3, 204–207.

Robinson, V., Brosseau, L., Casimiro, L., et al., 2002. Thermotherapy for treating rheumatoid arthritis. Cochrane Database Systematic Reviews (2), CD002826.

Scherder, E.J., Bouma, A., 1997. Is decreased use of analgesics in Alzheimer disease due to a change in the affective component of pain? Alzheimer Disease and Associated Disorders 11 (3), 171–174.

Scherder, E.J., Herr, K., Pickering, G., et al., 2009. Pain in dementia. Pain 145 (3), 276–278.

Shega, J.W., Ersek, M., Herr, K., et al., 2010. The multidimensional experience of noncancer pain: does cognitive status matter? Pain Med 11 (11), 1680–1687.

Siddall, P.J., Cousins, M.J., 2004. Persistent pain as a disease entity: implications for clinical management. Anesthesia and Analgesia 99 (2), 510–520.

Silverstein, F.E., Faich, G., Goldstein, J.L., et al., 2000. Gastrointestinal toxicity with celecoxib vs nonsteroidal anti-inflammatory drugs for osteoarthritis and rheumatoid arthritis: the CLASS study: A randomized controlled trial. Celecoxib Long-term Arthritis Safety Study. Journal of the American Medical Association 284 (10), 1247–1255.

Singh, N.A., Clements, K.M., Fiatarone, M.A., 1997. A randomized controlled trial of progressive resistance training in depressed elders. The Journal of Gerontology: Biological Sciences and Medical Sciences 52 (1), M27–M35.

Singh, N.A., Clements, K.M., Singh, M.A., 2001. The efficacy of exercise as a long-term antidepressant in elderly subjects: a randomized, controlled trial. The Journal of Gerontology: Biological Sciences and Medical Sciences 56 (8), M497–M504.

Sorkin, B.A., Rudy, T.E., Hanlon, R.B., et al., 1990. Chronic pain in old and young patients: differences appear less important than similarities. The Journal of Gerontology: Biological Sciences and Medical Sciences 45 (2), P64–P68.

Sullivan, D.H., Wall, P.T., Bariola, J.R., et al., 2001. Progressive resistance muscle strength training of hospitalized frail elderly. American Journal of Physical Medicine and Rehabilitation 80 (7), 503–509.

Takai, Y., Yamamoto-Mitani, N., Okamoto, Y., et al., 2010. Pain Management Nursing 11 (4), 209–223.

Teno, J., Chloe, B., Mor, V., 2003. The prevalence and treatment of pain in US nursing homes. Center for Gerontology and Health Care Research, Brown University.

Theiler, R., Spielberger, J., Bischoff, H.A., et al., 2002. Clinical evaluation of the WOMAC 3.0 OA Index in numeric rating scale format using a computerized touch screen version. Osteoarthritis and Cartilage 10 (6), 479–481.

Timonen, L., Rantanen, T., Timonen, T.E., et al., 2002. Effects of a group-based exercise program on the mood state of frail older women after discharge from hospital. International Journal of Geriatric Psychiatry 17 (12), 1106–1111.

Towheed, T.E., Maxwell, L., Anastassiades, T.P., et al., 2006. Glucosamine therapy for treating osteoarthritis. Cochrane Database Systematic Reviews; CD023654.

Towheed, T., Maxwell, L., Anastassiades, T.P., et al., 2009. Glucosamine for osteoarthritis. Online. Available: http://summaries.cochrane.org/CD002946/glucosamine-for-osteoarthritis, 7 Oct 2009.

Turk, D.C., Flor, H., 1999. Chronic pain: a biobehavioural perspective. In: Gatchel, R.J., Turk, D.C. (Eds.), Psychosocial factors in pain: critical perspectives. Guilford Press, New York, pp. 18–74.

Turk, D.C., Meichenbaum, D.H., 2000. A cognitive-behavioral approach to pain management. In: Melzack, R., Wall, P.D. (Eds.), Textbook of pain, third ed. Churchill-Livingstone, New York, pp. 1001–1009.

Turner, J.A., Keefe, F.J., 1999. Cognitive-behavioral therapy for chronic pain. In: Max, M. (Ed.), Pain 1999: an updated review (refresher course syllabus). IASP Press, Seattle, WA, pp. 523–531.

Van Spall, H.G., Toren, A., Kiss, A., et al., 2007. Eligibility criteria of randomized controlled trials published in high-impact general medical journals: a systematic sampling review. JAMA 297 (11), 1233–1240.

Ward, L., Wright, E., McMahon, S.B., 1996. A comparison of the effects of noxious and innocuous counterstimuli on experimentally induced itch and pain. Pain 64 (1), 129–138.

Washington, L.J., Gibson, S.J., Helme, R.D., 2000. Age-related differences in endogenous analgesia to repeated cold water immersion in human volunteers. Pain 89 (1), 89–96.

Weiner, D., Peterson, B., Keefe, F., 1999. Chronic pain-associated behaviors in the nursing home: resident versus caregiver perceptions. Pain 80, 577–588.

Weiner, D.K., Haggerty, C.L., Kritchevsky, S.B., et al., 2003. How does low back pain impact physical function in independent, well-functioning older adults? Evidence from the Health ABC Cohort and implications for the future. Pain Medicine 4 (4), 311–320.

Weiner, D.K., Rudy, T.E., Kim, Y.S., et al., 2004. Do medical factors predict disability in older adults with persistent low back pain? Pain 112 (1-2), 214–220.

Williamson, G.M., Schulz, R., 1992. Pain, activity restriction, and symptoms of depression among community-residing elderly adults. Journals of Gerontology A Biological Sciences and Medical Sciences 47 (6), B367–BB372.

Woods, B.M., Nicholas, M.K., Blyth, F., et al., 2010. Assessing pain in older people with persistent pain: the NRS is valid but only provides part of the picture. Journal of Pain 11 (12), 1259–1266.

Yong, H.H., Bell, R., Workman, B., et al., 2003. Psychometric properties of the Pain Attitudes Questionnaire (revised) in adult patients with chronic pain. Pain 104, 673–681.

Wood, B.M., Nicholas, M.K., Blyth, F., et al., 2010. The utility of the short version of the Depression Anxiety Stress Scales (DASS-21) in elderly patients with persistent pain: does age make a difference? Pain Medicine 11 (12), 1780–1790.

World Health Organization, 1990. Cancer pain relief and palliative care. (WHO Technical Report Series, 804). World Health Organization, Geneva.

Wynne, C.F., Ling, S.M., Remsburg, R., 2000. Comparison of pain assessment instruments in cognitively intact and cognitively impaired nursing home residents. Geriatric Nursing 21, 20–23.

CHAPTER 16

SEXUALITY, AGEING AND HEALTH PROFESSIONALS

Michael Bauer, Rhonda Nay and Elizabeth Beattie

Editors' comments

The importance of recognising older people as sexual beings and acknowledging the importance of sexuality in the lives of those with whom they care is a major challenge to health professionals. It is an area fraught with cultural, educational and social attitudes and beliefs that impinge on the way care is given to older people. Given the paucity of current research into this aspect of ageing, it is difficult for care staff to move beyond what they consider is best, based on their own knowledge and attitudes towards ageing and sexual expression. Self-reflection on one's own values, attitudes and beliefs is raised as a good starting point for discussion and clarification. Given that human beings seek meaning to create a quality of life it would seem that an expression of sexuality is an essential part of being human and something that cannot be ignored.

INTRODUCTION

Sexuality is a natural expression of human need and a key aspect of psychological health and wellbeing that continues throughout life and extends well beyond the reproductive years. Despite compelling evidence that refutes any notion that sexuality ceases to be of importance beyond a certain age, the subject is still largely ignored by many health professionals who fail to accept its significance to their practice. For health professionals working with older people, the topic of sexuality remains taboo and one of the last frontiers.

In this chapter we aim to raise the consciousness of the reader about sexuality and the sexual needs of older people. In doing so, we will explore a number of aspects related to sexuality that are significant to an understanding of this topic. Among these are the attitudes and beliefs we have about older people and sexuality, including myths and stereotypes, the factors that impact on older people's sexuality and sexual expression, and the role of health professionals. As has been noted elsewhere (Nay et al 2007), we are not advocating that all older people become 'sexy oldies' (Gott 2005b) or that health professionals encourage their clients to become more sexualised. What we urge is that all health professionals examine and confront their attitudes and prejudices, view the sexuality of older people as a legitimate area of consideration, and become more informed and more comfortable dealing with this topic.

 For health professionals working with older people, sexuality remains one of the last frontiers.

GRAPPLING WITH THE LAST FRONTIER: SOME CHALLENGES

As the population is rapidly growing older, the widely held view of ageing as a period of inevitable decline is giving way to a more positive discourse of ageing where older people are encouraged and supported to age well and age productively. Growing old is being aligned more with prosperity than paucity and government policy encourages older people to live happy, healthy and independent lives while also remaining actively engaged with the community. The new discourse on positive ageing attempts to redefine the popular belief that old age is sexless and tackles the traditional boundaries of what it means to be old by incorporating sexuality and sexual health as essential components for successful ageing (Brock & Jennings 2007, Henry & McNab 2003, Katz & Marshall 2003). According to Marshall (2010), sexual function is being increasingly taken to be an indicator of whether someone is ageing successfully.

 Sexuality and sexual health can be essential components for wellbeing in ageing.

For an older person, sexuality is a culmination of all the developmental processes and experiences in their life so far (Sharpe 2004). Given that increasing numbers of older people are living to be 100, sexuality will continue to be a factor of some significance for many years. For health professionals including doctors, nurses, social workers and other therapists, exploring this last frontier presents a number of challenges.

First, relative to other aspects of ageing, there is a dearth of empirical data about the sexual lives of older people, their sexuality needs (Brock & Jennings 2007) and how they conceptualise sexuality (Minichiello & Plummer 2004), with specific cultural or ethnic groups within the population still being particularly underrepresented in the research (Willert & Semans 2000). Over the past two decades we have seen some significant changes in society including shifts in social values, improvements in healthcare and increases in life expectancy. Stancil (2003) notes, for instance, that there are now more divorces among older people, and while marriage is still highly valued, changes in conservative attitudes have led to greater acceptance of a range of other lifestyle choices for people, including co-habitation, gay and lesbian relationships, and having multiple partners, in addition to not having a sexual partner at all. These developments, together with the increase in the longevity of people, challenge the relevance of much of the earlier research (Kinsey et al 1948, 1953, Masters & Johnson 1970, Pfeifer et al 1968, Pfeifer & Davis 1972) to the sexuality of older people today (Sharpe 2004).

Second, there is very little published material available to guide practice and policy in this area or guideline documents that can assist staff to address the sexuality needs of older people in the healthcare setting (including those with dementia) are rare and often inadequate (Bauer et al 2009, Everett 2007, Shuttleworth et al 2010). Many residential aged care facilities find it challenging responding to residents' sexuality and find it a source of concern, yet Australian residential aged care accreditation standards do not at this time require facilities to develop policies or provide staff training in this area. A survey of all Australian residential aged care facilities in 2011 found that 59% reported that their staff had never attended any education or training on sexuality or sexual health (McAuliffe et al, unpublished data). As a result, aged care staff often respond to older people's expressions of sexuality in an informal and ad hoc manner (Shuttleworth et al 2010).

There is also very little information available for older people who may be relocating to an aged care facility. A recent census of more than 800 residential aged care facilities was conducted in Victoria to uncover the prevalence of information about issues of sexuality, intimacy and the maintenance or establishment of relationships and how this information was couched (Bauer et al 2009). Less than 3% of facilities that responded were found to have any information available for prospective residents that addressed the issues of love, sex or intimacy in aged care.

The third reason why sexuality poses a challenge to health professionals is because talking about human sexuality is still largely taboo, even though depictions of sexuality are often very public in Western society. The majority of health professionals are reluctant to discuss sexuality issues with older people (Dyer & das Nair 2012) because of embarrassment, fear or discomfort (Andrews & Piterman 2007, Burd et al 2006, Gott et al 2004a, 2004b, Horden & Street 2007, Jones et al 2005, Magnan et al 2005). Many lack both knowledge and training in this area, so it is not surprising that the majority will avoid discussing this topic and will employ a range of avoidance strategies not to do so. If the subject does arise, many health professionals will try to limit the interaction to a level with which they feel comfortable (Horden & Street 2007).

Talking about human sexuality is still largely taboo, even though depictions of sexuality are often very public.

Fourth, professionals who work with older people are also influenced by societal views (Gunderson et al 2005, Hillman 2000) and many share the prevalent stereotypical and erroneous beliefs about sexuality and older people (McAuliffe et al 2007). These beliefs portray older people as either not having sexual needs, being interested but no longer capable, or having long outlived such desires (Walz 2002). Dyer and das Nair (2012) found that health professionals are less likely to initiate discussions about sexuality with older people, in part because of the widespread view that they are 'asexual'. It is arguable whether health professionals harbour such misconceptions because of the nature of their work, which exposes them on a regular basis to sick and disabled individuals, thereby contributing to a biased view of old age (Gibson 1992), or whether the association between ageing and death in our society is so strong that we fear and deny any aspect of old age (including sexuality) because it reminds us of our mortality (Nelson 2005). Gott (2005b) suggests that judgments about sexuality and older people are so entrenched in the fabric of society, and so powerful, that no one is immune from the influence. Even government policy agendas and health researchers, she notes, have been known to overlook the sexual views of older people.

 Judgments about sexuality and older people are so entrenched in the fabric of society, and so powerful, that no one is immune from the influence.

How, then, can health professionals begin to dispel any ageist attitudes they may harbour and become more comfortable with the notion of the older person as a sexual being? Brock and Jennings (2007) propose that a useful starting point is self-reflection of one's own values, attitudes and beliefs. To be able to respond to the needs of older clients and be non-judgmental, health professionals first need to become aware of their own feelings and attitudes. Consider the following questions (modified from Hillman 2000) and think about your attitudes and how you react. Would you feel any differently if these questions pertained to someone aged 20?

- How do you feel about your ageing parents or grandparents still having sex, or masturbating?
- How do you feel about an 85-year-old person pleasuring themselves and masturbating to orgasm?
- How would you react when, in the course of your work, you encounter an older person masturbating?
- How do you feel about an older man viewing images of a naked woman? An older woman viewing images of a naked man? Would you feel any differently if the naked man/woman was of the same age/younger?
- How do you feel about a couple aged 70 holding hands? Cuddling? Kissing? Deep tongue kissing? Giving and/or receiving oral sex? How would you feel if this couple were a gay or lesbian couple?
- Can you imagine an older couple making love and enjoying it?

- Would you feel comfortable initiating a discussion about sexuality and intimacy needs with an older person? How would you feel discussing sexuality if the person informed you he was gay?
- How do you feel about an older person who pays for sex, or who is paid for sex?
- Would you feel comfortable discussing the use of a vibrator with an older woman? An older couple? Would you feel comfortable discussing condom use with an older man? How would you react if you had to discuss these topics with an older person?
- Have you ever worked anywhere that had a policy related to sexuality and lesbian, gay, bisexual, transgender and intersex (LGBTI) people?

SEXUALITY: MORE THAN SEX

Sexuality is a term that means different things to different people (Bauer et al 2007). How we think about and experience our sexuality and how 'we "are" and "do" in relation to sexuality is socially, culturally and ideologically shaped' (Heaphy 2007 p 196). It is not uncommon to find the term used in the literature to refer to what is really only one aspect of sexuality—that is, intercourse or oral sex (Lindau et al 2007). Much of the research still uses intercourse as the gold standard by which to judge older people's sexuality (Gott 2005b). Without detracting from the significance of intercourse, sexuality is much more than this.

 Without detracting from the significance of intercourse, sexuality is much more than this.

According to the World Health Organization (WHO) sexuality is a broad construct that is 'experienced and expressed in thoughts, fantasies, desires, beliefs, attitudes, values, behaviours, practices, roles and relationships' (WHO 2006 p 5). Sexuality has many dimensions and includes intimacy, body image, self-esteem, romance, physical closeness, touch, cuddling, kissing, hugging, self-gratification and social relationships (National Ageing Research Institute 2002, Nay 2004), as well as sexual desire and gender-role identity (Zeiss & Kasl-Godley 2001). Older people have described sexuality as feeling masculine and feminine, looking nice through grooming and clothes, enjoying sexually explicit magazines or movies, and talking 'dirty', as well as spending time with the opposite sex (Nay 2004).

SEXUALITY AND HEALTHCARE

Sexuality is a legitimate area of concern for health professionals because it is a key component of quality of life (Robinson & Molzahn 2007) and is linked to our physical, emotional, mental and social wellbeing (WHO 2006). Sexuality is important to the maintenance of healthy interpersonal relationships, self-concept and sense of integrity (Zanni et al 2003) as well as self-esteem and physical health (Zeiss & Kasl-Godley 2001). It forms an essential component of how we feel about ourselves, even when close to death (Horden & Street 2007,

Lemieux et al 2004). A study by Lindau and Gavrilova (2010) involving more than 3000 adults aged between 57 and 85 years concluded that sexual partnership, frequency of sexual activity, a good-quality sex life and interest in sex were positively associated with health among older people.

Because the ability to express one's sexuality is so closely associated with quality of life, health professionals have been encouraged to adopt a health promotion approach in relation to sexuality and older people (Henry & McNab 2003). A health promotion focus is about acknowledging and recognising the role that sexuality may play in an older person's life and, where appropriate, incorporating this aspect of the person's life into the plan of care. This means enabling the older person to express their sexuality, where this expression does not infringe on the right of others. A failure to consider sexuality may potentially harm self-image, social relationships and mental health (Hajjar & Kamel 2003, Willert & Semans 2000) and moreover lead to inequities in care (National Ageing Research Institute 2002).

 Health professionals are encouraged to adopt a health promotion approach in relation to sexuality and older people.

REPRESENTATIONS OF SEXUALITY: IMAGES AND STEREOTYPES

We live in a highly sexualised society. Our language is replete with sexual references and sexual expletives (Goldman & Bradley 2004) and we are confronted by images of scantily clad women, and to a lesser extent men, on television, at the movies, in magazines, on billboards and on the backs of buses. The salacious images that we see, however, reinforce the notion that sexuality is the domain of youth, since sexuality is nearly always represented in the context of the active young man or woman. These images help to shape and reinforce the beliefs society has about older people (Minichiello et al 2005), make it difficult to imagine that sexuality could be associated with older people and that they may also have sexual needs and desires.

In the absence of positive narratives about the sexual lives of older people, stereotypes are known to fill the void (Walz 2002) and the research shows that ageism is widespread within the medical field, particularly against the very old and those residing in long-term care (Gunderson et al 2005). Kay and Neely (1982) long ago pointed out five key stereotypes that underscore how the sexuality of older people was and continues to be perceived:

- Older people do not have sexual desires.
- Older people are not able to have sex even if they wanted to.
- Older people are too fragile and might hurt themselves if they attempt to have sex.
- Older people are physically unattractive and therefore undesirable.
- The notion of older people engaging in sex is perverse and shameful.

According to Huffstetler (2006), these depictions are embedded in our history where sexual activities were once deemed by the church to be exclusively 'of the flesh' and a private matter for purposes of procreation. Sexual activity beyond menopause (or for men, past the age of 50) was once viewed as sinful and perhaps foolish at best (Huffstetler 2006), and for some unlucky women was likely to be associated with witchcraft, since no man could possibly find an older woman attractive by any other means (Hillman 2000). The idea that reproduction gives sexuality legitimacy is still ingrained in society today and, as Gott (2005b) reminds us, marginalises older people, since without the imperative of reproduction, sexuality in the context of older people is not seen to have any real purpose.

Sexual activities were once deemed by the church to be exclusively 'of the flesh' and a private matter for purposes of procreation.

Just as historical attitudes can influence societal attitudes (Huffstetler 2006), the way society views the sexuality of older people can, in turn, influence the way many older people themselves view their sexuality (Gott 2005b). For one, many older people in their 70s, 80s and 90s who were raised in an era of conservative Judeo–Christian values and social mores, may find it very difficult to openly discuss sexuality. This generation grew up at a time when open discussion of sexuality was not the norm, sexual knowledge was not freely available, and the only form of appropriate sexual pleasuring was thought to be sexual intercourse (Brock & Jennings 2007). Older gay men and lesbians, it should be noted, may find it difficult to discuss sexuality not only because there may still be some lack of acceptance of gay and lesbian people but because homosexuality was illegal when they were growing up and secrecy became a part of their way of life (Fannin 2006). It is also not uncommon for older people to internalise negative social attitudes and share the view that sexual needs and desires are unnatural and unnecessary in old age. Kass (1981) refers to this acceptance of the mainstream view by older people as *geriatric sexuality breakdown syndrome* since, when an older person subscribes to this view, over time their enjoyment of sexuality and arousal wanes, and in some cases disappears altogether. For health professionals this phenomenon may be significant, since it can in some older people lead to a loss of identity, social skills and self-esteem, and result in feelings of apathy, guilt and depression (Kass 1981).

SEXUALITY AND OLDER PEOPLE: AN EMERGING ISSUE

There is a growing public awareness of older people's sexuality and the once common image of the asexual older person is slowly being recast in a new light. This shift in culture is evident by the increasing popularity of films, television commercials and theatrical performances that portray older people as sexual beings. In 2007 a mainstream film about a woman with Alzheimer's disease who becomes romantically involved with another nursing home resident (*Away From Her*) was released. This was followed the next year by *Cloud 9,* a movie portraying a woman's sexual affair many years after menopause. Also at this time a home loan commercial depicting an older couple in various embraces and states of undress was aired on Australian public television, and a play (*Half Life*) about a couple who fall in love in a nursing home was performed in Melbourne. Stories about older people's sexuality are also becoming more common in mainstream newspapers. In 2012 *The Age* newspaper published a full feature article 'An age of desire', canvassing the issue of sexuality and older people living in residential aged care. In the United States (US), television advertisements for Viagra have become common (Huffstetler 2006), suggesting that advertisers at least believe older men are concerned about their sexual ability. These relatively recent portrayals paint older people as not only sexually desirable but also sexually active.

There is also a growing recognition of the need for further education for health professionals and older people alike in this area. Alzheimer's Australia and Family Planning New South Wales (NSW), for example, have both developed education programs that address the issue of older people's sexuality and sexual health. There are also myriad websites such as www.safersex4seniors.org aimed at providing information about sexuality to older people themselves.

There have been a number of catalysts for the emergence of older people's sexuality into the public arena. Marshall (2012) suggests that it is the increasing medicalisation of older people's sexuality that has propelled it into the mainstream. A focus on sexual dysfunction and the advent of highly successful pharmaceuticals such as Viagra, Levitra and Cialis to enhance male erectile function has restored men's sexual vigour and affirmed the possibility of sexual performance at any age. Kingsberg (2002) refers to this phenomenon as 'Viagratization'.

The other driving force that is beginning to shape future conceptualisations of older people and sexuality is the 'baby boomer' generation. Baby boomers were born between 1946 and 1964 and are frequently credited with bringing about the sexual revolution of the 1960s and 1970s (Chandler et al 2004). The baby boomers are now reaching retirement age and this generation is not known for passively accepting lifestyles handed down by previous generations (Kingsberg 2002). It is likely that individuals of this generation will be far less accepting of the social mores that governed sexual practices, sex outside marriage and multiple sexual partners than the current cohort of older people (Stancil 2003). While some will undoubtedly hold negative views about these topics, this generation grew up in a time when it was considered more acceptable to discuss sexuality among one's peers (Hillman 2000).

OLDER PEOPLE AND SEXUAL PRACTICES

Research has consistently shown that sexual activity remains important for many older people, including those living in residential aged care (Bauer et al 2007, 2012), even though there is a gradual decline in the frequency of activity compared with the younger years. Sexual desire and the capacity for sexual activity can exist well into the 90s (Bretschneider & McCoy 1988, Hyde et al 2010). It is beyond the scope of this chapter to review all the research in this area; however, we will highlight some of the key research findings in order to demonstrate the extent to which common societal attitudes reflect the actual sexual behaviours, activities and interests of the older population.

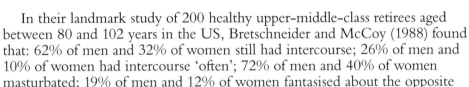

Research has consistently shown that sexual activity remains important for many older people.

In their landmark study of 200 healthy upper-middle-class retirees aged between 80 and 102 years in the US, Bretschneider and McCoy (1988) found that: 62% of men and 32% of women still had intercourse; 26% of men and 10% of women had intercourse 'often'; 72% of men and 40% of women masturbated; 19% of men and 12% of women fantasised about the opposite sex; and 53% of men and 25% of women had a regular sex partner.

Bergstrom-Walan and Nielsen (1990) surveyed 1574 randomly selected people between the ages of 60 and 80 (response rate 32.3%). They found that men were more sexual than women at all ages and that sexual interest and activity decreased significantly between 75 and 80 years of age. Despite this reported decline, they also found that a significant number of older people (approximately one-quarter of married couples aged 75–80 years) reported having intercourse at least 'sometime each month'.

In another study, Matthias et al (1997) conducted a telephone interview with 1216 people between the ages of 70 and 94. They reported that approximately one-third of the participants had participated in sexual activity in the last month and that two-thirds were 'satisfied' with their 'level of sexual activity'. The researchers also found that many older people were not aware about the physiological changes that accompany the ageing process and how these can impact on sexual function. Interviews with 3005 adults aged between 57 and 85 living in the community (Lindau et al 2007) also showed a decline in sexual activity with age. Many older people continued to be sexually active, however. Of the 75–85 age group, 54% of sexually active people reported having sex two to three times per month and 23% reported having sex once a week or more. Approximately one-third (31%) of this age group reported engaging in oral sex. Women were less likely to be involved in an intimate relationship with increasing age. An Australian study by Hyde et al (2010) involving 3274 men aged 75–95, similarly found that half the men considered sex to be important and one-third reported being sexually active.

Another study involving 474 women aged 40–80 years (Howard et al 2006), similarly demonstrated that while sexual interest and activity is likely to decline with age, some older women continue to have sexual thoughts and feelings. Of the 70–79 year olds participating in this research, the vast majority reported a declining interest in sex, although many women did not find this decline in desire and activity distressing.

Some studies, it should be noted, have reported the desire for more sexual activity by both older men and women (Ginsberg et al 2005, Hyde et al 2010, Wiley & Bortz 1996).

To be LGBTI, and to age into a system that offers marginal support for dealing with the consequences of discrimination, has historically been a harsh reality for LGBTI older Australians.[1] LGBTI-specific Community Aged Care Packages (CACPs), Extended Aged Care at Home (EACH) and Extended Aged Care at Home—Dementia (EACH-D) packages are available in some locales, but this is not a widespread trend. A recent Commonwealth Government initiative, the National LGBTI Ageing and Aged Care Strategy, designed to ensure that the needs of Australians who identify as LGBTI are addressed now and as they age was, at the time of writing, in community consultation (Department of Health and Ageing LGBTI 2012). While this is an essential undertaking it is occurring in an aged care health system that is struggling to acknowledge and accommodate the concept of sexuality and sexual expression in heterosexual older adults and the reality of attitude and system change is challenging.

In healthcare situations older adults are often assumed to be heterosexual—the presence of LGBTI older adults is not often considered a possibility. Further, ignorance and discrimination mean that assumptions and stereotypes about LGBTI older people result in many health professionals providing suboptimal care for LGBTI clients. Few services collect data on sexual orientation and gender identity, which prevents them from understanding whether LGBTI older people are being adequately served or if they remain isolated from the services they need and deserve. Such approaches makes invisible and ignores a sizeable group of Australians of diverse sexual orientation, sex identity or gender identity, as data sources indicate that up to 11% of the Australian population are LGBTI. In Australia there are examples of documents designed to appraise aged care providers of the need for greater sensitivity to LGBTI issues and service, for example, the Gay, Lesbian, Bisexual, Trans and Intersex Retirement Association (GRAI) LGBTI principles (GRAI and Curtin Health Innovation Research Institute 2010a) (see Box 16.1 for an example of the appropriate use of language).

However, it is unclear how widespread awareness and adoption of these principles is within the aged care provider community. An American online survey of the concerns of older LGBTI people around aged care housing options, while not conducted scientifically, found that the overwhelming majority (78%) would not be open with facility staff and 98% believed that staff would discriminate based on their sexual orientation (National Senior Citizens Law Center 2011). Other issues of concern raised included facilities' refusals to accept medical power of attorney, to use preferred names and to discourage visitors. All of these issues are either directly or indirectly concerned with sexual identity and the feeling of acceptance and integration, or the lack of, that older LGBTI people experience.

There is little domestic research that examines the experiences (Hughes 2007) or needs of older LGBTI people (Harrison 2006), making this group one of the least visible of all ageing Australians (ACON 2006). Garnets and Peplau (2006) indicate that there have been only two studies that have examined the

....
[1]Some individuals may identify as queer; however, this term is not used in the national LGBTI Ageing and Aged Care Strategy (Department of Health and Ageing 2012)

sexual issues for lesbians over the age of 60. An exploratory narrative study of older lesbians' and gays' experiences and expectations of the Australian health and aged care service delivery (n = 14; nine men and five women, mean age 56) identified the issues of healthcare agencies assuming heterosexuality and failing to address homophobic staff attitudes and practices, making the disclosure of LGBTI status difficult and uncomfortable (Hughes 2008). The issue of LGBTI retirement accommodation was addressed in a survey conducted by GRAI in 2009 that included questions relating to attitudes about sexuality and sexual expression, policy and staff training needs (GRAI and Curtin Health Innovation Research Institute 2010b). The idea of 'passing' as heterosexual as a response to discriminatory practices was also raised. A study focused on the end-of-life needs of LGBTI people noted that, despite legislation in all states and territories relating to decision making at end of life, LGBTI people report denials of their legal rights in the care of their partners and other important people in their lives, especially where advance care planning has not occurred (Cartwight 2012).

Box 16.1

Recommendations for LGBTI-sensitive language on healthcare forms

- Ask about 'relationship status' instead of 'marital status' to be inclusive of same-sex relationships that may not be legally recognised.

- Ask about sexual orientation identity (lesbian, gay, bisexual, and heterosexual). Consider using the term 'homosexual' with older adults, as this term may be more familiar to them.

- Ask if current and past sexual partners are/were female, male, or both.

- Ask the person about preferred name and pronouns.

- When asking about gender identity, offer options of female, male, and transgender.

- When asking about gender identity on forms, ask the person their sex assigned at birth and their current gender identity, including options for transwoman and transman.

  NOTE:

  Although sex and gender are often viewed as identical concepts, intake forms should distinguish between the anatomical status (preferences to be 'he' or 'she') and gender identity (female, male, transgender).

  All questions need to include 'don't know', 'not sure', and 'other' options to encourage discussion of matters not easily captured by predetermined categories.

These recommendations are adapted, in part, from the Gay and Lesbian Medical Association (2006).

Vignette

Louise (82) and Pat (76) had been in a monogamous lesbian relationship for more than 45 years when Lou had an unexpected stroke that resulted in paralysis on one side of her body and loss of clear speech. Pat cared for her partner at home for three years but, feeling the strain because of her own declining health, she sought to buy into an independent living unit in a retirement community offering 'ageing in place'. She visited more than 11 places and was met with discrimination when she stated that Lou was her 'life partner'. Eventually Pat found a place she found welcoming of LGBTI residents that seemed comfortable and affordable, and provided daily nursing support so she and Lou would be able to live together. Lou and Pat still shared a bed and engaged in touching, stroking, kissing and mutual masturbation. The first few months in their new home were pleasant and uneventful. Then one morning the new registered nurse (RN), a middle-aged man, came by to help shower Lou. The couple had not been told that the regular RN, Sandra, had moved areas and that Todd would now be caring for Lou.

Lou became visibly upset when Todd arrived. Todd was clearly surprised to find a lesbian couple and said, 'Oh, how long have you two ladies been together? It's very cute! Gay people don't usually have long relationships like you two. Are you married?' Both Pat and Lou found this conversation demeaning and Pat did not want Todd to provide personal care for Lou because she had never been seen naked by a man in her life. When Pat talked to the facility manager about the staff change the manager said, 'Don't take it too personally. Todd's a nice person. You'll get used to him.' This response sounded to the couple like the concerns Pat had raised were not taken seriously.

The heteronormative discourse that frames older people's needs (Heaphy & Yip 2006) raises some important issues about the preparedness of healthcare service providers and health professionals to engage with older LGBTI people (Hughes 2007).

 The predominantly heteronormative discourse that frames older people's needs raises some important issues about the preparedness of healthcare service providers and health professionals to engage with older LGBTI people.

It should be apparent from the above vignette that it is not possible to typecast older people when discussing sexuality. Not all older people are heterosexual, nor do all older people want to be sexually active. Those who do desire to be sexually active may choose to express their sexuality in a range of ways and not all will want to engage in intercourse. As people get older, they often redefine what 'sex' means to them (Gott 2005b). Many are happy to go without sexual intercourse because they have reprioritised the role of sex in their life. When intercourse is not preferred or possible due to illness or some other factor, alternative expressions of sexuality and physical intimacy, such as masturbation, cuddling and touching, holding hands, kissing, fondling and other displays of affection, can all assume importance and meet people's needs for sexual expression (Gott & Hinchliff 2003).

AGEING AND ILLNESS: EFFECTS ON INTEREST AND OPPORTUNITY

It is important for health professionals to understand the normal age-related changes to the body, the effects of illnesses and other medical interventions, and how these may impact on sexuality. The age-related physiological changes that can affect male and female sexual functioning have been well researched and are summarised in Table 16.1.

The changes listed in Table 16.1 need not prevent the continued enjoyment of sexual activity (Brock & Jennings 2007), although some adaptations may be necessary, such as spending more time on stimulating the partner and using lubricants to facilitate painless intercourse. The slower pace of sexual liaison that such adjustments can entail can be advantageous to lovemaking by prolonging sex and may explain why some older people say that sex gets better with age (Gott & Hinchliff 2003).

Many older people have a low level of knowledge about sexuality in later life (Minichiello et al 2000) and those who are not aware or prepared for these normal age-related changes may find sexuality and relationships challenging. Men are very erection-focused (Brock & Jennings 2007) and changes in the ability to achieve an erection can leave many feeling inadequate and impotent. Some may experience 'performance anxiety' as a result of not being able to meet previous levels of sexual performance. In some cases men may stop having

Table 16.1

Common sexual changes that occur with age

MEN	WOMEN
• More stimulation is needed to achieve an erection • Erections may not be as firm but usually sufficient for penetration • Force and volume of ejaculation is diminished • The time between erection and ejaculation (orgasm) is increased • The erection is lost more quickly after ejaculation • There is a longer time between erections • There may be more control over ejaculation and the need to ejaculate is not always felt	• More stimulation is needed to achieve an orgasm • There is a thinning of the lining of the vagina and vaginal lubrication is decreased • Sensations may be less intense • The ability to have multiple orgasms is not affected • The vagina narrows and shortens • The clitoris may become more exposed, sometimes causing irritation

Source: Nusbaum et al 2005, Trudel et al 2000

sex altogether (Hillman 2000). For people with a partner, satisfaction with the relationship is an important factor in the maintenance of sexuality (DeLamater & Moorman 2007). A demise in desire by one partner can leave the other partner feeling unattractive and undesirable (Hillman 2000) and therefore also unsatisfied with the relationship.

With increasing age comes increasing ill health and medical care and these factors commonly interfere with sexuality. Examples include the following:

- medications that interfere with sexual functioning, of which there are many—many drugs prescribed to treat chronic illness affect the autonomic nervous system and reduce responsiveness and sensitivity to stimulation; some of these can also interfere with sexual thought or fantasy (DeLamater & Moorman 2007)
- cardiovascular and other diseases that result in vascular insufficiency (Camacho & Reyes-Ortiz 2005)—heart disease can lead some men to give up sex for fear of angina or a heart attack (Henry & McNab 2003)
- impaired mobility due to rheumatoid arthritis or stroke (Henry & McNab 2003)
- depression leading to a loss of interest in sex (Kessel 2001)
- surgery that affects body image, or that involves sex organs (Messinger-Rapport et al 2003)
- arthritis, which may cause pain and limit sexual positions and endurance (Messinger-Rapport et al 2003)
- physical barriers such as catheters (Kessel 2001) and the presence of lower urinary tract symptoms (Camacho & Reyes-Ortiz 2005).

With increasing age comes increasing ill health and medical care and these factors commonly interfere with sexuality.

Gott and Hinchcliff (2003) are of the view that illnesses such as those listed above and the loss or absence of a partner are far more significant in explaining any decline in sexual activity in old age than any of the physical changes in Table 16.1. Other factors including caring for a sick partner, separation, divorce, bereavement and concerns that children or family would not approve may also explain a declining interest (Gott & Hinchliff 2003, Howard et al 2006, Hyde et al 2010).

Women can outlive men by 10 or more years, so the number of women who are unattached and not in a sexual relationship is hardly surprising. Women and men who do form new relationships on the other hand can often harbour feelings of guilt about another relationship with someone else. For men, this can lead to 'widower's syndrome' (Hillman 2000), a temporary inability to achieve an erection with their new partner.

AGEING AND SEXUAL HEALTH

Because older men and women engage in sexual activity, including with sex workers (Hillman 2000), they are at risk of sexually transmitted infections including HIV/AIDS. Older women in particular are at greater risk of infection than younger women due to the hormonal changes at menopause, which increase the likelihood of vaginal tears and abrasions during intercourse (Hillman 2007).

This should be of concern to health professionals since rates of sexually transmitted diseases such as chlamydia, gonorrhea and syphilis have doubled for people in their 50s, 60s and 70s in the past decade (von Simson & Kulasegaram 2012). Older people (in this case those aged over 50 years) represent approximately 10–15% of new AIDS cases reported to the Centre of Disease Control in the US (Emlet 2004). In NSW older gay men are estimated to represent 12–13% of new HIV infections (ACON 2006), although Cloud et al (2003) note the size of the problem in the older population is really not known. What is certain, however, is that the incidence and prevalence of sexually transmitted infections is likely to increase (Cloud et al 2003).

Older people are more likely to unwittingly engage in unprotected sex (Brock & Jennings 2007, Cloud et al 2003, Hillman 2007) and they are less aware than younger people of the risks of sexually transmitted diseases such as HIV (Hillman 2007). The AIDS prevention messages have been largely ignored by older people (Goodroad 2003), in part as a result of the failure of education programs to capture older people because of the stereotype that they are sexually inactive (Levy-Dweck 2005). Regrettably, many health professionals are unaware of the increased risks in the older population (Emlet 2004). This is at a time when the baby boomer generation, socialised at the time of the 'sexual revolution' (Gott 2005a) when there was no HIV, is reaching old age.

 Older people are more likely to unwittingly engage in unprotected sex.

SEXUALITY AND DEMENTIA

For older people who live with dementia the issue of sexual expression can become more complex. Sexuality is often constructed as a problem by health professionals, with the focus often narrowed to acts of sexual expression rather than encompassing a broader view that accounts for the need for physical contact, affection and intimacy (Ward et al 2005).

In residential care, the expression of sexuality by residents with dementia is often more easily dismissed by staff, and when it is addressed, it is often discussed in terms of 'managing' and 'regulating' 'challenging' behaviour. As Ward et al (2005) note, if a person has dementia, the level of surveillance and regulation they are subjected to is heightened. Staff often struggle with balancing residents' rights to express their sexuality with their duty of care. A significant and often vexed issue in aged care is the older persons' capacity to consent to sexual intimacy with another. Psychological barriers such as threats and punishment have been known to be used to control sexualised behaviour (Chandler et al 2004) and tranquillisers employed (Archibald 2003) to control what is constructed as a behavioural problem (Hajjar & Kamel 2003).

Archibald (2003) argues that disallowing sexual relationships between residents with dementia seems to be an attempt to manage 'scary' sexual situations. The issue of sexuality and dementia is complex in that it raises tricky ethical and legal considerations in relation to consent since care providers are accountable for the wellbeing of the older people in their care. It needs to be recognised that denying a person the expression of their sexuality may be an infringement on that individual's human right. It is also important to note that:

> *Allowing persons with dementia to make autonomous decisions about their sexuality may indeed expose them to some elements of risk such as emotional distress if a relationship ends; however, these are risks that any sexually active person faces throughout his or her life, and we should not confuse a bad or unwise decision with incompetence. Seeking to 'protect' individuals with dementia by not allowing them to express their sexual needs, thereby stifling their autonomy and personhood, is a far greater failure of duty of care.*

(Tarzia et al 2012 p 3)

 Denial of an individual's sexuality is an infringement on that individual's rights.

With supportive education and training, health professionals can also learn to communicate effectively and sensitively with families and assist them to understand that people with dementia may still have sexual needs, that they may no longer recognise their partner of many years, that the sexual relationship may change or have to cease, or that new sexual relationships may develop.

When assessing the sexuality needs of older people with dementia, health professionals should consider the person's quality of life, as well as their wellbeing and safety (Hajjar & Kamel 2003). Blanket judgments regarding competency to make informed decisions should be avoided. Rather, a person-centred (Ward et al 2005) and context-specific (Haddad & Benbow 1993) approach to decision making should be adopted.

SEXUALITY, HEALTH PROFESSIONALS AND PERSON-CENTRED CARE: THE NEED FOR CHANGE

A large number of older people are cognisant of the beneficial effects of expressing sexuality (Minichiello et al 2000, Walker & Ephross 1999) and, as embarrassing as the topic may be, many would welcome the opportunity to discuss aspects of sexuality with their health professional (Gott & Hinchliff 2003, Morerra et al 2005, Nusbaum et al 2004) and believe that issues related to sexual needs and function form a legitimate part of clinical care (Horden & Street 2007, Lemieux et al 2004). It must, of course, be acknowledged that not everyone will want to discuss sexuality. However, by being sensitive to older people's needs, giving people the opportunity to discuss sexuality, and providing information pertaining to sexuality (Henry & McNab 2003), health professionals are in a unique position to enrich an older person's life and give it more meaning (Pangman & Seguire 2000). Spending time during a consultation to sensitively enquire about social activities, loneliness and sexual health may provide an opportunity for the older person to raise concerns that they may otherwise be too embarrassed to mention.

> ## Spending time during a consultation to sensitively enquire about social activities, loneliness and sexual health may provide an opportunity for the older person to raise concerns.

It should be clear by now that if person-centred care is to be more than empty rhetoric then health professionals must overcome their own ageism and inhibitions in relation to discussing sexuality with older clients. The type of discussion will depend on the context and the conversation should be guided by the responses of the older person. For example, some older people will welcome the opportunity to talk frankly, some will need more encouragement to overcome long-held embarrassment and internalisation of societal attitudes towards older people and sex, and a small number may simply refuse to have the conversation.

Many health professionals indicate that they do not know 'how to commence the conversation' about sexuality and there appears to be little in the way of guidance in the literature, with many existing tools arguably stopping a discussion before it gets started! For example:

- Are you currently sexually active? If so, with one or more than one partner? Male or female partner?
- Do you have difficulty achieving erection (or orgasm)?
- Do you ever experience pain during intercourse? If so, what kind and under what circumstances?
- Do you have any questions or concerns about your sexual functioning? About your partner's sexual functioning? (Knutson 2008)

> ## Health professionals must overcome their own ageism and inhibitions.

As an alternative, the Australian Centre for Evidence Based Aged Care (ACEBAC) proposes the use of a script or 'conversation starter' as outlined in the following vignette.

Vignette

An older man regularly visits his GP. He has never raised the subject of sexuality despite it still being important to him. He feels embarrassed because, at 83 and 75, it seems he and his partner are alone in still being sexual at their age. This is complicated further by the fact that his partner is a local business woman and he is not sure if their partnership is known to be more than friends in business. On this day when he arrives there is a locum in the surgery because the usual GP is on leave. After the usual routine physical examination this GP introduces a new line of assessment that went something like this:

- Okay, we've talked about your bowel function and water works, and checked your heart and lungs, memory, hearing and eyesight.

- Often as we age, things can get in the way of us remaining as sexually active as we might like—things like pain, medications, loss of a partner, and so on. Most people feel a bit embarrassed talking about their sexuality, or having pap smears or prostate exams, and yet it can all be very important to our quality of life and relationships, so I just want to check with you if there are areas of your sexual expression causing you any concern.

- Ageing can, of course, slow us up a bit and leave us with some concerns and difficulties such as erection or dry vagina problems, so you may find taking more time and using lubricants can be a big help. With the arthritic pain, make sure you have your analgesics regularly and use some pillows to support painful arms or legs. (How you as the health professional respond here will depend on issues that may be raised—this could turn into a discussion around impotence, Viagra, vaginal prolapse, aversion to masturbation, safe sex or issues with the partner, and referral may be the most appropriate action.)

- A lot of people say their sex lives improve with age and we know it is good for reducing pain and depression so we need to keep you active!

- There are lots of books and other resources that older people have found useful—I can provide you with a list if you like.

This locum had in fact been using the ACEBAC sexuality assessment tool for health professionals, which also advises (Nay & Bauer, unpublished):

Because talking about sex is embarrassing for many people it is good to integrate the assessment into your overall workup—acknowledge it can be embarrassing, advise that it is perfectly normal to be sexually active (or not) in old age, and use a good dose of humour.

While broad use of this is yet to be tested, feedback has been positive. In addition to individual assessment and tailoring of treatment to reflect the older person's preferences, services for older people need to include information on sexuality.

CONCLUSION

Older people remain sexually interested and many active until death, and yet our society and health professionals continue to find this notion incomprehensible and even repugnant. The fallout is that sexuality is ignored, neglected, rarely if ever assessed and older people endure the consequences. These may be as simple as 'hiding' their sexuality or as damning as contracting and spreading HIV/AIDS. Mostly it is somewhere in the middle. For people living in their own homes managing their sexuality is less complex. For people in aged care it is very difficult. The environments that restrict privacy and staff and family morals, values and the entrenched attitudes that 'we know what is best' make the expression of sexuality almost impossible. If the older person happens to be anywhere on the LGBTI continuum the marginalisation is manifold. While there is increasing research and interest in removing the barriers and enabling the human right to express sexual identity, we have a very long way to go. Our firm hope is that in reading and reflecting on this chapter you have dared to recognise your own prejudices as a first step to changing practice.

Reflective questions

1. How do you feel when you think about your parents/grandparents having sex?

2. Have you ever actually assessed sexuality with an older person or even raised the subject?

3. How many of the medications that you administer in your practice may have an adverse effect on sexual expression?

4. People with dementia may act sexually in public spaces of a residential aged care facility. Should you prescribe/administer oestrogen so others are not offended? If not what else could you do?

References

Aids Council of New South Wales, 2006. Ageing disgracefully: ACON's healthy GLBT ageing strategy 2006–2009. ACON, Sydney.

Andrews, C.N., Piterman, L., 2007. Sex and the older man. Australian Family Physician 36 (10), 867–869.

Archibald, C., 2003. Sexuality and dementia: the role dementia plays when sexual expression becomes a component of residential care work. Alzheimer's Care Quarterly 4 (2), 137–148.

Bauer, M., Fetherstonhaugh, D., Tarzia, L., et al., 2012. 'I always look under the bed for a man.' Needs and barriers to the expression of sexuality in residential aged care: the views of residents with and without dementia. Psychology and Sexuality, DOI:10.1080/19419899.2012.713869.

Bauer, M., McAuliffe, L., Nay, R., 2007. Sexuality, health care and the older person: an overview of the literature. International Journal of Older People Nursing 2, 63–68.

Bauer, M., Nay, R., McAuliffe, L., 2009. Catering to love, sex and intimacy in residential aged care: what information is provided to consumers. Sexuality and Disability 27 (1), 3–9.

Bergstrom-Walan, M.-B., Nielsen, H.H., 1990. Sexual expression among 60–80-year-old men and women: a sample from Stockholm, Sweden. The Journal of Sex Research 27 (2), 289–295.

Bretschneider, J., McCoy, N., 1988. Sexual interest and behaviour in healthy 80 to 102 year olds. Archives of Sexual Behaviour 17 (2), 109–129.

Brock, L.J., Jennings, G., 2007. Sexuality and intimacy. In: Blackburn, J.A., Dulmus, C.N. (Eds.), Handbook of gerontology: evidence-based approaches to theory, practice, and policy. John Wiley & Sons, New Jersey, pp. 244–268.

Burd, I.D., Nevadunsly, N., Bachmann, G., 2006. Impact of physician gender on sexual history taking in a multispeciality practice. Journal of Sex Medicine 3, 194–200.

Camacho, M.E., Reyes-Ortiz, C.A., 2005. Sexual dysfunction in the elderly: age or disease. International Journal of Impotence Research 17, S52–S56.

Cartwright, C., 2012. Ethical challenges in end-of-life care for GLBTI individuals. Journal of Bioethical Inquiry 9 (1), 113–114.

Chandler, M., Margery, M., Maynard, N., et al., 2004. Sexuality, older people and residential aged care. Geriaction 22 (4), 5–11.

Cloud, G.C., Browne, R., Salooja, N., et al., 2003. Newly diagnosed HIV infection in an octogenarian: the elderly are not 'immune'. Age and Ageing 32 (3), 353–354.

DeLamater, J., Moorman, S.M., 2007. Sexual behaviour in later life. Journal of Aging and Health 19 (6), 921–945.

Department of Health and Ageing, 2012. National Lesbian, Gay, Bisexual, Transgender and Intersex (LGBTI) Ageing and Aged Care Strategy, Draft for consultation. Australian Government, Canberra.

Dyer, K., das Nair, R., 2012. Why don't health care professionals talk about sex? A systematic review of recent qualitative studies conducted in the United Kingdom. Journal of Sexual Medicine DOI: 10.1111/j.1743-6109.2012.02856.x.

Emlet, C., 2004. HIV/AIDS and aging: a diverse population of vulnerable older adults. Journal of Human Behavior in the Social Environment 9 (4), 45–63.

Everett, B., 2007. Ethically managing sexual activity in long-term care. Sex and Disability 25, 7–21.

Fannin, A., 2006. Gay and grey: Lifting the lid on sexuality and ageing. Working with Older People 10 (4), 31–34.

Garnets, L., Peplau, L.A., 2006. Sexuality in the lives of aging lesbian and bisexual women. In: Kimmel, D., Rose, T., David, S. (Eds.), Lesbian, Gay, Bisexual and Transgender Aging. Columbia University Press, New York, pp. 71–90.

Gay and Lesbian Medical Association, 2006. Guidelines for care of lesbian, gay, bisexual, and transgender patients. GLMA, Washington.

Gibson, H.B., 1992. The emotional and sexual lives of older people. Chapman & Hall, London.

Ginsberg, T.B., Pomerantz, S.C., Kramer-Feeley, V., 2005. Sexuality in older adults: behaviours and preferences. Age and Ageing 34, 475–480.

Goldman, J.D.G., Bradley, G.L., 2004. Sexuality information for older people in the technological age. Australian Journal of Primary Health 10 (1), 96–103.

Goodroad, B.K., 2003. HIV and AIDS in people older than 50: a continuing concern. Journal of Gerontological Nursing 29 (4), 18–24.

Gott, M., 2005a. Are older people at risk of sexually transmitted infections? A new look at the evidence. Reviews in Clinical Gerontology 14, 5–13.

Gott, M., 2005b. Sexuality, sexual health and ageing. Open University Press, Maidenhead, Berkshire.

Gott, M., Galena, E., Hinchliff, S., et al., 2004a. 'Opening a can of worms': GP and nurse barriers to talking about sexual health in primary care. Family Practice 21 (5), 528–536.

Gott, M., Hinchliff, S., 2003. How important is sex in later life? The views of older people. Social Science and Medicine 56, 1617–1628.

Gott, M., Hinchliff, S., Galena, E., 2004b. General practitioner attitudes to discussing sexual health issues with older people. Social Science and Medicine 58, 2093–2103.

GRAI (GBLTI Retirement Association Inc) and Curtin Health Innovation Research Institute, 2010a. Best practice guidelines. Accommodating older gay, lesbian, bisexual, trans and intersex (GLBTI) people. Online. Available: http://grai.org.au/wordpress/wp-content/uploads/2010/07/Best-Practice-Guidelines.pdf, 1 May 2013.

GRAI and Curtin Health Innovation Research Institute, 2010b. We don't have any of those people here: retirement accommodation and aged care issues for non-heterosexual populations. Curtin University. Perth, Western Australia.

Gunderson, A., Tomkowiak, J., Menachemi, N., et al., 2005. Rural physicians' attitudes toward the elderly: evidence of ageism? Quality Management in Health Care 14 (3), 167–176.

Haddad, P., Benbow, S., 1993. Sexual problems associated with dementia: Part 1. International Journal of Geriatric Psychiatry 8 (3), 547–551.

Hajjar, R., Kamel, H., 2003. Sexuality in the nursing home, part 1: attitudes and barriers to sexual expression. Journal of the American Medical Directors Association 4, 152–156.

Harrison, J., 2006. Coming out ready or not? Gay, lesbian, bisexual, transgender and intersex ageing and aged care in Australia: reflections, contemporary developments and the road ahead. Gay and Lesbian Issues and Psychology Review 2 (2), 44–53.

Heaphy, B., 2007. Sexualities, gender and ageing: resources and social change. Current Sociology 55 (2), 193–210.

Heaphy, B., Yip, A.K.T., 2006. Policy implications of ageing sexualities. Social Policy and Society 5 (4), 443–451.

Henry, J., McNab, W., 2003. Forever young: a health promotion focus on sexuality and aging. Gerontology and Geriatrics Education 23 (4), 57–74.

Hillman, J., 2000. Clinical perspectives on elderly sexuality. Kluwer Academic/Plenum Publishers, New York.

Hillman, J., 2007. Knowledge and attitudes about HIV/AIDS among community-living older women: re-examining issues of age and gender. Journal of Women and Aging 19 (3/4), 53–67.

Horden, A.J., Street, A.F., 2007. Constructions of sexuality and intimacy after cancer: patient and health professional perspectives. Social Science and Medicine 64, 1704–1718.

Howard, J.R., O'Neill, S.O., Travers, C., 2006. Factors affecting sexuality in older Australian women: sexual interest, sexual arousal, relationships and sexual distress in older Australian women. Climacteric 9, 355–367.

Huffstetler, B., 2006. Sexuality in older adults: a deconstructivist perspective. Adultspan 5 (1), 4–14.

Hughes, M., 2007. Older lesbians and gays accessing health and aged-care services. Australian Social Work 60 (2), 197–209.

Hughes, M., 2008. Imagined futures and communities: older lesbian and gay people's narratives on health and aged care. Journal of Gay and Lesbian Social Services, 20, 1–2, pp. 167–186.

Hyde, Z., Flicker, L., Hankey, G.J., et al., 2010. Prevalence of sexual activity and associated factors in men aged 75–95 years: a cohort study. Annals of Internal Medicine 153, 693–702.

Jones, M.K., Weerakoon, P., Pynor, R., 2005. Survey of occupational therapy students' attitudes towards sexual issues on clinical practice. Occupational Therapy Journal 12 (2), 95–106.

Kass, M.J., 1981. Geriatric sexuality breakdown syndrome. International Journal of Aging and Human Development 13 (1), 71–77.

Katz, S., Marshall, B., 2003. New sex for old: lifestyle, consumerism and the ethics of aging well. Journal of Aging Studies 17, 3–16.

Kay, B., Neely, J.N., 1982. Sexuality and aging: a review of current literature. Sexuality and Disability 5 (1), 38–46.

Kessel, B., 2001. Sexuality in the older person. Age and Ageing 30 (2), 121–124.

Kingsberg, S.A., 2002. The impact of aging on sexual function in women and their partners. Archives of Sexual Behavior 31 (5), 431–437.

Kinsey, A., Pomeroy, W., Martin, C., 1948. Sexual behavior in the human male. Saunders, Philadelphia.

Kinsey, A., Pomeroy, W., Martin, C., et al., 1953. Sexual behavior in the human female. Saunders, Philadelphia.

Knutson, M., 2008. Talking to older people about sex. Online. Available: www.medscape.com/viewarticle/444873, 1 May 2013.

Lemieux, L., Kaiser, S., Pereira, J., et al., 2004. Sexuality in palliative care: patient perspectives. Palliative Medicine 18, 630–637.

Levy-Dweck, S., 2005. HIV/AIDS fifty and older: a hidden and growing population. Journal of Gerontological Social Work 46 (2), 37–50.

Lindau, S.T., Gavrilova, N., 2010. Sex, health, and years of sexually active life gained due to good health: evidence from two US population based cross sectional surveys of ageing. BMJ 340, c810.

Lindau, S.T., Schumm, L.P., Olaumann, E.O., et al., 2007. A study of sexuality and health among older adults in the United States. New England Journal of Medicine 357 (8), 762–774.

Magnan, M.A., Reynolds, K.E., Galvin, E.A., 2005. Barriers to addressing patient sexuality in nursing practice. MedSurg Nursing 14 (5), 282–290.

Marshall, B.L., 2010. Science, medicine and virility surveillance: 'sexy seniors' in the pharmaceutical imagination. Sociology of Health and Illness 32 (2), 211–224.

Marshall, B.L., 2012. Medicalization and the refashioning of age-related limits on sexuality. Journal of sex research. 49 (4), 337–343.

Masters, W.H., Johnson, V.E., 1970. Human sexual inadequacy. Little Brown, Boston.

Matthias, R.E., Lubben, J.E., Atchison, K.A., et al., 1997. Sexual activity and satisfaction among very old adults: results from a community-dwelling medicare population survey. The Gerontologist 37 (1), 6–14.

McAuliffe, L., Bauer, M., Nay, R., 2007. Barriers to the expression of sexuality in the older person: the role of the health professional. International Journal of Older People Nursing 2, 69–75.

Messinger-Rapport, B.J., Sandhu, S.K., Hujer, M., 2003. Sex and sexuality: is it over at 60? Clinical Geriatrics 11 (10), 45–53.

Minichiello, V., Ackling, S., Bourne, C., et al., 2005. Sexuality, sexual intimacy and sexual health in later life. In: Minichiello, V., Coulson, I. (Eds.), Contemporary issues in gerontology: promoting positive ageing. Allen & Unwin, Sydney, pp. 78–104.

Minichiello, V., Plummer, D., 2004. Factors predicting sexual relationships in older people: an Australian study. Australasian Journal on Ageing 23 (3), 125–130.

Minichiello, V., Plummer, D., Loxton, D., 2000. Knowledge and beliefs of older Australians about sexuality and health. Australasian Journal on Ageing 19 (4), 190–194.

Morerra E.D.J., Glasser, D.B., Gingell, C., 2005. Sexual activity, sexual dysfunction and associated help-seeking behaviours in middle-aged and older adults in Spain: a population survey. World Journal of Urology 23, 422–429.

National Ageing Research Institute, 2002. The wellness project: promoting older people's sexual health. National Ageing Research Institute, Melbourne. Online. Available: www.mednwh.unimelb.edu.au/research/service_rac.htm, 22 Dec 2008.

National Senior Citizens Law Center, 2011. LGBT Older adults in long-term care facilities: stories from the field. Online. Available: http://www.nsclc.org/index.php/lgbt-older-adults-in-long-term-care-facilities-stories-from-the-field/, 1 May 2013.

Nay, R., 2004. Sexuality and older people. In: Nay, R., Garratt, S. (Eds.), Nursing older people: issues and innovations, second ed. Churchill Livingstone, Sydney, pp. 276–288.

Nay, R., McAuliffe, L., Bauer, M., 2007. Sexuality: From stigma, stereotypes and secrecy to coming out, communication and choice. International Journal of Older People Nursing 2, 76–80.

Nelson, T.D., 2005. Ageism: Prejudice against our feared future self. Journal of Social Issues 61, 207–2221.

Nusbaum, M.R.H., Lenahan, P., Sadovsky, R., 2005. Sexual health in aging men and women: addressing the physiological and psychological sexual changes that occur with age. Geriatrics 60 (9), 18–23.

Nusbaum, M.R.H., Singh, A., Pyles, A., 2004. Sexual healthcare needs of women aged 65 and older. Journal of the American Geriatrics Society 52 (1), 117–124.

Pangman, V., Seguire, M., 2000. Sexuality and the chronically ill older adult: a social justice issue. Sexuality and Disability 18 (1), 49–59.

Pfeifer, E., Davis, G.C., 1972. Determinants of sexual behavior in middle and old age. Journal of the American Geriatrics Society 20 (4), 151–158.

Pfeifer, E., Verwoerdt, A., Wag, H.S., 1968. Sexual behavior in aged men and women. Archives of General Psychiatry 19, 753–758.

Robinson, J.G., Molzahn, A.E., 2007. Sexuality and quality of life. Journal of Gerontological Nursing 33 (3), 19–27.

Sharpe, T.H., 2004. Introduction to sexuality in late life. The Family Journal 12, 199–205.

Shuttleworth, R., Russel, C., Weerakoon, P., et al., 2010. Sexuality in residential aged care: a survey of perceptions and policies in Australian nursing homes. Sexuality and Disability 28, 187–194.

Stancil, B.P.P., 2003. Sex and the elderly: no laughing matter in religion. Journal of Religious Gerontology 15 (1–2), 17–24.

Tarzia, L., Fetherstonhaugh, D., Bauer, M., 2012. Dementia, sexuality and consent in residential aged care facilities. Journal of Medical Ethics 10.1136/medethics-2011-100453.

Trudel, G., Turgeon, L., Piche, L., 2000. Marital and sexual aspects of old age. Sexual and Relationship Therapy 15 (4), 381–406.

von Simson, R., Kulasegaram, R., 2012. Sexual health and the older adult. Student BMJ 20, e688.

Walker, B.L., Ephross, P.H., 1999. Knowledge and attitudes toward sexuality of a group of elderly. Journal of Gerontological Social Work 31 (1/2), 85–107.

Walz, T., 2002. Crones, Dirty Old Men, Sexy Seniors: Representations of the sexuality of older persons. Journal of Aging and Identity 7 (2), 99–112.

Ward, R., Vass, A.A., Aggarwal, N., et al., 2005. A kiss is still a kiss? The construction of sexuality in dementia care. Dementia 4, 49–72.

Wiley, D., Bortz II., W.M., 1996. Sexuality and aging—usual and successful. The Journals of Gerontology Series A 51 (3), M142–M145.

Willert, A., Semans, M., 2000. Knowledge and attitudes about later life sexuality: What clinicians need to know about helping the elderly. Contemporary Family Therapy 22 (4), 415–435.

World Health Organization, 2006. Defining sexual health: Report on a technical consultation on sexual health 28-31 January 2002, Geneva.

Zanni, G.R., Wick, J.Y., Walker, B.L., 2003. Sexual health and the elderly. The Consultant Pharmacist 18, 310–322.

Zeiss, A.M., Kasl-Godley, J., 2001. Sexuality in older adults' relationships. Generations 25 (2), 18–25.

CHAPTER 17

INTERVENTION IN A SITUATION OF ELDER ABUSE AND NEGLECT

Susan Kurrle

Editors' comments

Elder abuse is another of the taboo topics that challenges health professionals from all disciplines. Recognition of abuse is difficult and, if suspected, there are few guidelines to assist action. Responses need to be sensitive, ethical and legal. This chapter takes a practical approach to raising awareness of the key issues.

INTRODUCTION

The purpose of this chapter is to explore the concept of elder abuse, identify prevalence rates, and examine the way in which practitioners might currently identify, respond to and effectively intervene in abuse situations. Several principles of practice for interventions in situations of elder abuse are elaborated and a guided decision model presented. A vignette will be analysed and discussed in conclusion.

DEFINITION AND OVERVIEW OF ELDER ABUSE

Abuse of older people is any behaviour that causes physical, psychological, financial or social harm to an older person (World Health Organization 2011). Abuse can occur within any relationship where there is an expectation of trust between the older person and the person who becomes the abuser. Abuse may involve a single act, repeated behaviour or a lack of appropriate action. It may occur when a vulnerable older person is persuaded to enter into a financial or sexual transaction to which he or she has not consented, or cannot consent.

Some forms of abuse of older people are crimes (Kurrle & Naughtin 2008, Lachs & Pillemer 2004, NSW Office for Ageing 2007).

IDENTIFYING ELDER ABUSE

One of the major problems in dealing with abuse is difficulty in recognition. It is necessary to be on the alert and be vigilant because symptoms and signs of abuse are often subtle and can be wrongly attributed to the ageing process itself.

One of the major problems in dealing with abuse is difficulty in recognition.

There are many symptoms and signs that may be suggestive of abuse and these are outlined below. However, it is also important to remember that the presence of one or more of the signs listed does not necessarily establish that abuse is occurring, as many of these symptoms are seen in frail older people with chronic disease. Ageing skin may bruise more readily, bones may fracture more easily due to osteoporosis, and falls may occur more often due to degenerative changes or disease in the musculoskeletal or central nervous systems. It is important to differentiate between those symptoms and signs that are due to physiological changes and those due to abuse (Wiglesworth et al 2009).

Types of abuse and recognisable signs and symptoms include:

- **Physical abuse:** the infliction of physical pain or injury, or physical coercion. Examples include hitting, slapping, pushing, burning, sexual assault, inappropriate use of medication and physical restraint. Signs include a history of unexplained accidents or injuries, bruising, burns, bite marks, abrasions, rope burns or fractures.
- **Sexual abuse:** the occurrence of non-consensual sexual intimacy or behaviour. Examples include sexual harassment, oral, vaginal or anal rape (including with objects) and inappropriate use of enemas or vaginal or perineal creams. Signs may include bruising or bleeding around genital or breast areas, evidence of sexually transmitted disease or reluctance to be undressed or bathed.
- **Psychological abuse:** the infliction of mental anguish involving actions that cause fear of violence, isolation or deprivation and feelings of shame, indignity and powerlessness. Examples include verbal intimidation, humiliation and harassment, shouting, threats of physical harm or institutionalisation and withholding of affection. Signs include fear and anxiety, apathy, resignation, withdrawal and avoidance of eye contact.
- **Financial or material abuse:** the illegal or improper use of the older person's property or finances. This would include misappropriation of money, valuables or property, forced changes to a will or other legal document and denial of the right of access to, or control over, personal funds. Signs include sudden inability to pay bills, loss of credit cards, bank books or cheque books, unexplained withdrawal of money from an account or transfer of money and improper use of a power of attorney.

- **Neglect:** the failure of a caregiver to provide the necessities of life to an older person. Neglect may involve the refusal to permit other people to provide appropriate care. Examples include abandonment, non-provision of food, clothing, shelter or medical care and poor hygiene or personal care. Signs include malnourishment, weight loss, dehydration in the absence of an illness-related cause, poor hygiene or skin care, inappropriate or soiled clothing and lack of aids such as spectacles, dentures, hearing aids or a walking frame (Kurrle 2004).

VULNERABILITY TO ABUSE

Older people may be particularly vulnerable to risk of abuse if they are:
- experiencing cognitive impairment and personality and behaviour changes because of progressively worsening conditions such as dementia (Wiglesworth et al 2010); they may experience confusion about their finances or environment
- in need of high levels of support and care from a family member because of dependence in activities of daily living due to frailty or illness (Homer & Gilleard 1990, Hughes 1997)
- women who have suffered domestic violence for many years (Jacobson et al 2006, Zink 2006)
- isolated from neighbours, family and/or community (Schaeffer 1999)
- relatively powerless because of diminished ability to advocate effectively for themselves or modify their environment (NSW Office for Ageing 2007).

PREVALENCE OF ELDER ABUSE

International studies of community-dwelling older people indicate that the prevalence of abuse varies between 1% and 6% of the population aged 65 or older (Podnieks et al 1994, Tinker et al 2007); however, Australia lacks reliable national data in this regard (Boldy et al 2005). Prevalence studies of older people presenting to aged care assessment teams (ACATs) in Australia show that approximately 5% of older people are victims of abuse (Kurrle et al 1992, 1997, Livermore et al 2001).

REASONS FOR THE EMERGENCE OF ELDER ABUSE AS A CONTEMPORARY SOCIAL ISSUE

There are several key reasons for the emergence of elder abuse as a contemporary social issue. First, the ageing of the Australian population means that more people are now surviving into late life, often with increasing frailty and with increasing incidence of conditions like dementia and stroke. Abuse can occur both within the community and in the residential setting, and may be perpetrated by family members, other carers or outside individuals. With more older people now entering residential care, as well as living on their own in the community, the opportunity for abuse has increased. There is also considerable pressure on care resources in ageing societies when families may live at some distance from their older relatives and may not be able to provide or monitor appropriate care because of their own work commitments; even if providing care, family members may experience the burden and stresses of care as overwhelming. Older generations today possess considerable wealth and substantial housing assets, which makes them vulnerable to financial manipulation both by family members and other external parties such as unscrupulous solicitors or financial advisors (Tilse et al 2003). Financial abuse is reported as one of the most significant forms of contemporary abuse in families partly because many adult children wrongly assume that their parents' assets are their assets (Field 1996, Lachs & Pillemer 2004, Wainer et al 2010).

 There are several key reasons for the emergence of elder abuse as a contemporary social issue.

GENERAL PRINCIPLES FOR ASSESSMENT

It is necessary to gain the consent of the person who has been abused for any assessment and while they may be happy to be interviewed and examined, there are often situations where they do not want any further action taken. Older people may be reluctant to report abuse by a family member or caregiver on whom they rely for their basic needs. There may be shame where a close family member is the abuser, or there may be fear of retaliation or fear of institutionalisation. If the person does not give consent to further action and is competent to make that decision then that decision must be respected (Anetzberger 2005, Dyer et al 2003, Kurrle et al 1997).

It is important to take a non-judgmental approach to cases of abuse and often it is most appropriate to look at the situation as one in which there are two victims, rather than a victim and an abuser. Attention must be paid to resolving the unmet needs of both the victim and the abuser rather than simply identifying abuse and punishing the guilty party (Kurrle 2004).

There are a number of ethical principles to be observed in relation to intervention in situations of elder abuse. *Beneficence* is the principle of doing good and ensuring that the best interests of the person are promoted. Harming or destroying a fragile family relationship that is important to the older person in the process of dealing with an abusive situation is not observing this principle. This may be averted by taking the non-judgmental approach described above. *Autonomy* is the principle of freedom of choice—the right of an individual to make decisions for themselves that are independent and made without coercion or undue influence. There are often major dilemmas involving our duty of care associated with the principle of beneficence and the victim's freedom of choice when we have a victim in a situation of abuse and clearly at risk who wishes to stay in that situation. If that person is competent to make that decision then that is their right (Kosberg et al 1996, 2005).

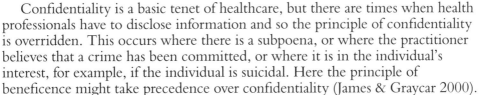

There are a number of ethical principles to be observed in relation to intervention in situations of elder abuse.

Confidentiality is a basic tenet of healthcare, but there are times when health professionals have to disclose information and so the principle of confidentiality is overridden. This occurs where there is a subpoena, or where the practitioner believes that a crime has been committed, or where it is in the individual's interest, for example, if the individual is suicidal. Here the principle of beneficence might take precedence over confidentiality (James & Graycar 2000).

It is absolutely imperative to know whether a person has mental capacity—that is, whether they are competent to make decisions. This is relevant from the taking of a history through to arranging appropriate interventions. If a person is incapable of giving an accurate history due to dementia or psychiatric illness, then involvement of others (family members, friends, service providers) is essential. It is important to remember that capacity is task-specific and a person with dementia may be quite able to make reasonable decisions about what they wish to wear or eat for dinner but may not be able to consent to a major surgical procedure or make financial decisions. While it is ultimately a legal decision as to whether a person is competent or not, the assessment of the health professional is very important. To the degree possible, the person suffering the abuse should be involved in decision making (Setterlund et al 1999).

OPTIONS FOR INTERVENTION

Ideally interventions seek to achieve freedom, safety, least disruption of lifestyle and include the least restrictive care alternatives (Department of Human Services 2009).

1. **Crisis care.** This might involve admission to an acute hospital bed or perhaps urgent respite care in a nursing home or hostel, depending on the needs of the victim. In cases of severe physical abuse, the victim often needs to be immediately separated from the abuser.
2. **Provision of community support services.** The full range of community services such as home nursing, housekeeping help, community options or linkage programs and Meals on Wheels can be used to alleviate situations where abuse is occurring. Assistance with shopping and transport is of practical help to the carer.
3. **Provision of respite.** This may be in-home respite, day-centre respite or institutional respite. It is particularly helpful when carer stress is a problem and where there has been a situation of neglect. If the victim is quite dependent, then often nursing home care is the only alternative.

4. **Counselling.** This is an important means of intervention. It may involve individual counselling or family therapy. The aim is to help the victim cope with his/her situation and find a way to be safe from the abuser. Group therapy may be utilised in situations such as carer support groups. In cases where domestic violence is the main cause of abuse, a referral may need to be made to services for victims of domestic violence.

5. **Alternative accommodation on a permanent basis.** Sometimes this may be necessary. Realistically it usually means institutionalisation, often nursing home placement, for the victim of abuse. However, in some situations where reverse abuse or carer abuse has occurred, it has been the abuser who has required nursing home placement.

6. **Legal interventions.** These are hopefully a last resort but may be the first line of intervention in cases of financial abuse or severe physical abuse where criminal charges may need to be laid. Guardianship Tribunal applications can be made where the victim is unable to make a decision because of cognitive impairment or psychiatric illness. Chamber magistrates or the police may need to be involved if a restraining order is being sought.

DECISION MAKING IN RELATION TO ELDER ABUSE

Several decision trees exist in relation to the identification of, and intervention in, situations of elder abuse. These frameworks are useful as guides and should be used together with local protocols or expert input of particular professionals. A typical protocol is presented in Figure 17.1.

A SITUATION FOR ANALYSIS

The next section gives a vignette for analysis and discussion, illustrating the need to carefully assess the presenting situation before deciding on action.

Vignette

Phase 1: Neighbours raise concerns

Mrs De Capprio is a 75-year-old Italian widow who lives with her daughter, son-in-law and their family of three children. The concerns of neighbours are raised when they hear Mrs De Capprio calling out from a locked garage during the day when the family is out.

Close neighbours communicate their concerns to Mrs De Capprio's daughter. The daughter explains that her mother has dementia, that they have a chair and a commode set up for her in the garage and provide sandwiches and cordial there but that they need to keep the garage door locked to prevent her wandering when they are out.

Strategies for intervention and management of elder abuse

Identification of above, neglect or exploitation in an elderly person.

- Take a history from the victim of abuse.
- Ensure performance of thorough physical examination and assess mental competence.
- Document any injuries, evidence of neglect, threats or allegation of violence.
- Interview the abuser separately, if possible.
- Liaise with family member and service providers to confirm details of abuse.
- Consider the need for immediate removal of the victim from the abuse situation.

Victim is **CAPABLE** of making decision

Victim is **INCAPABLE** of making decision

UNWILLING to accept intervention

- Assure the victim of continued support and provision of assistance when requested.
- Legal intervention may be necessary where criminal offence has been committed, or the victim's life or health are in danger.
- Arrange a follow-up and monitoring of the situation where possible — if not possible, document and withdraw.

WILLING to accept intervention

- Establish the needs of the victim.
- Provide information about abuse and arrange counselling where appropriate.
- Arrange appropriate community services.
- Encourage activities and contact outside the home situation.
- Assess the need for acceptance of respite care — in the home, day centre or institution.
- Explore the victim's desire or need for alternative accommodation.
- Assist with legal intervention if appropriate (e.g. guardianship, financial management, police restraining order).

UNWILLING to accept intervention

- Ensure the least restrictive intervention is considered.
- Arrange appropriate support services.
- Arrange monitoring and follow–up of situation.
- Guardianship — a legally appointed guardian has oversight of healthcare and treatment, accommodation and provision of appropriate services to the victim.
- Financial management.
- Comprehensive assessment by mental health services for crisis intervention.
- Involuntary psychiatric admission via the Mental Health Act.
- Restraining order.
- Police intervention in cases where serious crime has been committed.

Figure 17.1

Strategies for intervention and management of elder abuse

Reflective questions

1. What options do the neighbours have in responding to their concerns?

2. From where could Mrs De Capprio's daughter get assistance in better managing her mother's care?

3. Are there any specific cultural factors that might need to be considered in this case?

4. Should Mrs De Capprio be left unattended during the day? What alternatives are there?

Phase 2: Admission to hospital

Two months later, Mrs De Capprio is admitted to hospital with severe confusion, weight loss and urinary incontinence. She is diagnosed with Alzheimer's disease, malnutrition, dehydration and a urinary tract infection. However, she is very resistive to interventions and shouts at the staff, believing that they are trying to poison her. She is adamant that she wants to go home.

Mrs De Capprio is seen by a dietician who advises that she has been malnourished for some time and recommends supplements to improve her nutritional status and increased fluid intake. Mrs De Capprio, however, refuses to take drinks and becomes physically aggressive when staff attempt to insert a nasogastric tube.

Mrs De Capprio's urinary tract infection is treated with antibiotics and her incontinence is reduced. However, when left sitting in a chair for any length of time, she frequently becomes incontinent.

The hospital team assesses Mrs De Capprio as requiring long-term care because of her incontinence and Alzheimer's disease. They suggest to the daughter that she explore options for a dementia-specific residential care facility.

The daughter, however, insists that she wants to take her mother home and care for her as she has always done. She also states that the family has no money to place her mother into care, despite the fact that Mrs De Capprio owns the home in which they all live and receives the age pension.

Staff are concerned that Mrs De Capprio's safety and wellbeing will be at risk if she returns home. The daughter, however, has enduring power of attorney for her mother and believes she has the final say.

Reflective questions

1. How might the best decision for Mrs De Capprio be arrived at in this situation?

2. Who should participate in the decision making?

3. Was the tube insertion ill advised? What other options might have been tried?

4. What care plan needs to be put in place for Mrs De Capprio to return home?

5. Does the daughter's possession of enduring power of attorney override the authority of other decision makers?

Phase 3: Two possible decision pathways

(a) Referral home with a dementia community care package

As Mrs De Capprio has consistently expressed the wish to return home, the hospital decides to see if the daughter can continue to manage Mrs De Capprio at home. She is assessed by the local ACAT as requiring high-level care and is able to secure a dementia-specific Extended Aged Care at Home (EACH) package from a local ethno-specific agency. Her daughter is referred to Alzheimer's Australia for ongoing advice and support.

(b) Referral to the Guardianship Tribunal for appointment of a substitute decision maker

The hospital is sufficiently concerned about Mrs De Capprio's wellbeing that they decide to make an application to the Guardianship Tribunal. Investigation reveals that the daughter and her husband are experiencing major financial difficulties following the failure of the husband's business, and that they have been substantially drawing down on Mrs De Capprio's assets, including mortgaging her home.

Reflective questions

1. How should the first situation be monitored?

2. If financial abuse is substantiated, how might the second phase of the vignette proceed in terms of outcomes for Mrs De Capprio, her daughter and son-in-law?

DISCUSSION

While this vignette is fictional, it illustrates some common issues experienced by health professionals and by the community. For the neighbours confronted by their initial concerns, intervention is difficult. Depending on the relationship, they may approach the carer and express their concerns and perhaps discuss some ways to support Mrs De Capprio's daughter. For example, the neighbours may offer to check on Mrs De Capprio several times during the day. Discussions with the local GP and referral to the local aged care assessment service (ACAS) might be helpful in connecting the family with a day care program for several days per week, arranging in-home respite care or getting a referral to a local ethnic agency for access to an EACH package. Referral to the state association of Alzheimer's Australia could also assist Mrs De Capprio's daughter in managing ongoing care by providing advice and carer support.

From a cultural perspective it is important to understand the family dynamics and the expectations of care and filial responsibility (Kosberg et al 2005). It may be that Mrs De Capprio does not wish to leave the family home, despite the interpretation by others that the present circumstances are inappropriate for her care needs. Mrs De Capprio's daughter may feel the need to maintain her filial responsibilities and the restrictions on her mother's freedom are the only way she can deal with the situation because of her lack of knowledge of alternatives. Some specific ethnic outreach might be required to work with Mrs De Capprio's daughter in this regard.

As the vignette develops we can see that more questions are raised. There may be uncertainty among some health professionals as to whether or not this is abuse. It is important that all health professionals involved in the care process have an understanding of the individual and their family and maintain a person-centred approach while retaining a duty of care. Best outcomes for everyone require that all parties are involved in the discussions. It is important to listen to Mrs De Capprio's daughter and her perspective of what is happening and what she sees as the best outcome for her mother. It may be that the neglect of her mother was not done out of malice but from a lack of knowledge and understanding of the impact that dementia, and the subsequent poor nutrition, can have on an older person physically and mentally.

Given Mrs De Capprio's agitated state on admission, the decision to insert a nasogastric tube should be considered a last option. It is important that strategies are trialled that reflect Mrs De Capprio's preferences. Perhaps the liquids being offered were not to her liking or were not presented in a way that was familiar to her or reflect her previous experiences.

If Mrs De Capprio is returned home, then it is important that strategies are put in place to support and educate her daughter along the lines previously discussed.

Where someone who holds an enduring power of attorney is not seen to be acting in the best interests of the individual concerned, their authority can be challenged. However, it is important to clarify the implications of this and offer constructive solutions.

CONCLUSION

Identification of, and intervention in, situations of elder abuse requires knowledge of the signs and symptoms of the major types of abuse as well as knowledge of both the facility-level and wider system resources that can be brought into play in response to abuse. Many practice settings have now developed their own protocols to guide workers in their intervention decision making, but this may not obviate the need for specific consultancy around medical/legal or social impacts of the abuse.

References

Anetzberger, G., 2005. The reality of elder abuse. The Clinical Gerontologist 28 (1/2), 1–25.

Boldy, D., Horner, B., Crouchley, K., 2005. Addressing elder abuse: Western Australian vignette. Australasian Journal on Ageing 24 (1), 3–8.

Department of Human Services, 2009. With respect to age: practice guidelines for health services and community agencies for the prevention of elder abuse. State Government of Victoria, Melbourne.

Dyer, C.B., Connolly, M.T., McFeeley, P., 2003. The clinical and medical forensics of elder abuse and neglect. In: Bonnie, R. (Ed.), Elder abuse: abuse, neglect and exploitation in an aging America. The National Academies Press, Washington.

Field, A., 1996. Financial exploitation of older people in their homes (Government No. 0731088123). NSW Advisory Committee on Abuse of Older People. Department of Ageing and Disability, Sydney.

Homer, A., Gilleard, C., 1990. Abuse of elderly people by their carers. British Medical Journal 301, 1359–1362.

Hughes, M., 1997. That triggers me right off: factors influencing abuse and violence in older people's care giving relationships. Australian Journal on Ageing 16 (2), 53–60.

Jacobson, C., Pabst, S., Regan, S., 2006. A lifetime of intimate partner violence: coping strategies for older women. Journal of Interpersonal Violence 21 (5), 634–651.

James, M., Graycar, A., 2000. Preventing crime against older Australians. Australian Institute of Criminology, Canberra.

Kosberg, J., Biggs, S., Phillipson, C., et al., 1996. Elder abuse in perspective. Ageing and Society 16, 644–645.

Kosberg, J., Lowenstein, A., Garcia, J., 2005. Study of elder abuse within diverse communities. Journal of Elder Abuse & Neglect 15 (03), 71–89.

Kurrle, S., Sadler, P., Cameron, I., 1992. Patterns of elder abuse. Medical Journal of Australia 157, 673–676.

Kurrle, S., Sadler, P., Lockwood, K., et al., 1997. Elder abuse: a multicentre Australian study. Medical Journal of Australia 166, 119–122.

Kurrle, S., Naughtin, G., 2008. An overview of elder abuse and neglect in Australia. Journal of Elder Abuse and Neglect 20 (2), 108–125.

Kurrle, S., 2004. Elder abuse. Australian Society for Geriatric Medicine. Position Statement No.1. Australasian Journal on Ageing 23 (1), 38–41.

Lachs, M., Pillemer, K., 2004. Elder abuse. The Lancet 364 (9441), 1263–1272.

Livermore, P., Bunt, R., Biscan, K., 2001. Elder abuse among clients and carers referred to the Central Coast ACAT: a descriptive analysis. Australasian Journal on Ageing 20 (1), 41–47.

NSW Office for the Ageing, 2007. Inter-agency protocol on elder abuse. Dept of Disability Ageing and Home Care, Sydney.

Podnieks, E., McDonald, P., Hornick, J., et al., 1994. Elder abuse and neglect in Canada. Canadian Journal of Aging 13 (1), 123–126.

Schaeffer, J., 1999. Older and isolated women and domestic violence project. Journal of Elder Abuse and Neglect 11 (1), 59–73.

Setterlund, D., Wilson, J., Tilse, C., 1999. Substitute decision making and older people (No. 0642241422). Australian Institute of Criminology, Canberra, ACT.

Tilse, C., Wilson, J., Setterlund, D., 2003. The mismanagement of the assets of older people: the concerns and actions of aged care practitioners in Queensland. Australasian Journal on Ageing 22 (1), 9–14.

Tinker, A., O'Keffe, M., Hills, A., 2007. UK study of abuse and neglect of older people: prevalence survey report. National Centre for Social Research, London.

Wainer, J., Darzins, P., Owada, K., 2010. Prevalence of financial elder abuse in Victoria. Monash University, Melbourne.

Wiglesworth, A., Austin, R., Corona, M., et al., 2009. Bruising as a marker of physical elder abuse. Journal of the American Geriatrics Society 57, 1191–1196.

Wiglesworth, A., Mosqueda, L., Mulnard, R., et al., 2010. Screening for abuse and neglect of people with dementia. Journal of the American Geriatrics Society 58, 493–500.

World Health Organization, 2011. European report on preventing elder mistreatment. WHO Regional Office for Europe, Copenhagen. ISBN 978 92 890 0237 0230.

Zink, T., 2006. A lifetime of intimate partner violence. Journal of Interpersonal Violence 21 (5), 634–651.

CHAPTER 18

END-OF-LIFE DECISION MAKING FOR OLDER PEOPLE

Deirdre Fetherstonhaugh and Laura Tarzia

Editors' comments

This chapter deals with the increasing issues surrounding end-of-life decision making. As the life trajectory for older people changes, the need for open discussion about their health problems and treatment becomes more critical. Acceptance of the ageing process itself is often not easy so the matter of a good death is even more distressing for some people to consider. The vignette provides an excellent discussion on the need for open dialogue with the older person and their families, whether they are acutely ill or have chronic health problems. How a person wishes to be treated when quality of life is not going to improve, no matter what interventions are put in place, is essential in order for the care provided to be person centred. The issue of capacity/competency is one that must be determined before any decision is made by any person involved in care.

INTRODUCTION

Prior to the 20th century most people died suddenly of infections or injuries (Jones et al 2012). Today, however, most of us in the developed world will die well into old age after serious chronic disease and a substantial period of disability (Lynn et al 2000). Being able to have input into the process of our dying, whether that be through limiting or refusing interventions or determining how we are to be cared for, raises many ethical, legal and clinical issues. This chapter will examine end–of–life decision making with specific reference to older people who are no longer able to make an autonomous choice about their future care. We will introduce you to Charlie and explore the concerns his story raises to highlight some of the issues involved in end-of-life decision making. A discussion of the challenges of competency/capacity to make decisions will be provided. The final component of this chapter will examine advance care planning as a means by which the autonomous wishes of the older person (or people of any age) can be maintained, even when they are no longer competent to actively make their own decisions about future healthcare.

END-OF-LIFE TRAJECTORIES FOR OLDER PEOPLE

Life expectancy in Australia has increased dramatically over the last century, with a particular increase for those aged over 65 (Australian Institute of Health and Welfare (AIHW) 2012). Although statistically we can expect to live the majority of our lives in good health, it becomes more likely as we age that we will acquire a long-term condition that will affect our quality of life (AIHW 2012). In fact, in the most recent National Health Survey, nearly all people aged 65 years or older reported having at least one long-term condition, and over 80% of them reported having three or more long-term conditions (Department of Health and Ageing 2012). While these statistics include illnesses that are debilitating but not necessarily life-threatening, such as arthritis, in many cases chronic conditions can be fatal, such as ischaemic heart disease, cancer or diabetes. In recent years dementia has added significantly to the burden of serious chronic disease and has now become the third leading cause of death in Australia (Alzheimer's Australia 2012).

Lynn and Adamson (2003 p 8) have characterised the typical illness trajectories for people suffering from fatal chronic conditions in the following three ways:

1. Short period of evident decline (typical of cancer): the person is often able to maintain comfort and function for a relatively long period until a substantial decline in the last few weeks or days of life leads to death.
2. Long-term limitations with intermittent serious episodes (typical of heart failure): the person generally maintains a good quality of life, with occasional periods of decline as the disease overwhelms the body's processes. After a few such episodes, death may occur.
3. Prolonged dwindling (typical of dementia): multiple body systems become frail and the person slowly dwindles towards death over a period of years. Older people often fall into this category.

While these trajectories can be a useful guide in providing end-of-life care, there is still a great deal of uncertainty surrounding the experience of chronic illness and dying. In particular, issues concerning prognosis can complicate end-of-life decisions, such as inaccurate estimation of life expectancy by health professionals (Kwak et al 2011, Sampson et al 2011) and poor communication of the prognosis to family (Caron et al 2005). Research has shown that clinicians are reluctant to identify patients as dying (Kwak et al 2011) and tend to overestimate the person's survival time, which may mean that conversations about end-of-life care are postponed until it is too late. These issues are especially relevant for those in the prolonged dwindling category, primarily older people with dementia. When a person dwindles slowly towards death, it is difficult to assess exactly when they cease to be 'chronically ill' and begin 'dying'. As Lynn (2005 p S14) has described it, many older people 'are inching towards oblivion with small losses every few weeks or months', which makes it a challenge to identify when conversations about end-of-life care should take place.

Although managing one serious chronic illness is difficult enough, an even more complicated situation is when an older person has multiple chronic conditions (comorbidities). This is an increasingly common scenario among older people, and one that impacts significantly on the healthcare sector. Different conditions present with different symptoms and may follow different illness trajectories, which makes decision making around end-of-life care even more complicated. In a recent Australian study, for example, Caughey et al (2008 p 8) found that 'potentially for every elderly patient presenting to their GP with a chronic disease, one in two will also have arthritis or hypertension, and one in five will have a type of cardiovascular disease or diabetes'. In the case of an older person with a chronic illness that requires hospitalisation, management of any comorbidities forms an important part of end-of-life care, but who decides how they are managed?

The following vignette outlines the experience of Charlie, who has two chronic diseases, each with a differing illness trajectory. Charlie's story highlights the difficulties in providing appropriate end-of-life care when a person has multiple chronic conditions, particularly when the person's wishes for care are unknown. Despite the unpredictability of Charlie's medical conditions, however, as his story unfolds it becomes evident that safeguards should have been put in place to protect him from what eventually occurred and which would have provided more appropriate management at his end of life.

Vignette

Charlie was a 78-year-old man who had been widowed for 15 years, lived on his own, and had one married son who rarely visited him. Charlie had few medical problems until five years ago when a diagnosis was made of end-stage kidney disease requiring ongoing haemodialysis. He commenced dialysis in a satellite dialysis unit in the community. The ambulance transported him there. He had no problems or complications from the treatment until the nursing staff in the dialysis unit began to notice that he was becoming increasingly forgetful, confused and rather withdrawn. He started to send the ambulance service away in the mornings, denying that he had to go to dialysis, and became increasingly difficult for the staff to dialyse if/when he eventually arrived at the centre. Charlie's sister was worried about him living unsupervised at home. After much negotiation Charlie, although not very enthusiastic about the idea, finally agreed to move into a residential aged care facility.

Due to increasing frailty and behavioural problems, Charlie also had to move to the hospital for dialysis because he was no longer stable enough for the satellite unit. His mental capabilities began to diminish, he no longer spoke unless coerced, and he had to be prompted to eat, sometimes needing to be fed. He fell over in the residential aged care facility and fractured his femur, which was subsequently pinned. While he was being treated as an inpatient in hospital he was physically restrained to keep him in bed. During one episode of dialysis he pulled out one of his needles and lost several hundred millilitres of blood on the floor—subsequently both his arms were then tightly bound on either side of him to prevent a further such episode.

The nursing staff found it difficult to care for Charlie, especially because he had become totally uncommunicative and just sat with a vacant expression on his face. Many of the staff had known Charlie from when he started dialysis, when he was an avid reader, loved watching documentaries, and was quick to rise to a political debate at any time. The dialysis nurses thought that Charlie could probably feel pain because he pulled away and had to be held down while the dialysis needles were being inserted. The nursing staff were compromised in their care for Charlie and felt that dialysis was not in his 'best interests'. The medical staff, however, did not feel comfortable about withdrawing dialysis and Charlie's son (Michael), when finally contacted, would not discuss this option. Michael said that his father had made the decision to commence dialysis and that he 'could not' authorise the withdrawal of this treatment from Charlie. It was decided, however, by both Michael and the medical staff, that if Charlie fell over again he would not go to the operating theatre, and that if he got a chest infection intravenous antibiotics would not be given.

Charlie did fall over at the residential aged care facility after setting himself free from his restraints. This time he fractured his pelvis. He was transferred to hospital where he was kept in bed, given pain relief, and nursed to keep him as comfortable as possible. Charlie died 18 hours after he was admitted to the hospital.

Charlie's experience highlights several issues. Several years previously he had made a decision to undertake a life-sustaining treatment. He had not discussed with anyone whether or not he wanted the therapy to be maintained if he experienced a serious decline in his health status. Charlie had lived independently but then developed dementia, which impaired his decision-making capacity and necessitated his move into supported living accommodation. Increasingly it became apparent to those who provided his dialysis treatment that the continuation of this therapy, especially the way in which it seemed necessary to undertake it,[1] was burdensome for Charlie and even painful.

DECISION MAKING

Determining who should make decisions about care at the end of life is difficult. There is an expectation, especially in Western societies, that autonomy and the right of individuals to make autonomous choices should trump other ethical considerations when it comes to decision making. During the 20th and 21st centuries there has been increasing demand for control over one's body and medical destiny, especially in areas such as dying and reproduction (Parker & Cartwright 2005 p 57). Enhancing individual choice and supporting one's involvement in healthcare decisions has become a central theme of health ethics. This is reliant, however, on the person being competent to make, or having the capacity to participate in, these decisions. Alternatively, it is reliant on processes by which people can protect their autonomous decision making

....

[1]It was deemed necessary to restrain Charlie from both the perspective of 'safety' for him, so that he wouldn't bleed to death if he pulled out the needles, and for infection control for nearby patients.

for a time when they themselves are no longer able to explicitly express their wishes. Older people who have a disease such as dementia where there is deterioration and permanent cognitive impairment, or who have experienced some catastrophic health event that renders them temporarily cognitively impaired, may find themselves in a situation where they are no longer able to decide or determine what is in their best interests and what will happen to them. They lack decision-making capacity.

> ## Enhancing individual choice and supporting one's involvement in healthcare decisions has become a central theme of health ethics.

COMPETENCE

Competence, thought of as the capability to consent, is generally acknowledged as a legal determination while its clinical counterpart is known as 'decision-making capacity' (Singer 1992 p 1236). In the literature, however, the two terms are often used interchangeably (Biegler & Stewart 2001, Miller & Martin 2000). For the purposes of this discussion both these terms will be taken to have a similar meaning—that is, whether a person is cognitively able to make an informed decision about their healthcare, and specifically in the context of this chapter, about the care/interventions to be provided (or not to be provided) towards the end of life. Competence or capacity to make healthcare decisions go to the heart of the concept of informed consent (Miller & Martin 2000) and decision making. According to Parker and Cartwright (2005 p 61), capacity is 'a primary arbiter of social life, and the inclusion of certain members of society from standard decision making rights and practices on the basis of capacity is one of the clearest social-ethical distinctions we make'.

> ## Competence or capacity to make healthcare decisions go to the heart of the concept of informed consent.

In general, a person is presumed to be competent to make decisions and the burden of proof lies with others to prove that they are not. Since competence is commonly understood to mean the ability to perform a task (Biegler & Stewart 2001), the 'criteria of particular competencies [can] vary from context to context because the criteria are relative to specific tasks' (Beauchamp & Childress 2009 p 112). Whether someone is competent or not depends on the person's ability to meet the demands of a particular task or situation. Competence or incompetence should be the conclusion about the match or mismatch between the person's ability and the decision-making demands of the situation they face—a functional approach (Parker & Cartwright 2005 p 63). In the context of healthcare decisions, competence means being able to consent to, or refuse, medical treatment and make decisions about that treatment.

Health professionals' judgments of a person's incompetence may lead to overriding that person's decisions, turning to surrogates,[2] applying for the appointment of a guardian or seeking involuntary institutionalisation for the person whose competence is questioned. Given these implications, it is therefore important that all factors are considered when a determination of cognitive incompetence is made.

In Charlie's case, the health professionals perceived his increasing lack of understanding and insight about the fact he needed to have dialysis if he wanted to stay alive as evidence of cognitive decline and, therefore, an increasing lack of decision-making capacity. The staff determined that this lack of insight was initially demonstrated by his turning away of the ambulance, and then later by his removal of the dialysis needles and his inability to sit still while the needles were being inserted. It must be said, however, that Charlie's behaviour could also have been an indication of his desire not to continue with dialysis. This was not explicitly explored as a reason for his behaviour. The assumption by the health professionals that Charlie's removal of the dialysis needles was a sign of incompetence highlights an important ethical issue in determining decision-making capacity. Whether a person is competent or has the capacity to make a decision should not be determined by the *outcomes* of the decision because this implies that 'competent decisions conform to some specified content ... since it dictates conformity with some authority external to the individual' (Parker & Cartwright 2005 p 62). In other words, a decision should not be labelled as irrational just because it is not judged as the right decision by others (Brock & Wartman 1990). Using compliance or noncompliance with the opinion and conclusions of health professionals as the barometer to question competence is an outcome approach. The outcome of the decision has been deemed more important than the process by which the person reached the decision (Caplan 1992 p 214). In real-life clinical situations, when someone reaches a decision that is not commensurate with what the health professionals or family would have decided, then the competence of the person to make that decision has been known to be questioned, as was the case with Charlie. Alternatively, another approach is to use the person's status as the criteria to determine decision-making capacity—that is, the competent are separated from the incompetent along conventional social lines such as age or the existence of an illness (Parker & Cartwright 2005 pp 62–63). This approach, however, like that of only reviewing the outcome, does not look at the content of the decision and immediately classifies older people with dementia into the incompetent category without taking into account the cognitive ability of the individual to make a particular decision at a particular time.

Grisso and Appelbaum (1998) define competence as the ability to *reason* with relevant information so as to engage in a logical process of weighing treatment/care options. A determination of competence also involves being able to express

---

[2]In the case of Victoria this person refers to the appointment of a medical enduring power of attorney (MEPoA).

a choice about the treatment options (Grisso & Appelbaum 1998). It could be argued that Charlie was unable to verbally and coherently indicate what course of treatment/care he desired. However, given that his story is true, it must be noted that there was no effort made to try other methods of communication besides the active asking of questions with the expectation that he would, or should, appropriately respond. A lack of ability to express a preference can become apparent in the course of routine attempts to talk with a person (Grisso & Appelbaum 1998). Medical conditions that can affect a person's cognitive capacity include mental illness, dementia and delirium, and an assessment is needed to determine whether any of these are present. Health professionals sometimes perform clinical assessments using validated tools, dementia ratings or neuro-psychological testing to help determine general competence. These tests, however, are not definitive in their ability to determine whether or not someone is competent to make a *specific* healthcare decision. In short, there is no acceptable 'gold standard' test for determining competency to make decisions. While the health professionals suspected that Charlie had dementia, no formal screening was undertaken to assess whether he was competent to make a specific decision about the continuation of his dialysis.

Determining competence

So how should health professionals determine whether a person is competent? Health professionals generally should informally assess a person's competence during several interactions with them (Parker & Cartwright 2005). According to Biegler and Stewart (2001), the treating doctor is the person best placed to assess a person's competence as they are likely to know the facts of the case. In particular, they are likely to know whether any of the factors that may impair competence are present. Moye et al (2006) also recognise that clinical judgment is still the best way to make a capacity determination, although they admit that it can be unreliable. Parker and Cartwright (2005 p 79) advocate a simple, practical method for assessing capacity to make decisions, which could consist of the following steps:

1. Ensure a valid indication for assessing capacity is present.
2. Inform the person about the assessment.
3. Discuss with the person and other relevant people the relevant indications and circumstances.
4. Provide good communication processes and relevant information for decision making.
5. Assess the person's understanding of the issues and consequences of the options available.
6. Act according to results of the assessment.

Decision-making capacity can fluctuate according to time and the presence of illness (Skene 2004 p 154). It could be argued, therefore, that the greater the potential risk to the person, the more stringent the standard of competence needs to be (Kerridge et al 1998, Miller & Martin 2000). It has also been argued, however, that if a risk-related scale is accepted, then levels of capacity may differ for treatment refusal compared with consent (Parker & Cartwright 2005), especially if the probable outcome of no treatment is death.

Furthermore, to accept such a scale would mean that the criteria used to determine capacity depends on the likely outcomes of the decision, rather than the processes used to make the decision (Parker & Cartwright 2005). This smacks of paternalism and, as mentioned earlier, essentially becomes an outcome approach because it allows health professionals to use their own value judgments about what is the 'right' decision in a particular instance.

Cognitive capacity is essential for engagement in any sort of healthcare decision making. Even though no formal assessment was undertaken, Charlie evidently did not have the capacity to engage in healthcare decision making. There was not any discussion about what he would have wanted had he thought about the possibility of his current situation when he had been cognitively capable. No one had been appointed to act and make decisions on his behalf. In hindsight and after reflecting on Charlie's situation, it probably would have been appropriate if someone (probably one of the health professionals caring for Charlie) had made an application for a guardian to be appointed who could act on his behalf. The following section will discuss advance care planning, something that if undertaken in Charlie's situation could potentially have improved his experiences.

ADVANCE CARE PLANNING

People have a fear of dying. They do not want to die in pain or undergo overly burdensome treatment, especially if the benefits are likely to be non-existent and the prognosis poor. Having some control over what treatments are instigated, continued or never commenced is one way for a person to have some input into the management of their dying. In Australia every competent adult has the legal right under common law (and in some states and territories under statute law) to accept or refuse any healthcare or treatment including life-saving treatment (Cartwright 2011 p 14).[3] The protection and exercise of this right for people who are no longer competent and cannot communicate their choices can be facilitated through a process called advance care planning.

Advance care planning can describe any activity that involves thinking about preferences for future care (Aw et al 2012). Specifically, advance care planning is a process by which a person can plan and make decisions in advance about their healthcare by discussing their preferences with family, health professionals and significant others. Advance care planning can also involve discussion and determination about: where the person might like to be when they die; the environment in which they would like to die; funeral arrangements; the people they most want around them; whom they wish consulted about their care, and other aspects that might make the end of their life as peaceful as possible.

The process of advance care planning provides insight into a person's wishes before they lose capacity to make their own decisions and can be seen as an ethically desirable extension of a person's right to make autonomous choices (Singer et al 1998). Ideally, it involves ongoing discussions about healthcare preferences between the person for whom the advance care planning is being

....
[3]For example, in Victoria a Refusal of Treatment certificate under Section 5 of the *Medical Treatment Act 1988* (Vic).

undertaken and their family, health professionals and significant others, and then documentation of these preferences (Blackford & Street 2012, Van Leuven 2012). Advance care planning can help people avoid unwanted, non-beneficial or futile life-prolonging treatments or physical states that are considered by some to be without dignity. Advance care planning should not be static. Once the discussion has been initiated, it should be regularly revisited. This is especially important when the person has a chronically progressive disease such as dementia. People do not 'become demented overnight' and in most cases the gradual progression of the disease allows for adaptation and a shift in response (Hertogh 2011 p 513); an ongoing advance care planning process recognises this.

 Advance care planning should not be static. Once the discussion has been initiated it should be regularly revisited.

Ideally, advance care planning is best initiated at a time when the person retains capacity. For those people (and especially those who are older) who are in receipt of ongoing medical treatments, advance care planning should be part of routine care. Malcomson and Bisbee (2009) advocate that discussions about advance care planning should be separate consultations with no distractions from other issues. Discussions should be undertaken by people who know the person well and they should be documented. Advance care planning reduces the burden of decision making placed on families.

Types of advance care planning

The formal legal components of advance care planning involve advance directives. These can be classified into two categories: treatment directives and proxy directives. A treatment directive, known as a living will in many jurisdictions, refers to a document specifying what kind of treatment the person would have desired under specific conditions in the event of incapacity, while a proxy directive empowers another person (healthcare proxy, surrogate decision maker or power of attorney) to make decisions on behalf of the person (Hertogh 2011). The existence of a living will or written advance directive enables the person to exercise their precedent or prospective autonomy (Hertogh 2011) and prioritises the person's past preferences over what may now be their best interests. The living will or written advance directive presumes that the person writing the directive is currently in a better position to decide how healthcare decisions should be made for a time in the future when they no longer have capacity (Hertogh 2011). There are many arguments that debate why past preferences and thereby precedent autonomy should be prioritised and these include:

- *The belief that such preferences are likely to be carefully thought through, and reflect the person's whole approach to their life, what they value, and the kind of person they are or would like to be.*
- *The importance of permitting people to exercise control over their future (incapacitated) lives.*

- *The belief that the preferences of the person who no longer has capacity do not have the same status as their past preferences, because they cannot be the result of a rational decision making process.*
- *The practical difficulties inherent in interpreting the preferences of people who are no longer able to communicate clearly.*

(Nuffield Council on Bioethics 2009 p 82)

Written advance directives are usually characterised in the form of: '1) a negative advance directive (negative treatment directive) that stipulates which kinds of treatments are not to be applied in specified circumstances; and 2) a positive advance directive which describes what treatments or actions the author of the advance directive would wish for under certain circumstances' (Hertogh et al 2007 p 50). It may be argued, however, that people may not be the best judges of what is in their own best interests in circumstances they have never encountered (Dworkin 1986), such as certain disease states or as recipients of some medical treatments such as dialysis. A living will or written directive, therefore, may protect a person's best interests better if it states what a person decides is an acceptable outcome—that is, what they are willing to accept in respect to their ability to communicate or function physically or cognitively—rather than a list of treatments or health states they would or wouldn't accept (Silvester & Detering 2011). Providing a list of treatments is problematic because people cannot accurately predict what they might be able to endure in the future and treatments need to be evaluated in context. A person might say they don't want to be kept alive with artificial ventilation, but this statement does not consider specific circumstances—short- versus long-term treatment, good versus bad prognosis of recovery, short versus long life expectancy (Levi & Green 2010).

The second type of advance directive, the legal appointment of a surrogate decision maker, is potentially far more flexible and can be reactive to the progression of chronic illness states and the potential adaptation that the person may make to those illness states. Surrogate decision making can have advantages over directives documented when the person is well; the most apparent being the fact that the surrogate decision maker can keep up with changing wishes and thereby is better positioned to know what is in the current best interests of the person. In the state of Victoria surrogate decision making is legally recognised in the form of an agent with enduring power of attorney (medical treatment) (MEPoA) and this person(s) can agree to, or refuse, medical treatment and can also consent to participation in medical research on behalf of the person who no longer has capacity (Office of the Public Advocate 2009). The surrogate decision maker is usually appointed by the person when they still have capacity. Surrogate decision makers should: act in the best interests of the person who no longer has capacity; wherever possible make the same decision that the person would have made; and avoid situations in which there is a conflict of interest (Office of the Public Advocate 2009). Surrogate decision making allows for respect for the precedent autonomy (past preferences) of the person who no longer has capacity, while also taking into account what the person's current best interests and preferences may be. In a situation such as Charlie's, where the person has dementia or cognitive impairment, recognition of present preferences means acknowledging:

- *... that a person with dementia, however cognitively impaired, has a perspective that is valid, even though it is rooted in the present moment rather than in the past ...*
- *... that people with dementia remain 'valuers' and that cognitive impairment does not prevent people from holding and expressing values, if need be through gesture and facial expression ...*
- *... people should not be 'held to ransom' by their past beliefs and assumptions especially as such attitudes may change radically when facing major life events ...*
- *... once the individual with dementia can no longer remember their past beliefs and wishes, they are no longer the same 'person' as they once were, and hence should not be bound in any way by those past beliefs.*

(Nuffield Council on Bioethics 2009 p 82)

The determination of best interests on behalf of someone else who does not have capacity to articulate them cannot be prescriptive. There are, however, several considerations that should be taken into account and these may include:

- *the person's past and present wishes, feelings and preferences in regard to healthcare—these may have been documented or just discussed*
- *the beliefs and values that would be likely to influence the person's decisions if they had capacity. This may have been documented or in many cases be something that significant others such as family and friends who have had a relationship with the person for a long time know*
- *other factors they would be likely to consider if they were able to do so*
- *the views of a number of others concerned with the person's welfare as to what action would be in the person's best interest where practical and appropriate.*

(Nuffield Council on Bioethics 2009 p 78)

Another consideration in the determination of best interest should be the current distress and/or pleasure of the person who no longer has capacity to articulate their preferences. For example, in Charlie's case, had he discussed his wishes with his son, he may have stipulated that if he were to develop dementia he would not want to continue the dialysis or be given any other life-sustaining treatment. Considering that Charlie's experience with dialysis was not a positive one once he developed dementia, it may have been fairly evident that to follow his wishes (evidenced by his behaviour) would have been the right course of action. But what if Charlie had appeared to enjoy a *good* quality of life after he developed dementia? What if he appeared to enjoy the experience of living in residential care and did not have any problems with the dialysis? Would it be right to stop dialysis and let Charlie die, even though he still seemed to be enjoying life?

Some issues to consider ...

Incorporating advance care planning as a component of healthcare provision gives anyone, especially older people with multiple comorbidities, the best opportunity to make informed decisions. Research has shown that advance care planning can successfully be embedded into organisational structures and routine practices (Blackford & Street 2012), and therefore it should be introduced into public education programs, national healthy ageing policies, residential aged care facilities, funding and accreditation streams and into healthcare culture and routines to assist health professionals to facilitate informed decision making with older people. We need to remember, however, that formalised advance care planning may not be suitable for all or may need to be tailored to suit an individual's requirements. Australia is a multicultural society, and therefore the influence of a person's culture and ethnicity needs to be explored in relation to advance care planning. Research shows that culture plays a significant part in determining how individuals 'perceive, experience, and practice health' (Johnstone & Kanitsaki 2009 p 406), as well as shaping a person's fundamental values about life and death. In Australia, the uptake of advance care plans is low amongst individuals from culturally and linguistically diverse (CALD) backgrounds (Johnstone & Kanitsaki 2009), often due to a difference in the way a particular culture views the core values embedded in the advance care planning process. As mentioned earlier in the chapter, in the Western world the mainstream culture promotes autonomy and self-determination, and advance care planning is seen as a way of preserving these values. Many ethnic minorities, however, emphasise group consensus and family decision making as the preferred option. A participant in a study on Korean-American older people's attitudes towards end-of-life care, for example, explained that:

> Even if I had completed an advance directive and left it with my children, they will be the one[s] who will make the decision through family discussion. After all, the final decision will be made based on love and trust for each other ...

(Kwak & Salmon 2007 p 1869)

Furthermore, issues surrounding truth-telling can be a barrier to advance care planning. As discussed earlier in this chapter, knowledge about a person's prognosis is an essential part of effective end-of-life care. As Johnstone and Kanitsaki (2009) have pointed out, however, many cultures believe that to inform a person of a bad diagnosis is fundamentally inappropriate for a number of reasons:

- Talking about death is considered to be akin to wishing death on someone.
- Family members are expected to be 'gatekeepers' of bad news to avoid the patient becoming distressed and losing hope.
- Bad news must be delivered the right way, through the right people.

Health professionals need to take these cultural factors into account when raising the issue of advance care planning. Phrasing the discussion around what could be done to make the person more comfortable during their stay in hospital, for example, might be a better way to approach the issue, rather than asking what care they would like at the 'end of life'.

CONCLUSION

In this chapter we have highlighted the complexities surrounding end-of-life decision making for older people, particularly those living with dementia or other cognitive impairment. The centrality of informed consent to healthcare and end-of-life decision making means that, in some cases, an older person with dementia will no longer be capable of making a reasoned choice and understanding the implications of their decisions. In these cases, as we have suggested, advance care planning—either in the form of a discussion with family and friends, a documented advance directive or the appointment of a surrogate decision maker—can be a way of protecting the older person's autonomy and ensuring that treatment decisions are made in their best interests. It is important to remember, however, that advance care plans need to be regularly reassessed to ensure that they continue to comply with the person's current circumstances and preferences. Furthermore, advance care planning needs to have the flexibility to incorporate a range of cultural and religious beliefs so that all Australians have the opportunity to maintain control over healthcare and end-of-life decisions.

Reflective questions

1. The matter of determining competency/capacity is a difficult issue for healthcare providers. How does your workplace deal with this issue?

2. Advance care planning is increasingly being adopted in healthcare organisations and residential aged care facilities but it is not as prevalent in the community. How could you improve the uptake of this process in community care?

3. Reflect on how you would want to be cared for if you were 80 years old and had just been diagnosed with early-stage dementia. Write your care plan now.

References

Alzheimer's Australia, 2012. National facts and figures 2012 Online. Available: http://www.fightdementia.org.au/understanding-dementia/statistics.aspx, 25 Oct 2012.

Australian Institute of Health and Welfare, 2012. Australia's health 2012 Australia's Health Series no.13 (Vol. AUS 156). AIHW, Canberra.

Aw, D., Hayhoe, B., Smajdor, A., et al., 2012. Advance care planning and the older patient. Quarterly Journal of Medicine 105 (3), 225–230.

Beauchamp, T., Childress, J., 2009. Principles of biomedical ethics, sixth ed. Oxford University Press, New York.

Biegler, P., Stewart, C., 2001. Assessing competence to refuse medical treatment. Medical Journal of Australia 174, 522–525.

Blackford, J., Street, A., 2012. Is an advance care planning model feasible in community palliaitve care? A multi-site action research approach. Journal of Advanced Nursing 68 (9), 2012–2033.

Brock, D.W., Wartman, S., 1990. When competent patients make irrational choices. New England Journal of Medicine 322, 1595–1599.

Caplan, A., 1992. If I were a rich man could I buy a pancreas? Indiana University Press, Indianapolis.

Caron, C.D., Griffith, J., Arcand, M., 2005. End-of-life decision making in dementia. The perspective of family caregivers. Dementia 4 (1), 113–136.

Cartwright, C., 2011. Planning for the end of life for people with dementia. Paper 23. Part 1. Alzheimer's Australia, Scullin, ACT.

Caughey, G.E., Vitry, A.I., Gilbert, A.L., et al., 2008. Prevalence of comorbidity of chronic diseases in Australia. BMC Public Health 8, 221–234.

Department of Health and Ageing, 2012. Chronic disease. Online. Available: http://www.health.gov.au/internet/main/publishing.nsf/Content/chronic#, 3 Dec 2012.

Dworkin, R., 1986. Autonomy and the demented self. The Milbank Quarterly 64 (Suppl.2), 4–16.

Grisso, T., Appelbaum, P.S., 1998. Assessing competence to consent to treatment: a guide for physicians and other health professionals. Oxford University Press, New York.

Hertogh, C.M.P.M., 2011. The misleading simplicity of advance directives. International Psychogeriatrics 23 (4), 511–515.

Hertogh, C.M.P.M., de Boer, M.E., Droes, R.-M., et al., 2007. Would we rather lose our life than lose our self? Lessons from the Dutch debate on euthanasia for patients with dementia. The American Journal of Bioethics 7 (4), 48–56.

Johnstone, M.-J., Kanitsaki, O., 2009. Ethics and advance care planning in a culturally diverse society. Journal of Transcultural Nursing 20 (4), 405–416.

Jones, D.S., Podolsky, S.H., Greene, J.A., 2012. The burden of disease and the changing task of medicine. New England Journal of Medicine 366 (25), 2333–2338.

Kerridge, I.H., Lowe, M., McPhee, J.R., 1998. Ethics and law for the health professions. Social Science Press, Katoomba NSW.

Kwak, J., Allen, J.Y., Haley, W.E., 2011. Advance care planning and end-of-life decision making. In: Dilworth-Anderson P., Palmer M.H. (Eds.), Annual review of gerontology, vol. 31. Springer Publishing Company, New York.

Kwak, J., Salmon, J.R., 2007. Attitudes and preferences of Korean-American older adults and caregivers on end-of-life care. Journal of the American Geriatrics Society 55 (11), 1867–1872.

Levi, B.H., Green, M.J., 2010. Too soon to give up: Re-examining the value of advance directives. The American Journal of Bioethics 10 (4), 3–22.

Lynn, J., 2005. Living long in fragile health: the new demographics shape end-of-life care. In: Jennings B., Kaebnick G.E., Murray T.H. (Eds.), Improving end of life care: why has it been so difficult? The Hastings Centre, New York.

Lynn, J., Adamson, D.M., 2003. Living well at the end of life: adapting health care to serious chronic illness. RAND Health, California.

Lynn, J., Schall, M.W., Milne, C., et al., 2000. Quality improvements in end-of-life care: insights from two collaboratives. Joint Commission Journal on Quality Improvement 26 (5), 254–267.

Malcomson, H., Bisbee, S., 2009. Perspective of healthy elders on advance care planning. J Am Acad Nurse Pract 21 (1), 18–23.

Miller, S.S., Martin, D.B., 2000. Assessing capacity. Emergency Medicine Clinics of North America 18 (2), 233–242.

Moye, J., Gurrera, R., Karel, M., et al., 2006. Empirical advances in the assessment of the capacity to consent to medical treatment: Clinical implications and research needs. Clinical Psychological Review 26 (8), 1054–1077.

Nuffield Council on Bioethics, 2009. Dementia: ethical issues. Nuffield Council on Bioethics, London.

Office of the Public Advocate, 2009. Enduring power of attorney (medical treatment). Planning ahead for future medical treatment decisions. Online. Available: http://www.publicadvocate.vic.gov.au/file/file/Powerofattorney/Enduring%20Power%20of%20Attorney%20(Medical%20Treatment)%20-%20Print%20-%2021_07_09.pdf, 1 May 2013.

Parker, M., Cartwright, C., 2005. Mental capacity in medical practice and advance care planning: Clinical, ethical and legal issues. In: Collier B., Coyne C., Sullivan K. (Eds.), Mental capacity: powers of attorney an advance health directives. The Federation Press, Leichhardt NSW. pp. 56–92.

Sampson, E., Burns, A., Richards, M., 2011. Improving end-of-life care for people with dementia. British Journal of Psychiatry 199, 357–359.

Silvester, W., Detering, K., 2011. Advance care planning and end-of-life care. Medical Journal of Australia 195 (8), 435–436.

Singer, P.A., 1992. Nephrologists' experience with and attitudes towards decisions to forego dialysis. The end-stage renal disease network of New England. Journal of the American Society of Nephrology 2 (7), 1235–1240.

Singer, P.A., Martin, D.K., Lavery, J.V., et al., 1998. Reconceptualising advance care planning from the patient's perspective. Archives of Internal Medicine 158 (8), 879–884.

Skene, L., 2004. Law and medical practice: rights, duties, claims and defences. Butterworths, Sydney.

Van Leuven, K.A., 2012. Advanced care planning in health service users. Journal of Clinical Nursing 21 (21–22), 3126–3133.

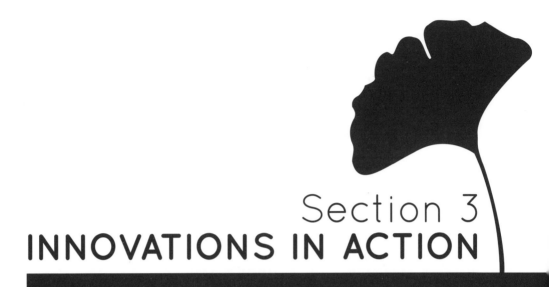

Section 3
INNOVATIONS IN ACTION

CHAPTER 19

SELF-ESTEEM, DIGNITY AND FINDING MEANING IN DEMENTIA

Sally Garratt and Patricia Baines

Editors' comments

This chapter raises the issues involved in maintaining self and feelings of control when confronted with loss of cognitive abilities. Shared living environments can erode the sense of self as control over day-to-day activity is lost. Behaviour can change when the sense of self is threatened and responses are often labelled by others as difficult, aggressive, rude or other descriptors. Often the threat to self is caused by the actions of staff that create dependence and loss of control by using a task-oriented approach to care delivery. Gaining trust is central to feelings of belonging and these feelings drive self-esteem. Trust is earned over time, which means getting to know the other person and their way of finding meaning in their life. In this chapter Baines and Garratt also reflect on some of their personal experiences with people with dementia.

INTRODUCTION

Since the focus on person-centred care has become the prime principle in age care there has been an effort to understand exactly what this means. It is described as client-directed care, person-first care, client-inclusive care and many other ideological concepts. Whatever definition is used there are key person-related indicators that accompany, and make sense of, person-centred care. These indicators or concepts relate to feelings of worth, self-esteem, dignity, finding meaning in life, contributing and social inclusion. Without these concepts being understood by care staff, either in the community or in residential aged care facilities, person-centred care cannot occur. Person-centred care is more than physical care.

As Kimble (2003 p 31) explains: 'By examining the lived worlds of persons with dementia, expressions of meaning can be found in their feelings, actions and values'. A holistic exploration of the person means moving past the biological, psychological and technological realms to a realisation that even though memory may be damaged the humanity and social worth of the person remains.

THE CONCEPT OF SELF

To discover a meaningful life in dementia care there must be an understanding of self. We all have various ways of presenting ourselves depending upon the situation we find ourselves in. Self is what makes each person unique and we should celebrate these differences instead of labelling all people who have a dementia as having the same responses and behaviours (Kitwood 1997). There are variations on the perception of self, largely due to attitudes, beliefs and values learnt throughout life. The person who dislikes other nationalities may be called a racist, a bigot or another derogatory name. Attitudes leading to such beliefs are often taught by family values or community perceptions. By the time we are 80 years old our value system has been well established and our sense of self secure, as long as we remain in control of our life. We display our values by our responses to others and act in ways that demonstrate what those values are.

When dementia affects our abilities to retain control we react in ways to maintain it. When there are threats to our sense of self we react by using the defence systems we have used all our lives. We may use anger, argumentative and emotional outbursts, and retreat to ritualistic behaviour, denial and withdrawal. Dementia threatens our sense of self because it attacks our memories of who we are. Scherer (1995) suggests there are six ways to check the integration of self:

- identity—who am I?
- abilities—what can I do?
- relationships—how do I relate to important others?
- current reality orientation—where am I and why am I here?
- memory—has all this arisen from my past?
- self-esteem—what am I worth?

Dementia threatens our sense of self because it attacks our memories of who we are.

Personhood is both an act of self-affirmation (who I see myself to be and my perception of my value as a human being) and an accordance of recognition (how others behave towards me). It is both subjective and interactive. Feeling that one's dignity is regarded and receiving respect are responses to actions—that is, to how a person is treated. While a sense of self-esteem or self-worth may be a subjective self-evaluation, it is dependent on the external environment of the person. The stigmatisation of the condition 'dementia' clearly works against self-esteem, just as the judgments of those who are not living with dementia do. The sense that to lose one's cognitive abilities would be terrible/shameful and would make one a burden, may work against one's feeling of worth (McIntyre 2003).

When the sense of self is fragile—when the person feels stigmatised by their diagnosis of dementia and may have lost pride and self-confidence—to be treated with dignity is a pathway towards restoring positive self-regard. McIntyre (2003), in an article intended to rebalance the concept of the 'burden of care' towards 'the privilege' of caring for someone with dementia, wrote: 'Revising the narrative of dementia by placing dignity as the guiding value in relationship shifts the emphasis from fear and distance to a shared humanity of creativity in connection' (p 473). McIntyre's work (2003) is grounded in Kitwood's seminal concept of person–centred care to which she has added the ideas of Pullman (1999) about 'basic dignity', which should be accorded to all humans simply because they are human beings, and 'personal dignity', which is socially constructed and mediated. While a belief in the value of each and every person should then be a 'guiding principle' (McIntyre 2003 p 475) of care, an experience of having one's dignity as a person respected develops from the quality of interactions.

Meaning in our life is affected by any attack on the integration of self. An attack can be either a changed environment, staff that react unfavourably to dementia, infantilisation or loss of control and freedom of choice. A study by Garratt (1984) revealed the attack on self in residential aged care was often due to the attitudes/values of the care staff and management policies and demands. Feelings were expressed in either a positive or negative dialectic and were influenced by the way staff communicated and acted. At any point in time the person feeling under threat may swing from one feeling to another during the day and show the negative responses (see Table 19.1) more as they become increasingly stressed.

To interpret feelings and make sense of how the person with dementia is acting requires careful analysis and knowledge of the person. The following stories help to reveal some of the reasons why people act the way they do.

Table 19.1

The polarised concepts influencing self

POSITIVE	NEGATIVE
Autonomy	Dependence
Hope	Hopelessness
Faith	Fear
Calmness	Anxiety
Achievement	Frustration
Optimism	Pessimism
Worth	Worthlessness
Certainty	Uncertainty
Giving	Receiving
Peace	Grief
Comfort	Pain
Creativity	Boredom

Vignette

Gladweena Westward is in her mid-80s and has lived with advanced dementia for some time. She is still living at home with the support of professional caregivers and her family but has returned that morning to the art therapy group she has been attending for some months, having just spent two weeks in respite in an aged care facility. In the past Glad had always greeted other participants, not by name but with expressions of familiarity (e.g. 'How are you, darling?'), enquiring after their health. On this particular day, Glad arrived as usual, beautifully dressed but eyes glazed. 'Who am I?' she asked, then, 'Where am I?'

She turned to the woman sitting next to her, 'Are you my sister, Millicent?'

'No, I'm Constance from Ulverstone.'

'Who am I?' Glad asked again.

The other participants in the group repeated her name to her and reassured her that they knew her. Glad smiled with evident relief.

Slowly Glad began to write in small, neat handwriting, 'Gladweena Cook. Gladweena Cook. Gladweena Cook'.

She was in fact writing her maiden name.

When it was later suggested to her that her married name was 'Gladweena Westward' Glad said that she had no memory of that name. 'Was that Bill? I loved Bill. I still love Bill. I really love my father, James Cook'. She began to write 'James Cook. I love my father, James Cook'.

The disorientation, which follows after a period in respite care, is common. Scherer's (1995) model cited above, would suggest that Glad's sense of self was fractured on this particular day. The time spent in respite in an aged care facility had, it appears, confused her. The writing of her name appeared to be a strategy for reaffirming her identity. In the same way looking for members of her family for orientation (i.e. for her sister and father) was again seeking to locate her identity in a familial framework. This leads on to ways in which selfhood is maintained and ways in which it can become unsettled or damaged.

Anecdote

On another occasion Patricia Baines spoke to the art therapy group about their impending trip overseas. Glad responded with an invitation to come to the casino. 'We're all going on a trip. I'm inviting you all. The queen's coming and Princess Margaret Rose is too. We're going to the casino. You can stay for as long as you like. It won't cost you anything. My father's paying.' The group thanked her warmly for her generous invitation and she glowed with pride.

Baines recalls another woman, Hermione, who lived in an aged care facility, who would tell other residents that she had been a nurse in the Crimea (so, by suggestion, with Florence Nightingale). When her son remonstrated with her saying that her story was not true, she had told him that 'in here' she could claim to have been anything she liked.

These accounts do not suggest memory loss and confusion, as much as the need to be someone of worth, someone who knows important people and who is making an important contribution. Perhaps the question about the ability to distinguish between fact and fiction is present, even a poor sense of an historical timeline, but the words give an overwhelming sense of name dropping. The underlying message is clearly that the speaker is an important person. The issue of self-esteem and feeling valued is then, for people living with dementia, not a peripheral but a central issue; dementia is a stigmatised condition in which individuals are said to suffer memory loss and loss of 'capacity' and insight. The label, which comes with the diagnosis, threatens their sense of worth. These responses are imaginative and creative ways to restore self-esteem.

It is noticeable in aged care facilities how many residents living with dementia are looking for a parent or parents. This may be more than the strength of early memories over recent ones. In adulthood most people have been responsible for others. Ageing within Western societies, especially when individuals have been deemed 'at risk' and 'in need of care', has often involved not just the loss of a home but also of a meaningful existence. An individual has 'gone into permanent care'. The terminology needs to be considered carefully as it may in fact be less positive than it suggests. People who have cared for others are now recipients of 'care'. It suggests dependency and helplessness.

Ageing within Western societies, especially when individuals have been deemed 'at risk' and 'in need of care', has often involved not just the loss of a home but also of a meaningful existence.

Maintaining self-esteem is difficult to achieve in environments that foster dependency by offering 'care' to the 'aged'. Person-centred care needs to be combined with opportunities to contribute to communal life, to offer support to others, and to fill time with meaningful activities. Unstructured time is not necessarily restful but stressful.

Vignette

'Well, what happens now?' Marilla asked.
Baines was packing away the art and writing materials so that the tables could be prepared for the evening meal.
'What are you doing? They're here now. What are we going to do? Let them be!' Marilla continued, clearly annoyed that the group activity was coming to an end.

For a slice of time residents had been gathered together; some had been painting, others writing or looking at art or poetry books. The activity gave the space of the dementia unit a focus. Other residents came and sat and watched, sometimes picking up a pen or a brush, sometimes tidying everything around them, and then getting up and walking on, only to return a few minutes later. Now the space was no longer held by meaningful activity. People started to pace. Some were guided to a seat facing the television, but, when living with advanced dementia, television may be a mixed blessing. The boundaries between 'on the television' and 'in the room with me' may be shaky, and some events and people on the television may not be comfortable in one's life space.

In subsequent sessions, Baines found ways to ease the transition by singing well-known songs with the group or holding a conversation on a topic of interest (e.g. catching rabbits during the Great Depression, making jam and so on), as she packed things away.

Having nothing meaningful to do may remind residents of other places, which have seemed liminal. A woman with advanced dementia in a long narrow communal space with rooms off it kept asking when the ferry would arrive in Devonport. She was clearly feeling in transit. Residents seated doing nothing in particular appeared to recall Bass Strait journeys to her. Locked doors may lead residents in a dementia unit to believe that they are in prison. Memories of wartime fears of capture and incarceration may resurface.

A woman recently admitted to an aged care facility began declaring loudly that she wanted to go home 'right now'. She had tried every door into the dementia unit and walked through the enclosed courtyard garden, looking for an exit. She had returned to where residents were sitting, her hands now shaking, and her tone shifting between pleas and an expression of indignation. 'This is ridiculous,' she said, 'I live at 9 Paradise Court. I've got the key here. Now show me the way out.'

Another long-term resident with advanced dementia came up and said quietly, 'It's hard. You do feel trapped in here.'

It is the lucidity of people living with advanced dementia and their compassion that may be both moving and confronting. On one occasion Baines asked two women in a dementia unit to tell two visiting secondary school students what it was like living in an aged care facility. The two women looked at each other and said in unison, 'Boring'.

Feeling constrained against one's evident wishes and feeling bored work against maintaining a sense of positive identity. A duty of care is certainly necessary for individuals living with advanced dementia, but what this means needs to be examined carefully.

Returning to Garratt's (1984) research, it showed that both positive and negative feelings are extremes that fluctuate according to the way the caregiver acts on any day. For example, the ability to choose one's dress, the encouragement of bathing oneself as much as possible, being able to chose food, having personal space that nobody invades, ensuring privacy and recognising discomfort, all contribute to how the day proceeds and aids autonomy. Having a caregiver who rushes in and hurries the shower, is abrupt and makes the person feel like a nuisance, puts the attack on self into the negative pole and leads to an unpleasant day.

When a person who has dementia has unpleasant feelings their behavioural responses may be recognised as 'being difficult' or 'aggressive'. Labels such as these lead to loss or distortion of understanding and no attempt is made to identify why it occurred. Carers often state they never understand why a person's behaviour changes from one hour to the next, but rarely do they stop to examine why or what may have triggered the changes.

The question asked by Dr Bruce Miller (2005) thinking about people with frontotemporal dementia is valuable: 'What is this person still able to do well or better than before?' Rather than seeing people with dementia as having deficits, one should ask the other question about abilities. Professor Gene Cohen (2000) has introduced the useful concept of 'potential beyond problems'. 'It is only when problems and potential are considered together that health is best promoted and illness best cared for' (Cohen 2000 p 14). While reminiscing is valuable and honouring what an individual has been is valuable, people living with dementia want to be valued and cherished as they are in the present.

Rather than seeing people with dementia as having deficits, one should ask the other question about abilities.

AUTONOMY

Autonomy means making one's own choices; in other words, independence, the right of self-government, and freedom from external control or influence. The argument that people who have a dementia are not capable of making choices may be valid as the disease enters the final stages of life but not in the early or more severe stages. Even the latter assumption may not be entirely true. The Alzheimer's Society, based in London, UK, interviewed people living with the later stages of dementia in a project written up as 'My name is not dementia' (2010) and found that by using images on cards, they could indeed obtain meaningful responses to questions about quality of life.

There seem to be several intertwined issues in this discussion because self-worth is not just simply the way a person feels about themself but is an interaction with how other people treat them and regard them. It is connected with self-respect and being offered respect—that is, being respected. It is said that people living with dementia have or may have low self-esteem. The interactive question is whether they are esteemed by others.

The Government of Scotland has produced a Charter of Rights for People with Dementia and their Carers in Scotland (2011). It is a document that enshrines many of the 'best practice' recommendations of the 21st century. To quote just a portion of the Charter, it says:

> People with dementia and their carers have the right to be able to enjoy human rights and fundamental freedoms in every part of their lives and wherever they are, including full respect of their dignity, beliefs, individual circumstances and privacy.

> and

> People with dementia will be valued and treated at all times as a person, with dignity and respect.

(Charter of Rights for People with Dementia and their Carers in Scotland 2011, p 5)

There is growing recognition now that those living with dementia are able to share their views and that self-esteem is raised and dignity maintained when there is genuine consultation. It seems therefore not just impertinent but a failure in respecting human rights to speak about people living with dementia without asking at least some of them what their thoughts are about self-worth and human dignity. Many members (*n* = approximately 70 individuals in total) of the various art therapy groups who were asked responded with serious interest. Participants were in nine different groups, six of which were in dementia units in various parts of Tasmania. All the people who spoke about the concepts 'self-esteem', 'dignity' and 'hope' or who wrote down their thoughts, had lived with dementia for some time (so were not in the early stages of the various diseases causing dementia but were in that rather nebulously defined time called 'the middle' or sometimes were living with advanced dementia). Just over two-thirds of the people who responded were living in aged care facilities; a little less than a third of the number, were still living at home. In return for their giving permission to gather their thoughts together and share them, they were guaranteed that their individual identities would not be revealed (Baines 2012).

When the participants were asked how they felt when shown respect, a number of positive adjectives were used: lovely, great, proud, happy, good, worthwhile, uplifted, warm, satisfied, really heartened, pleased with myself, appreciated. Someone wrote: 'It puts a smile on your face'. Another person wrote: 'My chest comes out and it makes me feel important'. Yet another person wrote, 'Humble and of worth'. No one suggested it was not good to be shown respect, although one person said that respect was something you had to earn. One person said that for her it was evidence that she had 'contributed'. She went on to add that being shown respect was 'highly necessary'. Another person added the reciprocal dimension: 'It makes me prone to be really nice to other people'.

Explaining the concept of 'human dignity' was avoided by some people or was met with silence. It is a more abstract concept. However, some individuals provided statements:
- 'Caring for other people and showing compassion. [It] would be to listen to other people's outlook on life.'
- 'Understanding other people's weakness and that they understand mine.'
- 'It's if other people know what you can do and what you're capable of and respect that. Respect for what you are and who you are.'
- '[Human dignity is] our gift. We should have respect for all humans.'
- 'Someone who makes you feel welcome and respected.'
- 'Being treated equal.'

What is interesting about these responses is the 'angle' or viewpoint of the response—that is, whether the person is thinking about their own human dignity or of the human dignity of other people. The distinction made between 'basic dignity' and 'personal dignity' is also evident. What also stands out in the responses is that human dignity is often linked with the idea of respect and being respected (Baines 2012).

Baines asked what things gave the person a sense of self-worth. There was an overwhelming agreement among respondents that contributing in various ways, helping and doing things for others were what elevated people's sense of worth. A number of people said that family was what gave them a sense of worth. When asked to elaborate, individuals spoke about bringing up their children.

To cross-check the answer about self-worth Baines asked what contributions the individual saw him or herself as having made. Again the importance of having helped others was by far the strongest response; those who had been given assistance included family, strangers or simply other people.

This raises the question of whether people with dementia are shown respect for what they have done or for what they now are. Many people living with dementia are living in situations in which they seem to have very little opportunity now to contribute or help others. In fact they may be confined to a wheelchair or held in a lounge-style reclining bed. They wait for others to come to them and their requests for help may be delayed because of staffing shortages. They live in a situation of dependency. However, even the most physically and cognitively dependent person may have things they are able to share. Opportunities need to be created for this, for to negate autonomy and the chance to contribute to the lives of others is to encourage dependence that, in turn, lowers self-esteem and dignity.

To negate autonomy is to encourage dependence that, in turn, lowers self-esteem and dignity.

People living with dementia are often able to make contributions to the life of others. Comforting, encouraging, praising, explaining, thanking and praying are all ways in which people living with dementia are able to help other people and affirm their own sense of worth. These acts of kindness and understanding are seldom recalled afterwards but happen moment by moment in response to immediate human needs. Beneath the inability to recall names there is another kind of recognition. We may be greeted by verbalisations such as 'You're plus, plus', or simply, 'You' that indicate recognition with a smile and sometimes a hug. There are any number of reunions in the space of an hour as someone with advanced dementia meets you yet again 'for the first time'. This formal greeting and re-meeting appears to create a sense of goodwill in the living space and the repetitions may be a satisfaction of our earliest responses to smiling human faces.

HOPE

When feelings of hopelessness affect people, these feelings can lead to depression. Not being able to see a future free of pain, unable to make personal choices and living with others who are ill all contribute to low self-esteem. The ability to maintain hope in the face of an uncertain future must be fostered by families and staff (Harder 2002).

An older resident of a nursing home told Sally Garratt that her hope was she would not die like Mrs B, her friend, who she could hear rasping for breath down the corridor. She knew she would die in the home but hoped her end would be quick. This hope was always in her mind but did not alter her day-to-day activity. To destroy this hope would be an act of violation of her self-esteem and cause more anxiety. While a guarantee of how another would die is not possible, the reassurance that pain can be alleviated and the presence of another being with her at all times maintains hope that all may be well.

The nature and complexity of hope is outlined in Harder's work (2002 p 2) as observances, but as she states, 'hope has been seen as a determinant of healing but science has no language to describe it'. One observance is that hope is a crucial antidote to fear. One may not know the future, or may see the future as being grim, but the presence of hope will allow potential for benevolence and less focus on limitation.

Vignette

Bonnie, who is in her late 80s, has been a resident in an aged care facility for just over a year. As the dementia progresses, she has become uncertain of where she is living. She called Baines over. 'I shall need a bed for the night,' she said confidentially. Reassurances of a room that was always hers and only a few metres away only comforted Bonnie for a short time until she was given an art book to look at. In fact Bonnie had, with caregivers' patience and encouragement, made some progress. When she first moved in she had remained in her bedroom most of the time, probably in fear that she would never locate it or her possessions again. When brought out for a meal, she would ask repeatedly to be taken back to her room. She would whisper that she didn't know where her room was and, although it was actually within sight, Bonnie could not recognise it or see her name in large letters on the door. Now Bonnie has enough trust in those caring for her to share the communal living space, although her interactions with other residents remain polite enquiries after their health. Her asking for a bed for the night and yet remaining in a shared space is then evidence of the trust she has placed in others.

Snyder (2002 p 10) has attempted to develop a theory of hope. In this work hope is defined as 'the perceived capacity to devise pathways to desired goals, and motivate oneself via agency thinking to use those pathways'. From this theoretical perspective Bonnie is using her capacity to interact with another person to ensure her own future wellbeing. Indeed she demonstrates both hope and trust in seeking a bed for the night (and demonstrates an understanding that she should remain in this place). Many residents in aged care facilities seek to go 'home', although this may be a childhood home or a place of residence of many years before.

Hope and trust are affected by a person's internal dialogue—their self-assessment. 'I've had a good life. A very good life,' Morgan said emphatically.

'We were poor in terms of money but we had plenty of love.' Marilla looked thoughtful as she spoke and then smiled and nodded affirming her conclusion.

These positive affirmations—self-affirmations—are critical to ongoing wellbeing, and caregivers can both reinforce them and repeat them back to people living with dementia.

Yet hope and trust may be fostered and encouraged by the way day-to-day living is carried out. The research findings of Cohen-Mansfield et al (2010) into the use of various stimuli in American aged care facilities to reduce agitation (verbal agitation, physical agitation—such as pacing, fiddling with things, repetitive agitated gestures) are illuminating. They conclude, first, that 'exposure to any type of stimulus is preferable to current nursing home standards of care,' and second, that 'providing stimuli offered a proactive approach to preventing agitation in persons with dementia'. However, some planned interventions were more successful than others in reducing agitation. Giving an individual things to do that related to the person's 'most salient self-identity' had the greatest impact in reducing the actions that indicated fearfulness, boredom and the gamut of possible negative emotions. What this means is that people living with dementia respond most intensely to being offered activities that have meaning in terms of their own life histories and that confirm a sense of worth and value. A homemaker may then enjoy helping with domestic tasks, such as folding linen; an accountant may enjoy being given a ledger. Baines recalls a retired school teacher living with the later stages of dementia accepting pages with incomplete sentences on them (the sentences were themselves intended to confirm positive thoughts). The teacher would complete the sentences and then mark the sheet, adding comments like 'Good work. Keep it up!'. Cohen-Mansfield et al (2010) also found that social interaction and music (the noise level was important and excessive noise was shown by their other research to be distressing) also helped to reduce agitation. An environment that maintains a sense of hope and provides for the development of trust can be created by well-trained caregivers.

The work of Cameron Camp (1999), who developed Montessori rehabilitative therapy, is relevant here. In Australia, Anne Kelly, who works with Alzheimer's Australia (Tasmania), has been introducing and teaching Camp's therapy after receiving a Churchill fellowship to study it. As the name suggests the therapy works to re-teach/rehabilitate basic skills to and in people living with advanced dementia, so they may resume feeding themselves and do as much for themselves as possible. The most important feature in relation to this chapter is that the Montessori rehabilitative therapy seeks to give each person a role within their immediate residential aged care facility. Having found something the person is still able to do, caregivers train and assist that person with picture prompts and written prompts to carry out the task. One person may be 'the table setter', another 'the bringer of jugs of water' to other residents, a third person may be 'the welcomer' when guests visit. The aged care facility may also set up labelled areas where various meaningful activities are available, so a place for putting flowers in vase, a nursery with life-size baby dolls, a mirror with hats and make up and so on. The aim of all these activities is to rekindle self-esteem and gain respect for the individual.

BOREDOM

It is easy to interpret walking up and down corridors as a symptom of dementia rather than as a need for activity. People living with dementia do need exercise, and opportunities for physical movement are important, but people with a dementia may be walking up and down because there is no focused activity for them to engage in and they are bored. Living with advancing dementia the person may find it difficult to initiate satisfying activity themselves, or the means of achieving meaningful activity may be out of sight or out of reach.

'Good. Something to do.' Davina, who has lived with Alzheimer's disease for six years, says smiling, as art materials are placed on the table directly in front of her. For some people living with dementia it is enough to supply the means for activity. For others, initiating the activity may be necessary. Modelling the activity and then letting the person do it for themselves may be needed to begin activity. A sense of worth comes from doing. Boredom is lack of activity that is meaningful and worthwhile to the person. Passive observation is no substitute for active participation in which the process of doing is more important than the end result. This adds to the importance of person-centred care plans and of care staff having detailed knowledge of their client's interests (Department of Health 2011).

CREATIVITY

The aesthetics of the immediate environment does not feature in family carers' assessments of what gives quality to life, although, in all fairness, there are many family carers who arrive in dementia units with bunches of flowers from their gardens. Even in the later stages of dementia, most people respond to beauty. Flowers almost always produce a response. A large print version of Wordsworth's *The Daffodils* placed on the table in an art therapy group in a dementia unit together with bunches of the same flowers led to multiple, unsolicited reading aloud of the poem (six or seven times with annotations from one of the readers). Other people spoke aloud that they knew that poem and chimed in to create a group recital. Although the rereads are perhaps because the readers no longer recall having already read the poem aloud, the appreciation of words and rhymes did not falter. In fact, whenever poetry has been provided on A3 sheets in large print, some group members living with dementia have been moved to read the poetry aloud. An aesthetic response was included in the D-QOL questionnaire, which was developed by Karim et al (2008) to evoke qualitative responses about quality of life by individuals living with dementia (intended for mild and moderate dementia rather than advanced dementia). Baines (2007) has documented examples of aesthetic responses in individuals living with advanced dementia in her Alzheimer's Australia publication, *Nurturing the heart*.

> *The potential for creativity is ageless; it need not wane as life goes on.*

(Goleman et al 1992)

We all have some form of creative spirit within us, some form of pleasure from doing something that brings intrinsic reward. Sometimes our need for creative expression is not fostered by parents, teachers or work requirements, but the need remains and the potential for expressing ourselves remains. The truck driver who enjoyed his watercolour painting sessions was starting to produce strong memories from his past on paper and was proud of his achievements. His wife, however, saw this as childlike behaviour and something he would never usually do, so refused to let him take them home. His ability to create something was therefore limited to his time in art groups at the day centre where his work was put on a board for all to see and enjoy. Understanding how creativity is essential for self-expression and identity links to self-esteem and dignity and, even though the creative work may not be seen as great artistic development, it is nevertheless meaningful and important to the person engaged in doing it.

Person-centred care focuses on the needs of the person, but rarely does the need for giving and gaining trust and respect get written on a care plan. Respect is a right of all human beings and is instilled in professional care, but trust must be earned. Trust between two people develops over time and carers who understand the positive concepts of self will gain trust from the person who has dementia. This trust brings hope, joy and a sense of control into the caring process and life has meaning (Kimble 2003).

Person-centred care focuses on the needs of the person, but rarely does the need for giving and gaining trust and respect get written on a care plan.

All people have a need to belong. Belonging means you are valued and recognised as a person. Entering a care facility threatens the sense of belonging because there is no recognition of the self being in control. Decisions are made for the person, schedules must be followed, the ability to choose is reduced and staff take over what was once the person's way of life. Self-esteem is developed through a sense of belonging so small wonder when dementia is present there is a confused perception of meaning in life.

Vignette

A group of older ladies who lived in the nursing home had a history of quilt-making. They continued to meet to discuss their past sewing experiences and to make a quilt from scraps of material they had collected. Over time they made several quilts that were raffled to generate funds for the home. Unfortunately, one by one they either died or lost vision and the group was disbanded. The last person could not find the energy to continue to sew by herself and was quite distressed because she felt she was no longer helping to raise money for the home.

This need to contribute was related to reciprocity and a need to belong. She said, 'They do everything here, cooking, cleaning and looking after us, and I can't do anything in return.'

The lady came from a small farming community that would share whatever they had between members of the community and hold church fetes, raffles and dances to raise funds for community enterprises or to help others in need. The need for reciprocal action was strongly influencing her sense of self and belonging.

This need continued after her dementia became really noticeable and she would wander looking for something to do.

Vignette

The second occurrence that indicated a need for belonging relates to the lady who hoarded food. She had lived through a war and the depression and food was a very important feature of her existence. Staff would clean out her caches of mouldy bread, fruit and other food and she would become very distressed. Finally her son revealed she made cheese from sour milk to give to her family and was considered to be the family's best cook. This explained the collection of sour milk in bowls on the window sill and the hanging of stockings filled with the curdled milk in the bedroom. The strong smell originating from her room was unpleasant and any attempt to remove her collection was strongly resisted. Once the explanation of her behaviour was identified staff began to find ways she could occupy herself to meet her need to reciprocate and feel useful.

Reflective questions

1. How is the need for belonging related to reciprocity?

2. Discuss the nature of personal control and self.

3. Can feelings of self-worth and dignity be fostered in a nursing home? How can this be done?

4. How could you substitute feelings of belonging that arise through giving and hoarding food without reducing the need for self-esteem?

5. Creating a meaningful life for people who have dementia requires knowledge of the person and their sense of self. Discuss how this can be achieved.

CONCLUSION

This chapter discusses the need for self-esteem, belonging and identity to create a meaningful life when dementia distorts reality. To understand the person the carer must know about their life, their values and beliefs and to be non-judgmental of behaviour.

The understanding of 'self' is the foundation for person-centred care and the way to ensure positive feelings are as important in care as physical comfort. Behaviour is often the way in which a person with dementia expresses threats to self and generally, with analysis and an attempt to discover links between feelings and expression, a reason for this can be found.

References

Baines, P., 2007. Nurturing the heart: creativity, art therapy, and dementia. Quality dementia Care No. 3. Alzheimer's Australia, Canberra.

Baines, P., 2012. Anecdotal reports from practice. Alzheimer's Association Tasmania.

Camp, C. (Ed.), 1999. Montessori-based activities for persons with dementia. Menorah Park Center for Senior Living, Beachwood, OH.

Charter of rights for people with dementia and their carers, 2011. The Scottish Government, Edinburgh.

Cohen, G.D., 2000. The creative age: awakening human potential in the second half of life. Harper Collins, New York.

Cohen-Mansfield, J., Marx, M.S., Dakheel-Ali, M., et al., 2010. Can agitated behavior of nursing home residents with dementia be prevented with the use of standardized stimuli? Journal of American Geriatric Society 58 (8), 1459–1464.

Department of Health, 2011. Dementia-friendly environments. State Government of Victoria, Melbourne.

Garratt, S., 1984. unpublished thesis We just need a little love: caring needs of institutional older people. University of Colorado, Boulder.

Goleman, D., Kaufman, P., Ray, M., 1992. The creative spirit: companion to the PBS television series. Penguin, New York.

Harder, A.F., 2002. The nature and complexity of hope. Online. Available: http://www.learningplaceonline.com.illness/hope/nature.htm, 22 Sep 2012.

Karim, S., Ramanna, G., Petit, T., et al., 2008. Development of the dementia quality of life questionnaire (D-QOL): UK version. Aging and Mental Health 12 (1), 144–148.

Kimble, M., 2003. chapter 3 The whole person. In: Hudson, R. (Ed.) Dementia Nursing: a guide to practice. Ausmed, Melbourne.

Kitwood, T., 1997. Dementia reconsidered: the person comes first. Open University Press, Buckingham.

McIntyre, M., 2003. Dignity in dementia: person-centred care in community. Journal of Aging Studies 17, 473–484.

Miller, B., 2005. Grandad is an artist: Dementia and the creative mind. Online. Available: www.abc.net.au/allinthemind/stories/2005, 22 Sep 2012.

Pullman, D., 1999. The ethics of autonomy and dignity in long-term care. Canadian Journal of Aging 18 (1), 26–46.

Scherer, S., 1995. The psychological bases of dementia. In: Garratt, S., Hamilton-Smith, E. (Eds.), Rethinking dementia: an Australian approach. Ausmed, Melbourne.

Snyder, C.R., 2002. Hope theory: rainbows in the mind. Psychological Inquiry: An International Journal for the Advancement of Psychological Theory 13 (4), 249–275.

CHAPTER 20

ACCREDITATION: COMPLIANCE OR THE PURSUIT OF EXCELLENCE?

Mark Brandon

Editors' comments

Accreditation of healthcare services has had an interesting history in Australia. It has long been used by the acute healthcare system and rarely 'hits the press'. When it was introduced to aged care the industry saw it as a major imposition and complained about lack of consistency and an officious approach to the inspection of facilities, often with the 'assessors' having no knowledge of aged care; the aged care standards and accreditation agency (ACSAA) was seen as spying on them. Over time, with improvements in the capacity to demonstrate consistency, education and a partnership approach to quality improvements, this has changed. No one knows more about these and international changes than Mark Brandon. We asked him to provide a sketch of his experiences.

INTRODUCTION

This chapter has been written from the perspective of a person whose responsibility as chief executive officer of the Aged Care Standards and Accreditation Agency ('Accreditation Agency') is to promote high-quality care in the Australian residential aged care sector. The key tools available are the accreditation scheme prescribed by government and an industry education program designed to promote high-quality care through providing information, education and training. There is a strong consumer and provider perspective of the accreditation program as the assessment of quality.

In my view, the concepts of regulatory compliance and the pursuit of excellence are not mutually exclusive. Regulatory compliance is not a sinister term. It simply means that one must comply with a set of rules or regulations.

Of course the underlying assumption is that the regulations are fit for purpose; they reflect the wishes and expectations of the community and are achievable.

ACCREDITATION

We need first to understand what external evaluation is and what it is not. Accreditation is one of the forms of external evaluation that exist in the health and aged care sectors around the world. Others include certification against the International Organisation for Standards (ISO) standards and regulatory requirements. Generally these are forms of risk management and quality assurance schemes that set assessable performance expectations and, in doing so, aim to mitigate the risk of a poor outcome for a service user.

Accreditation systems are forms of risk management and quality assurance schemes that set assessable performance expectations and, in doing so, aim to mitigate the risk of a poor outcome for a service user.

The Australian Commission on Safety and Quality in Health Care in its 2006 discussion paper *National Safety and Quality Accreditation Standards* states there are two conditions for accreditation. They are an explicit definition of quality (i.e. standards) and an independent review process aimed at identifying the level of congruence between practices and quality standards.

ACCREDITATION, OF ITSELF, WILL NOT STOP BAD THINGS HAPPENING

The accreditation and other third party evaluation schemes in acute care have been well established since the 1950s. The Australian Council on Healthcare Standards (ACHS) was established in 1974. ACHS remains the largest hospital accreditation provider in Australia.

Health sector accreditation schemes tend to be member-based where participation is voluntary, the members set the standards, and the member-owned accreditation body assesses performance against the standards. The members of such schemes tend to be hospitals that have a high proportion of staff with tertiary-level qualifications, and patients who have increasingly short stays and whose health status improves as a result of their stay. Reports of performance against the standards are not usually made available to the public. This is despite the high level of taxpayer contribution to the publicly funded acute hospital system.

General practitioners in Australia seeking to receive Practice Incentive Payments (PIP) from the Australian Government must subject themselves to accreditation against standards developed by the Royal Australian College of General Practitioners. Reports of these assessments are not available to patients.

This can be contrasted with long-term residential care for older people (residents). Residents tend to stay in aged care facilities for extended periods of time, their health status will generally deteriorate during the stay and the relative percentage of staff who have tertiary-level qualifications is low.

Internationally, in long-term residential care for older people, participation in an external evaluation program is often mandatory for those organisations that wish to provide residential aged care services. In some countries where accreditation is linked to government subsidies (e.g. Australia) it forms part of the quality assurance and oversight framework. In other countries compliance with care standards is simply a regulatory requirement of government. Failure to comply may lead to enforcement action by the regulator. The reasons for these differences might be tracked to the legal construct of the jurisdictions, for example, the Australian Government cannot legislate for quality of care directly; however, the promotion of quality is linked to meeting government requirements in order to qualify for subsidies. England has no such constitutional hurdles.

 Internationally, in long-term residential care for older people, participation in an external evaluation program is often mandatory.

While we refer to some schemes as 'accreditation' it is more broadly third-party evaluation where one party (usually government) sets performance expectations, called standards or regulatory requirements; another party delivers the services and the external evaluator (called the accreditation body) assesses performance against standards. Increasingly the reports of the external evaluator are made public. The limited research in this area indicates that accreditation does drive quality improvement. There is evidence to suggest public reporting can stimulate quality improvement activities. Chen's (2010) review found substantial evidence of significant increased quality-improvement activities associated with public reporting in a range of different settings.

The lack of quantitative research has not dissuaded governments from implementing external evaluation schemes for long-term care for older people in countries such as Australia, New Zealand, Ireland, Canada, Denmark, Germany, England, Scotland, the United States and the Netherlands. There is continuing interest and ongoing development in the European Union. The schemes mentioned all require long-term care providers to participate in (or accept) the regulation as a condition of being approved to provide services.

We know there is interest in developing accreditation as a form of risk mitigation and quality assurance in Asia because of the requests organisations such as the Accreditation Agency receive to brief government representatives and take part in conferences. The longest established accreditation scheme in Asia is the voluntary scheme conducted by the Hong Kong Association of Gerontology.

The third-party evaluation arrangement we have in Australia for residential aged care is not unique to Australia. Increasingly, in high-income countries around the world there is a growth in external evaluation programs auspiced by government in relation to long-term care for older people. A review of the membership of the International Society for Quality in Healthcare's (ISQua) accreditation federation reveals that the vast majority of members who are engaged in evaluating the performance of aged care services for older people have some link to government. Universally the performance expectations are reflected in accreditation standards or regulations prescribed by government and the evaluating organisation is a government-related entity such as in England, Scotland, Ireland, the US (some states), the Netherlands, Germany and Australia, or has been authorised to undertake the work by a government department such as in New Zealand, Denmark and the US (some states). The publication of audit assessment reports is a widespread practice.

The publication of audit assessment reports is a widespread practice.

STANDARDS

Clarity of the meaning of standards and their purpose are the lynchpin of a robust accreditation scheme. In this context standards can be a generic term for any performance expectation. Poorly understood or incomplete standards do not contribute to positive outcomes for residents. In fact they will misguide aged care managers.

External evaluation of aged care services is a relatively recent innovation. Most sets of standards and regulations are based on the Donabedian (2005) framework, consisting of standards that are either structure-, process- or outcome-based:

- structural standards—the existence of structures that enable a process such as suitably qualified personnel and equipment
- process standards—structures of themselves will not enable quality outcomes—there needs to be processes that are followed
- outcome standards—what is achieved.

In the Australian residential aged care standards the standards are commonly referred to as expected outcomes. In fact they are a mix of structure, process and outcome standards.

Most sets of standards and regulations are based on the Donabedian framework consisting of standards that are either structure-, process- or outcome-based.

Among external assessing bodies there is a view that standards drive performance. Therefore, standards and regulations must be fit for purpose in that they encompass the range of performance expectations and do not lead to unexpected outcomes. In Australia the *Aged Care Act 1997* makes it clear that the purpose of accreditation is to promote high-quality care and protect the health, safety and wellbeing of residents. It is also the policy intent of Parliament that the accreditation scheme exists explicitly for the benefit of residents. The legislation mandates engagement with residents as part of the assessment process by the Accreditation Agency.

RESIDENTS

Residents are the people best placed to tell us what is happening in the facility in which they live. Obtaining that information has its challenges, particularly for those who have a cognitive impairment. They cannot communicate easily and those who say they will report for them are often their children. The family of the resident and the person identified as the 'representative' have a well-defined role in the Australian residential aged care sector. Can we be confident the children of a resident can, and will, reflect the expectations, feelings and views of their parent? Does the son/daughter reflect their own view/expectation rather than those of their parent? We certainly see situations where there may be several children who all have views on the same topic but their views are quite different. On balance, one must question whether relatives are reliable informants concerning the wishes and expectations of older people who are themselves not able to communicate their wishes.

On balance, one must question whether relatives are reliable informants concerning the wishes and expectations of older people who are themselves not able to communicate their wishes. Who are reliable sources and can more effort be put into understanding the wishes of the resident?

The other consideration in obtaining information from a son or daughter is whether it was they who made the decision to admit their parent to the facility. The question then is: Is a criticism of the facility a criticism of their earlier selection of the facility? We then need to further consider the challenges in obtaining information about care and services from residents.

Why would a resident be reluctant to criticise the aged care facility? There is no single or simple response, but the reasons may include:
- fear—they are vulnerable and in the hands of their carers
- dependency on carers who they rely on for physical, emotional, spiritual and psychical needs
- being part of a generation that has more of a sense of gratitude than entitlement
- cognitive, language or other impairments that can inhibit communication
- cultural norms, gender or socioeconomic status.

When we consider quality of life we must see it through the eyes of the resident. Relatively little has been researched in the area of quality of life. From my perspective the essential domains of quality of life go well beyond merely being alive and breathing. In an older person's life there is much more and a good system recognises the quality of life aspects that include food, hygiene, privacy, dignity, respect and the right to take risks and make choices.

In developing standards in Australia we have long taken the view that a person entering an aged care facility does not lose their rights as a citizen.

COMPLIANCE WITH REGULATIONS OR THE PURSUIT OF EXCELLENCE?

Generally speaking regulations are themselves a form of performance standard in that we are required to comply with or meet them in our daily lives. For example, speed limits on roads are a standard. Additionally, the requirement that a driver must drive in a safe manner is set out in most traffic Acts. So, similarly to the residential aged care standards, we have a tension to be managed. You can drive at 100 km an hour but you have a duty of care to others not to drive in an unsafe manner. Aged care providers have a duty of care, but in the context of the rights of residents too many things, including choice and decision making, need to be considered. A person does not lose their rights as a citizen because they have been admitted to a nursing home.

Regulations tend to be a combination of what is required and what is proscribed—what you must do and what you must not do. The key to successful service delivery is actively managing these tensions. We ignore regulations at our peril—but what role should regulation play in daily management of a residential aged care service?

Put simply one could say that a 'regulatory compliance' approach to aged care service delivery is a minimalist approach. The provision of quality care, or a higher order approach in the form of the pursuit of excellence, is more likely to meet the legal requirements and at the same time deliver a standard of services that the community expects for older people. Some commentators argue that the community does not generally consider aged care services until they need them. This can be contrasted with the responses of speakers at the Accreditation Agency Better Practice conferences, who are quite clear about their expectations of the sector now and into the future. Based on those comments, there will be challenges in aligning the expectations with what is possible.

 A 'regulatory compliance' approach to aged care service delivery is a minimalist approach.

What then is the relationship between regulations, quality and the pursuit of excellence?

REGULATION

'Regulation' is arguably the easiest to define. It is simply a set of rules established by the Parliament by which we are required to comply. If we don't comply we may get caught and there may be some form of penalty. The existence of regulations will drive behaviour. Well-conceived regulation provides a framework and the right number of rules necessary to do the job. Of course poor regulation is a burden that may drive poor outcomes. The same can be said of accreditation standards.

Accreditation standards are best described as performance expectations in the same way regulations set out expectations to do or not do something. In healthcare, standards set out requirements to achieve certain outcomes or to have structures and processes in place to support service delivery. These process and structure standards are important because they provide the infrastructure for sustained performance.

In the context of service delivery one cannot assume that because nothing 'bad' has happened that the systems and processes are robust. It may simply be that an accident is waiting to happen.

QUALITY

There is no universal definition of quality in healthcare and certainly none internationally accepted in long-term care for the older people (Irwin 2012). Runciman (2006 p 297) defines quality as 'the extent to which a health care service or product produces desired outcome/s'.

While the word 'quality' is a neutral word it is now commonplace in aged care for commentators, including Runciman (2006), to use it as a positive adjective. Increasingly a service is described as a 'quality' service, meaning it is good. In external evaluation we say we assess the quality of the aged care service against performance expectations (regulations or standards).

In aged care stakeholders tend to talk about concepts of quality of care and quality of life. In Australia this may well be because the narrative surrounding the introduction of the Aged Care Act regularly referred to the 'homelike environment' in relation to government-subsidised residential aged care, thereby recognising that older people living in residential aged care have a range of needs that go beyond clinical care and go to life and lifestyle. This construct is reflected in the accreditation standards, which include standards relating to living environment, privacy/dignity, leisure interests/activities and cultural and spiritual life alongside standards that encompass medication management, clinical care and palliative care.

Residents of nursing homes have a range of needs that go beyond clinical care and go to life and lifestyle.

There are different views about the relationship between quality of care and quality of life. Some commentators view them as different concepts, while others argue that the two concepts overlap and that the degree of overlap depends on the health status of the individual. The latter view suggests the more impaired an individual's health the more likely quality of care is a factor that influences their quality of life (Department of Health and Ageing (DoHA) 2007 pp 49–50).

Older people living in residential aged care generally receive care for an extended period of time and experience increasing dependency and decline in their health status. The integration of the two concepts, quality of care and quality of life, is therefore regarded as being essential in the residential aged care sector (DoHA 2007 p 46). In contrast, in the acute care sector, where the emphasis is largely placed on healthcare interventions and their safety and outcomes, quality of life is seldom a part of the measurements of quality.

While some residential aged care services use more sophisticated assessment tools to assess the quality of life of residents, using a resident survey as a piece of source information is quite widespread. Those that are most successful seem to be the ones that encourage residents to express their concerns and positive feedback in freeform text, ensuring the resident is in a position to 'have their say' rather than merely respond to what the facility's management wants to know.

Could an aged care provider simply self-define quality and ignore the regulations? Such an approach would be high risk. The number of regulations to which a residential aged care provider is subject is extensive. They are set by all levels of government and in some cases across a number of departments of state.

Definitions of quality from the internet (BusinessDictionary.com 2013) include:

- level of excellence, an attribute that differentiates
- the absence of a defect (from a manufacturer)
- to be at a high degree of excellence
- essential characteristic of a good tea (from a tea-maker)
- characteristics by which stakeholders judge an organisation.

Stakeholders include residents, relatives, community, government and anyone else who seeks to be stakeholder. So, maybe the 'characteristics by which stakeholders judge an organisation' without trying to further define stakeholders and their relative worth or influence is as good a definition as we are going to get.

Quality in the aged care context is concerned with achieving positive outcomes for each and every resident who relies on the aged care service for support. There must also be an approach to service delivery in that the outcomes are sustained over time. But of course the challenge is to ensure that the desire for consistency, which is an underlying business need, does not get stifled because process is put ahead of outcomes and the institution's convenience ahead of residents.

But so many of these notions of 'quality' are different things to different people. Moreover an individual's view will likely change over time. We can consider the newly admitted low-care resident who has little or no interest in pain management and a big interest in bus trips and 'how will I fill in my day?'. That person will have a personal definition of quality. 'Why are you telling me about pain management and palliative care?' they might say.

Twelve months down the track their health status may have declined markedly and advanced cancer has been diagnosed and their expectations and interests will almost certainly have changed. The immediacy of their condition will dictate their view of quality.

There was also an interesting outcome from a study conducted by Campbell Research (DoHA 2007) in relation to what is considered important in defining quality services. The response themes in focus groups were:

- residents—issues based, relationships, food
- Aboriginal and Torres Strait Islander people—respect for traditions, staff sensitivity
- culturally and linguistically diverse respondents—communication, food, language

- families of residents—staff support
- nurses—physical and emotional needs, staffing numbers, homelike environment
- care staff—appropriate and timely support to residents, homelike environment
- aged care managers—opined care is what they do; life is what residents experience
- owner/operators—best possible service, evidence-based care, individual needs met
- doctors—good healthcare for residents
- peak provider organisations—safety, security, care and comfort
- accreditation assessors—resident focus, leadership, importance of staff.

This variety of themes from different stakeholders is consistent with the research about quality in health around the world and reinforces the thing we know: Quality is a multidimensional concept and residents are multidimensional. In the end, however, the community expects aged care facilities to deliver high-quality resident-focused care and services in a homelike environment. That is not their language but rather the bureaucratise that heralded the introduction of the Aged Care Act. I think people are much simpler in their approach. They just want to have the best life they can and they will measure that in whatever way they want.

 But in the end the community expects aged care homes to deliver high-quality resident-focused care and services in a homelike environment.

On balance, I believe residents are typically more inclined to form their own view of their experience in the home than rely on the views of an accreditation assessor. So we know there is a challenge to deliver quality services when each player has a view as to what constitutes quality and the government also has a view. Some of the submissions to the recent *Productivity Report – Caring for Older Australians* (Productivity Commission 2010) expressed the view that the funding arrangements were not consistent with community expectations of service. That remains a point of contention because, like many things in aged care, there is a huge diversity of opinion.

In the broader context of quality we must not lose sight of the point that a person's perception of quality is founded on their experiences of life and expectations. The Accreditation Agency has anecdotes of people who complained when the accreditation of the home in which they lived was revoked because they were 'happy with the care' but sometime after relocation came to the realisation that the care had not been up to standard.

As we seek to measure quality absolutely there are some cautionary thoughts and questions.

- Can we actually assign a rating?
- There are differing views as to what constitutes quality.
- We need to be cautious in how we set quality measures or indicators because standards and measures do drive performance. We need to

ensure they are comprehensive without becoming an end in themselves. But beware: what gets measured gets done (e.g. a focus on simply counting falls might have unintended consequences). Chemical and physical restraint will reduce the number of falls; however, there are negative consequences with such an approach.

We tend to see indicators as numbers only. However, in our daily lives we use instinctive or observational indicators—that is, we notice changes in the weather (not numbers) and they cause us to take action. You do not need to know the temperature to know to put on a coat. Using these types of observational indicators cannot be understated in long-term care. A care worker who simply observes a resident's change in demeanour and acts on that is gold.

We should also question the utility of institutional scores. They do provide some commentary about how the aged care service is performing against the government standards, but do they have meaning for residents? Not if you are in the minority 2% who had an adverse event that could have been avoided or you are unhappy with things.

Indicators, observations and monitoring are all useless unless they translate into action for individuals.

In relation to indicators I want to make a couple of further comments. People frequently talk about indicators variously known as quality indicators, performance indicators, key performance indicators (KPIs) and benchmarking. Indicators are not measures of quality. They are exactly as they say— 'indicators'. Individual indicators viewed alone are a great risk creator. We have many indicators in the clinical aspects of aged care but much work needs to be done in regard to the 'life' things residents report as important to them. To be effective, indicators must be a comprehensive set and viewed in the same way as the 'balanced score card'.

Indicators can be useful in benchmarking institutional performance. The important thing in comparing performance is the like-with-like comparison. The alternate is to undertake significant risk adjustment to create the like-with-like comparison. That is the real challenge in aged care and there can be significant costs in collecting the baseline data. The true value of a comprehensive set of indicators is their use in trending a facility's performance over time. Even then the information must be considered in context. But remember indicators inform the creation of the hypothesis for further investigation. They are not the hypothesis.

EXCELLENCE

This now brings me to the notion of excellence. I think excellence is the Holy Grail in service delivery in any industry. Similarly, like many words, the word 'excellence' has many meanings. A search of the internet turns up:

- the quality of excelling
- possessing good qualities in high degrees
- the state or quality of excelling
- the quality of being excellent.

The same word is the name of a fictional robot, a magazine about Porsche cars, a word processor for the Amiga computer and a Swedish pop group.

But some words of caution: This section is about the pursuit of excellence rather than being excellent.

This section is about the pursuit of excellence rather than being excellent.

In considering the concept of excellence I will take some thoughts from the Chief Justice of Queensland (2001), who in a speech titled 'In Pursuit of Excellence' encapsulated the notion of the pursuit of excellence extremely well. He said: 'The pursuit of excellence is a quest without end. As with wisdom or humility, we should never rightly see ourselves or our organisation as truly "excellent"—although we may note such a quality in others.'

So 'in pursuit of excellence' means we want to demonstrate 'the quality of being exceptionally good'. But is this possible? Maybe the linking of pursuit (i.e. to chase with no obvious reference to catching) is not so out of line or defeatist as one might have first thought or implied.

Could I suggest that if you had an objective to 'provide excellent service', that objective is self-limiting. You might simply decide you were already providing excellent service and then stop trying to improve and remain static. We cannot ignore that many corporate mission and vision statements include phrases about providing excellent service. Such statements may be more about marketing and promotion than a reflection of approach or vision.

True excellence requires more than skill, ability, intellect, effort and accomplishment. All those qualities are without value if they exist in a moral or ethical vacuum. This is particularly true in aged care. It may be no accident that charitable or not-for-profit organisations manage a large percentage of residential aged care bodies in Australia.

In fact history is littered with brilliant figures who might have been considered to embody excellence had they only used their talents for good. Being very, very good at something (otherwise described as technically sound) can only be considered heading to excellent if it is in the right context or in the context of right! Excellence in aged care encompasses more than documents, systems and processes. It is about people, and a pursuit for the benefit of others.

In aged care it is the residents who are the ultimate judges and it is against their standards, their values and what they rate as important that the people and organisations that provide services should be judged. I also suspect that residents place greater credence on their assessments than they do on those of government inspectors and accreditation assessors. However, the absence of a true market and the practical incapacity of a resident to relocate means they are more than a customer (who may chose to go elsewhere). This very feature justifies the involvement of government in the setting of standards and creating a quality assurance scheme of accreditation.

So should we just leave it to residents to decide whether the quality of care and services is appropriate? I must say I don't see any government or the community agreeing to that proposition when we are talking about the frail, the vulnerable, the elderly and the disempowered.

Some respondents to the Campbell research opined that care and services is that which residents receive and quality of life is the outcome of that.

TO BRING THIS TOGETHER

- **Regulations** are the law! It is the rules of the game set by a third party.
- **Quality** is something we try to measure in many ways.
- **Excellence** is something we pursue with the full and complete understanding that if ever we feel we have attained the status of excellent … we have not!

So … should aged care providers be focusing on regulations, quality indicators and accreditation standards when they are developing systems and recruiting and training staff, or should they be building systems to meet people's ever-changing needs and wants, then deciding how to measure performance? Or, put another way—do they behave in accordance with the intention and spirit or letter of the law?

This is in the context that well-framed regulations will not impede innovation and delivery of quality services. Among accrediting bodies the question concerning the level of prescription that should exist in standards is vexed. It is true that there is a range of views concerning detail. The Accreditation Agency experience is that there is no unity of view among aged care managers. Some expect extensive guidance concerning the expectations that lie under the expected outcomes under the accreditation standards. Others suggest that the headline will suffice. My view is that the more detailed the standard, the less arguments there will be among accredited assessors. However, that is more than counterbalanced by my view that detailed standards will stifle innovation and straitjacket service delivery.

If one has an eye only for the letter of the law, and is managing only to comply with the regulations, then one risks missing the opportunities that the broader approach of an eye for the spirit offers. From my perspective using the letter of the law to get out of trouble with the authorities is probably not a bad call. But we should not look to regulations as lighting the way to deliver high-quality services.

MY EXPERIENCE 2003–2012

I doubt that many people in aged care deliberately flout the many rules and regulations. I think that what happens in most cases, particularly where the level of failing to meet a standard is low, is that the journey to failing to meet the standard has been only a little faster than a glacier and is only noticed when it tips over the edge. This can be prevented by good information management systems. The recent history from the Accreditation Agency demonstrates that failing to meet the standards related to having effective information management systems in place is among the highest predictors of risk. However, having said that, there is little one can do to eliminate the fact that a staff member will have a bad day once in a while. That happens in all organisations. Most are more forgiving than aged care.

Notwithstanding any of that, compliance with regulations is something with which we are all bound. This can also be quite complex for the people responsible for governance in your organisation. While the business of aged care is inherently risky (as are other businesses), the risks are exacerbated by the type of service, nature of the clientele and work organisation structures where one or two people direct the traffic in the aged care facility.

So what are the risks if an Australian aged care provider is found not to meet the minimum requirements? The most immediate risk is a visit from the regulating DoHA. Outcomes following that visit may include:

- that residents' health, safety and wellbeing has been put at risk/compromised
- Commonwealth subsidies cease or are reduced
- other revenue and support wanes
- costs associated with mitigation/repair are increased
- the organisation's reputation is damaged thus affecting the capacity to recruit
- staff morale sags
- the career/reputation of management is damaged
- the organisation becomes risk averse and being risk averse is a significant risk in itself to innovation.

I must ask you to also consider the risk to achieving excellence if on achieving the minimum required by law to obtain subsidies you simply stop and rest on your 'achievement'.

CONCLUSION

The accreditation standards reflect what Parliament believes align with the expectations of residents and their families, overlayed with a view of community expectation, a notion of good practice and the cloak of 'the state knows best'. The current review of the standards (at the time of writing) is an important piece of work because it creates an opportunity to reflect the vast increase in knowledge about residential aged care service delivery over the past 12 years and changes in industry practices. The other challenge is to meet the diversity of quality between providers.

The challenge in setting accreditation standards is to go far enough, but not too far such that the level of detail ends up prescribing processes and structures rather than requiring the existence of process and structures to support the services that provide outcomes for residents.

I also think we need to remember that generally regulations tend to be directed at protecting the community and thereby the focus in application is on those perceived to be poor achievers. I think it is true that the overall quality of residential aged care in Australia has improved since the introduction of accreditation in 1997. Many commentators suggest it is superior to that generally available in other countries. It has been suggested that, because of this improvement, it is time to relax the regulatory framework related to quality. Such an approach represents a risk to residents because at this time we cannot say that the reason the quality has improved is not directly attributable to the existence of the quality framework.

In aged care we aim to protect health, safety and wellbeing and promote quality. Many other countries are more focused on protection; their approach assumes physical safety and protection is more relevant than the broad range we consider in the Australian accreditation scheme. It does beg the question as to whether the accreditation standards are performance or quality indicators. I think they are at best a proxy for measuring quality in the absence of anything else. That is why standards must be fit for purpose. At the same time an accreditation program can be characterised as a risk mitigation strategy and one that provides some assurance to the community.

The other thing I would add is that accreditation standards compliance scores tend to be institution measures. As a concept excellence in service is not about aggregating and saying 'well, 95% of people are happy; ain't that grand?'. Excellence is about the 100% and the experience of each individual. Who would volunteer to be in the 5% unhappy group?

The accreditation standards are not a management system. In their pure form they are a measure of the effectiveness of those systems. It concerns me when I read that some providers use the standards as a management system.

How does one position for excellence? That is a huge topic that goes to book size. Consequently I will talk about what not to do. Let me use the radio telescope at Parkes to illustrate my point. That piece of equipment is very powerful and very expensive. However, it has no mind of its own and looks only in the direction it is pointed. The information the scientists get back relates only to where they point the telescope. An aged care manager does not have the luxury to be looking only in one direction. A spotlight highlights what it sees but the rest is concealed. If the corporate telescope is pointed at achieving accreditation only, the home will pass the accreditation test on the day but will almost certainly fail its residents over time. If the 'quality telescope' uses the wide lens and is focused on residents and their needs and wants, the provider has the opportunity to provide excellent care. You just need to look and act. You will breeze through accreditation if you act on what you see.

Good systems and focused people will deliver your accreditation as a byproduct. Continued and sustained excellent performance is not a one-off. It is a habit that entails effort and commitment. In regard to systems and processes, it is systems and processes that provide the support structures for service delivery. It is the people who use those support structures that influence the outcomes for residents as they adopt and adapt the systems to meet the individual needs of residents.

Systems and efforts should be focused on residents and accreditation will happen. Aged care services need to:

- have systems that deliver quality services through well-trained and motivated people—the Accreditation Agency research shows a common theme for noncompliance is inadequate supervision and under-training
- be alert to but not alarmed by the regulations
- keep their eye on the 'care' ball
- remember accreditation is the check (exam if you like); it is not the goal
- develop their systems and measures to meet residents' needs, not to impress assessors.

In the end it all gets down to one thing, which can be said in a number of ways. Do you strive to provide high-quality care and chase excellence or do you just want to be accredited with no detected failure to meet an expected outcome? In any event, what does full compliance with the accreditation standards at your aged care service mean for each individual resident?

Do you say 'yes, got accredited' or do you say 'we delivered high-quality care'? These are questions to ask yourself and not necessarily for public consumption. Despite what you say, how do you act? While achieving a 44/44 score probably means you've got your board off your back and staff have settled back into the routine and management still has a job, does this mean that residents have the best quality of life that can be provided or they deserve?

Full compliance with the accreditation standards says you passed the examination at that point in time. The elusive excellence of service is approached when the services are delivered consistently at a high level and in a moral and ethical framework.

In closing I will share some advice from Orison Swett Marden (1850–1924). Dr Marden was an American writer associated with the new thought movement. He said, and given he was a doctor and a successful publican he must be right,

People who have accomplished worthwhile work have had a very high sense of the way to do things. They have not been content with mediocrity. They have not confined themselves to the beaten tracks; they have never been satisfied to do things just as others do them. They always pushed things that came to their hands a little higher up, this little farther on—that counts in the quality of life's work. It is constant effort to be first-class in everything one attempts that conquers the heights of excellence.

(Khalid 2013)

I say, 'notwithstanding all the difficulties, complexities and hurdles, it is up to you'. Do you just want to get a tick from the accreditation body? Or do you want the satisfaction of knowing you are providing near excellent service.

Vignette

In 2004 SummitCare recognised that 'excellence' in its full embodiment would lead to a point of difference in what has been a highly regulated and immature aged care market. Its strategic goal was to deliver a whole-of-business approach to excellence and not merely a focus on a minimum standard to inform the deliverables to its customers.

As a result, it identified the Australian Business Excellence Framework (ABEF) as the ideal frame of reference to inform the organisation's direction. It used the accreditation standards to inform the minimum resident-related requirements but recognised that the ABEF drive a focus around the entire business.

SummitCare operates nine residential aged care services delivering a mix of high, low and extra service delivery options. Today its revenue exceeds $70 million and it employs more than 900 staff. Testament to the experience SummitCare has, in every instance, it exceeded its accreditation requirement. The quality systems enable achievement of the 44 expected outcomes as a byproduct rather than as a core focus.

SummitCare achieved silver in 2009 and built on this result to become the only aged care business in Australia to achieve 'gold' in 2012. This is especially significant given the framework was enhanced and the scoring matrix reinforced with emphasis on 'success and sustainability' (300 of the 1000 available scores). SummitCare CEO Cynthia Payne comments: 'We always knew that we needed a whole business approach to focus on excellence and that we are a sum of all of our parts. The accreditation standards directly informed part of the quality systems for the customer experience, on their own they are not enough to stimulate a focus on Excellence. The Australian Business Excellence Standard is a recognized international standard and has placed our organization in strong position for all regulatory requirements' (personal communication).

Reflective questions

1. Do you think external evaluation of health/aged services does anything to improve quality?

2. Think as a client rather than a health professional—would you feel safer if you knew the service you were using had passed an external evaluation?

3. What do see as the benefits—or otherwise—of having mandatory compliance expectations?

4. Should this be linked to taxpayer/government funding?

5. What views do you have on making audit reports public?

6. Does the public good have precedence over the organisation's right to privacy?

7. Think about person-centred care and pain—see if you can come up with a list of structures and processes that would need to be in place to ensure the approach to the person in pain is person centred; see Chapters, 7 and 15 for some ideas.

8. Most families would argue vehemently that they 'know what Mum/Dad wants. Do you think they do? Read also Chapters 8 and 10 to see what evidence they provide on this issue.

9. What then is the relationship between regulations, quality and the pursuit of excellence?

10. What would you see as most important if you/a family member were living in a nursing home? The clinical knowledge? Environment? Comfort? Or something else? How would you measure it?

References

Australian Commission on Safety and Quality in Health Care, 2006. Discussion Paper National Safety and Quality Accreditation Standards p 5. Online. Available: http://www.acipc.org.au/about-us/partnerships-affiliated-organisations-and-links/acsqhc, 1 May 2013.

BusinessDirectory.com, 2013. Definition of 'quality'. Online. Available: http://www.businessdictionary.com/definition/quality.html, 1 May 213.

Chen, J.C., 2010. Public reporting of health system performance: Review of evidence on impact on patients, providers and healthcare organisations: An Evidence Check. Rapid review brokered by Sax Institute for the Bureau of Health Information.

Chief Justice of Queensland, 2001. 'In Pursuit of Excellence'. Speech. University of Queensland Commencement Service, Sunday 25 May 2001—Mayne Hall.

Department of Health and Ageing (DoHA), 2007. Evaluation of the impact of accreditation on the delivery of quality of care and quality of life to residents in Australian Government subsidised residential aged care homes, (Campbell report). Commonwealth of Australia, Canberra.

Donabedian, A., 2005. Evaluating the quality of medical care. Milbank Quarterly 83, 691–729. doi: 10.1111/j.1468-0009.2005.00397.x

Irwin, L., 2012. Quality indicators in long-term care and health services. unpublished.

Khalid, H.R., 2013. Book of famous quotes. Online. Available: http://www.famous-quotes.com/topic.php?page=4&total=147&tid=418, 6 Mar 2013.

Productivity Commission, 2010. Submissions: Productivity Report—Caring for Older Australians. Online. Available: http://www.pc.gov.au/projects/inquiry/aged-care/submissions, 1 May 2013.

Runciman, W.B., 2006. Shared meanings: preferred terms and definitions for safety and quality concepts. Medical Journal of Australia 184 (10), S41–S43.

CHAPTER 21

ENVIRONMENTS THAT ENHANCE DEMENTIA CARE: ISSUES AND CHALLENGES

Richard Fleming and Kirsty Bennett

Editors' comments

The beneficial effects of a well-designed environment on older people who have dementia have become increasingly clear over the past 30 years. They include a reduction in confusion, agitation and depression, along with an increase in engagement with activities and social interaction. The characteristics of environments that are helpful to people with dementia are well enough known for the quality of the environments to be measured and this is leading to an increase in our understanding of the interrelationship between the physical environment and the quality of life of residents. However, the application of our knowledge is patchy and much remains to be done to ensure the next generation of buildings reflects the learning that has taken place. The key to applying the knowledge resides in the awareness of the principles of design by the architects and managers of the residential care facility, often nurses, who between them are responsible for the design process and the development of a philosophy of care that ensures that the design of the building is in harmony with the model of care. When the philosophy of care includes a commitment to person-centred care the likelihood of people with dementia finding meaning and pleasure in their lives is increased.

INTRODUCTION

THE SCOPE OF THE PROBLEM

In 2009–10 it was estimated that there were more than 84,000 people with dementia in residential aged care facilities across Australia (Australian Institute of Health and Welfare (AIHW) 2011) and the demand for these places is estimated to grow at 4% per annum between now and 2029 (AIHW 2011). This reflects a worldwide phenomenon. The number of people with dementia in the United Kingdom (UK), for example, is currently estimated at 700,000 and will double within 30 years (Knapp & Prince 2007). The scale of the demand for residential facilities for people with dementia, and the evidence of the positive contribution that the environment can make to the care of people with dementia, directs attention to the need for these facilities to be well designed.

THE EVIDENCE BASE

Since 1987 there have been a number of attempts at defining the characteristics of good design for people with dementia. In an early Australian paper Fleming (Fleming & Bowles 1987) identified eight principles of good design: (1) small size; (2) provision of domestic facilities; (3) easy access to local community; (4) reduction of unhelpful stimulation; (5) highlighting of helpful stimuli; (6) good visual access—that is, residents able to see where they want to go; (7) provision of a clear pathway that guides residents from inside to outside and back again without obstacles and opportunities for passing interaction; and (8) familiar furniture, fittings and décor. While not explicitly described these principles were also addressed in the development of small, homelike facilities by Brian Kidd (1987).

Five years later in the United States (US) Cohen and Weisman (1991) described nine goals for the environment: (1) ensure safety and security; (2) support functional ability through meaningful activity; (3) maximise awareness and orientation; (4) provide opportunities for stimulation and change; (5) maximise autonomy and control; (6) adapt to changing needs; (7) establish links to the healthy and familiar; (8) provide opportunities for socialisation; and (9) protect privacy. Cohen and Wiesman's book provides specific suggestions for planning and building to achieve these goals by using photos, floor plans, and guides with examples of how the specific aspects of the environment achieves the therapeutic goals. However, the examples given seem very institutional by contemporary Australian standards.

Some 10 years later Marshall (2001) provided a synthesis of the principles, promoting facilities that: (1) are small in size; (2) are domestic and homelike; (3) provide scope for ordinary activities (unit kitchens, washing lines, garden sheds); (4) have unobtrusive safety features; (5) have rooms for different functions, with furniture and fittings familiar to the age and generation of the residents; (6) have a safe outside space; (7) have single rooms big enough for a reasonable amount of personal belongings; (8) have good signage and multiple cues where possible; (9) use objects rather than colour for orientation; (10) enhance visual access; and (11) control stimuli, especially noise.

Two reviews, published 10 years apart, analyse and discuss studies that have investigated empirical research on the effects of specific environmental features (Day et al 2000, Fleming & Purandare 2010). Day et al's review (2000) focuses on research from 1970 to 1999 and features mostly positive effects from these environmental interventions, while Fleming and Purandare (2010) critically evaluate studies from 1980 to 2009, giving each study a rating of strong, moderate or weak based on an analysis of the methodology. The results of this later review are used in the description of the principles of design below.

The field of designing for people with dementia is also an area of practice and much can be learnt through critically evaluating built examples and the interrogation of the brief and the philosophy of care that led to the finished result. There are a variety of books providing case studies of good design and practical advice for its implementation (Calkins 1988, Judd et al 1998). The evidence base has also been used as the basis for recommending modifications to the homes of people with dementia to facilitate ageing in place (van Hoof et al 2010) and for designing hospital wards (Dementia Services Development Centre 2012b, Fleming et al 2003, King's Fund 2012).

There is a strong evidence base that we can use to inform our designs.

ASSESSING THE PHYSICAL ENVIRONMENT

The development of this evidence base has been paralleled by the development of tools that allow us to evaluate the environment. The published research on the evaluation of environments for people with dementia has been dominated by three scales and their variations: the MEAP, the TESS and the PEAP.

The Multiphasic Environmental Assessment Procedure (MEAP) (Moos & Lemke 1984), developed in 1984, has been described as 'the most established instrument' (Sloane et al 2002). It has a number of components, only one of which, the Physical and Architectural Features Checklist, is concerned with the physical environment. The scales of this procedure were designed to assess planned residential environments for older people ranging from congregate housing to nursing homes. The physical-feature categories were derived from an *a priori* theoretical model with nine dimensions: physical amenities; social-recreational aids; prosthetic aids; orientational aids; safety features; architectural choice, space availability; staff facilities; and community accessibility. It is a very detailed assessment that is not suitable for use by non-researchers. Its scoring is biased towards larger, more institutional settings, and it is compiled at the facility level rather than at the unit level (Moos & Lemke 1984).

These limitations were addressed in the development of the Therapeutic Environment Screening Survey for Nursing Homes (TESS-NH) (Sloane et al 2002). First developed in 1990, the TESS-NH has undergone several stages of development. The TESS-NH contains 84 discrete items plus one global item that cover 13 domains. These domains include exit control, maintenance, cleanliness, safety, orientation/cueing, privacy, unit autonomy, outdoor access, lighting, noise, visual/tactile stimulation, space/seating and familiarity/homelike environment. It takes 30–45 minutes to complete and is intended for use by researchers. The TESS-NH instrument and instructional manual are available at <www.unc.edu/depts/tessnh>. It has been further modified to improve its application in a residential, rather than clinical, setting (Zimmerman et al 2005), but the reliability and validity of the new scale, the TESS-RC, has not been established.

The Professional Environmental Assessment Protocol (PEAP) (Lawton et al 2000) was developed in 2000 to supplement the TESS by providing an assessment of a set of conceptual dimensions. It is designed to be completed by raters who possess substantial knowledge and expertise in person–environment design research.

The PEAP consists of five-point ratings of nine dimensions, each of which represents a desired outcome of 'quality' environments: maximising awareness and orientation; maximising safety and security; provision of privacy; stimulation and coherence (regulation); stimulation and coherence (quality); support of functional abilities; provision of opportunities for personal control; continuity of the self; and facilitation of social contact. Each dimension is defined, with an expanded conceptual discussion of its meaning, followed by a rater's guide to what to observe and enquire about at the time of the walk-through. Each point of the scale is described in such a way as to highlight the differences among the five points. The time taken to complete the PEAP during the validation study was 45–90 minutes.

The choice between these scales is reasonably clear when the environment being assessed is a residential unit for people with dementia. The MEAP does not address some of the environmental issues that are considered to be important in dementia care; its scoring is biased towards larger, more institutional settings. The PEAP requires a sophisticated and experienced rater able to devote a considerable amount of time to the assessment. The TESS-NH yields results that correlate well with the PEAP, takes half the time and can be used by a research assistant after eight hours of training (Sloane et al 2002). So the TESS-NH has a practical edge over the PEAP.

However, the TESS-NH has some severe limitations. While the 84 items cover a wide variety of relevant environmental features, they do not combine to form a scale and therefore do not enable a simple summary of the quality of the environment to be obtained. This is left to a single-item global rating scale. The TESS-NH is also heavily influenced by the North American style of care for people with dementia.

While not so extensively used in the research literature there are two more recently developed scales that warrant consideration for use in the Australian context. They are the audit tool designed to be used in conjunction with the *Best Practice in Design for People with Dementia* booklets published by the Dementia Services Development Centre (DSDC) in Stirling, Scotland (Cunningham 2008, DSDC 2008) and the most recent version of the Environmental Audit Tool developed in a New South Wales Department of Health project on adapting wards in small, regional hospitals for long-term use by people with dementia (Fleming et al 2003). The Scottish tool will be referred to as the Stirling Environmental Audit Tool (SEAT) and the Australian tool as the Environmental Audit Tool (EAT).

The SEAT (Cunningham 2011) comprises 194 statements describing the features of the environment. The descriptions are designed to focus attention on design features that are recognised in the literature or in good practice as being significant for the wellbeing of people with dementia (Cunningham 2009). They are divided into two categories: 'essential' (81 items), described as 'essential criteria, based on research and expert opinion'; and 'recommended' (113 items), described as 'based on current evidence and international best practice' (p 5).

An example of an 'essential' item is: 'The colour of the toilet seat contrasts with both the toilet bowl and the floor'. A related 'recommended' item is 'cisterns are traditional in appearance' (p 29).

The items are organised by location so that the SEAT can be completed by walking through a facility area by area. Each item is scored on a three-point scale with 0 indicating standard not met, 0.5 indicating standard partially met and 1 that the standard has been fully met. The final score is weighted according to category. The 'essential' percentage makes up 30% of the overall rating and the recommended percentage makes up 70%. The reliability and validity of the SEAT were assessed in a study carried out for the Principal Dementia Collaborative Research Centre based in The University of New South Wales (Fleming 2010) and found to be very satisfactory. A new version of the SEAT has recently been published but there is no information yet available on its reliability or validity (DSDC 2012a).

The EAT comprises 72 items that have been selected to exemplify 10 design principles supported by the literature (Fleming & Bowles 1987, Fleming & Purandare 2010). The reliability, validity and ease of use of the EAT have been investigated and found to be very satisfactory (Fleming 2011, Smith et al 2012).

The SEAT and the EAT differ primarily in the detail of the questions and the way in which they are organised. The SEAT has more detailed questions and organises them around locations. The EAT organises observations around a set of principles and is the easiest of the audit tools to use. While the SEAT and the EAT have developed in different countries, they share a common approach to the design of environments for people with dementia and are designed to provide an understanding of the strengths and weaknesses of the environment that leads to positive changes.

The 10 principles contained in the EAT, and the evidence for them, are described below.

 There are tools available to identify the strengths and weaknesses of our environments.

THE PRINCIPLES OF DESIGN

The principles are presented with a brief label followed by a short description of the need that the principle meets and a summary of the evidence base supporting the principle.

UNOBTRUSIVELY REDUCE RISKS

People with dementia require an internal and external environment that is safe, secure and easy to move around if they are to make the best of their remaining abilities. However, obvious safety features and barriers will lead to frustration, agitation and anger, and so potential risks need to be reduced unobtrusively.

The confusion that accompanies dementia determines the need for a variety of safety features to be built into the environment. Among other things, they often include the provision of a secure perimeter (Rosewarne et al 1997). It is important to note that residents may respond negatively to a safety or security measure if it obviously impedes their freedom (Low et al 2004, Torrington 2006). This can be mitigated by providing these unobtrusively (Annerstedt 1997, Zeisel et al 2003). In the case of a perimeter fence, for example, shrubbery can be used to hide a fence that prevents someone wandering off.

There are varying attitudes to the provision of this type of security. In some countries, Norway for example, it is illegal to lock people up simply because they have dementia. The security of the person is protected by providing a sufficient number of staff so that a person who wishes to leave can be accompanied. In Japan there has been a great deal of effort put into training millions of volunteers to recognise a person with dementia and to provide assistance if they are lost in the community (Lancioni et al 2010).

These variations in approach raise the issue of the dignity of risk and illustrate the constant tension between the desire to protect a person with a problem and the rights that that person has to lead as normal a life as possible—a life that contains risk (Nay 2003). This is an integral part of the person-centred care approach (Woods 1999).

PROVIDE A HUMAN SCALE

The scale of a building will have an effect on the behaviour and feelings of a person with dementia. The experience of scale is determined by three factors: the number of people that the person encounters, the overall size of the building and the size of the individual components, such as doors, rooms and corridors. A person should not be intimidated by the size of the surroundings or confronted with a multitude of interactions and choices. Rather the scale should help the person feel in control.

The development of special care units for people with dementia has been influenced by the view that larger facilities increase agitation and are confusing for residents (Hagglund & Hagglund 2010, Sloan et al 1998), and that high-quality care is easier to provide in small groups (Annerstedt 1993, Reimer et al 2004). However, the findings reported in the literature are hard to interpret as there is no accepted definition of small, which has been defined as up to 150 beds (Leon & Ory 1999). Small size is almost always accompanied by particular approaches to the delivery of care, such as providing a homelike environment (Verbeek et al 2012). This may contribute to the contradictory findings. Zeisel et al (2003), for example, found less social withdrawal in larger units and a large, recent study found no link between small size and neuropsychiatric symptoms (Zuidema et al 2009). The evidence tends to suggest that the best outcomes occur when the resident lives in a small unit but has access to a larger social network.

ALLOW PEOPLE TO SEE AND BE SEEN

The provision of an easily understood environment will help to minimise confusion. It is particularly important for people with dementia to be able to recognise where they are, where they have come from and what they will find if they head in a certain direction. When they can see key places, such as a lounge room, dining room, their bedroom, kitchen and an outdoor area, they are more able to make choices and find their way to where they want to go. Buildings that provide these opportunities are said to have good visual access. Good visual access opens up opportunities for engagement and gives the person with dementia the confidence to explore their environment. It can also enable staff to see residents from where they spend most of their time. This reduces their anxiety and the anxiety of the residents.

Confusion may be reduced by caring for the confused person in a simple environment. The simplest environment is one in which the resident can see everywhere that she wants to go to from wherever she is; being able to see the kitchen, dining room, lounge room and the person's own room is particularly important. This principle defined the plans of the units for the confused and disturbed elderly built by the NSW Department of Health in the late 1980s, which were shown to improve self-help, socialisation and behaviour (Atkinson 1995, Fleming & Bowles 1987), and is associated with improved orientation (Marquardt 2011, Passini et al 1998). Disorientation has been found to be less pronounced in L-, H- and square-shaped units where the kitchen, dining room and activity rooms were located together (Elmstahl et al 1997), and where the straight layout of the circulation system, without any change of direction, provided good visual access (Hagglund & Hagglund 2010).

Good visual access also provides benefits for the staff. If staff can see the residents from the places where they spend most of their time, this reduces their anxiety. At the same time the visibility of the staff to the residents helps them to feel supported.

Evidence of the importance of being able to see what you need to see when you need to see it is provided in a study that investigated the effects of making the toilet visible rather than hiding it away (Namazi & Johnson 1991a). This increased visits to the toilet eightfold, which is good evidence for the effectiveness of making things visible but might be too much of a good thing as far as spending time in the toilet is concerned.

REDUCE UNHELPFUL STIMULATION

Because dementia reduces the ability to filter stimulation and attend to only those things that are important, a person with dementia becomes stressed by prolonged exposure to large amounts of stimulation. The environment should be designed to minimise exposure to stimuli that are not helpful. The full range of senses must be considered. Too much visual stimulation, for example, is as stressful as too much auditory stimulation.

Because people with dementia experience difficulties in coping with a large amount of stimulation, the environment should be designed to reduce the impact of stimulation that is unnecessary for their wellbeing (Cleary et al 1988). There is strong evidence that residents are less verbally aggressive where sensory input is more understandable and where such input is more controlled (Zeisel et al 2003). Aggressive behaviours increase with high noise levels (Cohen-Mansfield & Werner 1995). Busy entry doors pose particular problems for staff and residents because they are a constant source of over stimulation and offer a temptation to escape. These problems can be significantly reduced by reducing the stimulation (Dickinson et al 1995, Namazi et al 1989). The goal is to provide residents with an optimum level of stimulation. This is well illustrated by using two wardrobes to increase independence, one containing the majority of the resident's clothes the other containing a manageable number of clothes. The larger wardrobe is camouflaged and secured, while the smaller wardrobe is highlighted and the door handle is accessible to the resident. When the resident opens the door of this wardrobe they are not confronted with a confusing, over-stimulating mess of clothing, shoes, bags, ties, belts, etc. but a level of stimulation that they can deal with (Namazi & Johnson 1992). The person-centred approach can be seen when the staff have worked with the resident the evening before to choose the selection of clothing in the small wardrobe.

OPTIMISE HELPFUL STIMULATION

Enabling the person with dementia to see, hear and smell things that give them cues about where they are and what they can do can help to minimise their confusion and uncertainty.

Consideration needs to be given to providing redundant cueing—that is, providing a number of cues to the same thing, recognising that what is meaningful to one person will not necessarily be meaningful to another. A person may recognise their bedroom, for example, because of a view, the presence of furniture, the colour of the walls, the light fitting and/or the bedspread. Cues need to be carefully designed so that they do not become unhelpful stimulation.

The reduction in unnecessary stimulation should be balanced by highlighting stimuli that are important to the residents. Providing signs and other aids to wayfinding is integral to the design of many environments for people with dementia (Grant et al 1995, Passini et al 2000) and have been associated with a reduction in behavioural symptoms (Bianchetti et al 1997). The placement and nature of the signs is important; signs placed low and using words rather than pictograms are most effective (Namazi and Johnson 1991b). There is some evidence that the use of colour to distinguish the doors to residents' rooms has a beneficial effect (Lawton et al 1984); the display of personal memorabilia outside the room may also be of some benefit (Namazi et al 1991, Nolan et al 2001).

Personalised signs and cues are often used. They can take the form of a glass-fronted box immediately outside of the person's bedroom door. Personal objects and photos can be placed in it, preferably with the relatives helping the resident to choose and place them. These provide a unique and familiar reminder to the resident that this is their room.

SUPPORT MOVEMENT AND ENGAGEMENT

Aimless wandering can be minimised by providing a well-defined pathway, free of obstacles and complex decision points, that guides people past points of interest and gives them opportunities to engage in activities or social interaction. The pathway should be both internal and external, providing an opportunity and reason to go outside when the weather permits.

Wandering is sometimes a feature of the behaviour of people with dementia. Providing a walking path has been shown to be associated with lower levels of agitation (Zeisel et al 2003). Access to an outside area is associated with reduced sadness and increased pleasure (Cox et al 2004). However, providing a walking path alone does not reduce neuropsychiatric symptoms (Zuidema et al 2009); it is necessary for someone to interact with the residents while they are outside for benefits to occur (Wood et al 2005).

A well-designed garden can be a pleasant place for residents and staff to spend a little time (Cochrane 2010). They can also provide a place where relatives, and most importantly their children, can spend time with the residents. In this way, the environment contributes to fostering intergenerational relationships (Edwards et al 2012).

CREATE A FAMILIAR SPACE

People with dementia are more able to use and enjoy spaces and objects that were familiar to them in their early life. The environment should afford them the opportunity to maintain their competence through the use of familiar building design (internal and external), furniture, fittings and colours. This will involve an understanding of the personal background of the people living in the environment.

The involvement of the person with dementia in personalising the environment with their own familiar objects should be encouraged.

The person with dementia recalls the distant past more easily than the recent past. This may explain the beneficial effects associated with them being in an environment similar to that of their early life. The opportunity to increase the familiarity of the surroundings by the resident bringing in their own belongings has been associated with the maintenance of activities of daily living and reductions in aggression, anxiety and depression (Annerstedt 1997).

While it is possible for people with dementia to learn to use new technologies this is not easy and requires a great deal of support from skilled staff (Lekeu et al 2002). It is much easier, more practical and, possibly, more pleasant for the person with dementia to be provided with fittings, for example taps, that they are familiar with because their use is recorded in their long-term memory.

People with dementia who come from other cultures are at particular risk of finding themselves in an unfamiliar environment. A detailed knowledge of their heritage, customs and beliefs is required to provide an environment that will help them make the most of their abilities (Day & Cohen 2000).

PROVIDE OPPORTUNITIES TO BE ALONE OR WITH OTHERS

People with dementia need to be able to choose to be on their own or spend time with others. This requires providing a variety of spaces, some for quiet conversation with one or two others and some for larger groups, as well as spaces where people can be by themselves. These internal and external spaces should have a variety of characters, such as a place for reading, looking out of the window or talking, to cue the person to what is available and stimulate different emotional responses.

The provision of rooms for different functions has been shown to be a hallmark of dementia-specific units in a survey involving 436 Minnesota nursing homes (Grant et al 1995). The strongest evidence for its importance comes from Zeisel et al's (2003) well-controlled study, which indicated that residents with the opportunity to enjoy privacy were less anxious and aggressive, and those who had access to a variety of common spaces with varying ambiance were less socially withdrawn and depressed. The time residents spent in active behaviour has also been shown to be associated with the provision of a variety of spaces (Barnes 2006).

PROVIDE LINKS TO THE COMMUNITY

Without constant reminders of who they were, a person with dementia will lose their sense of identity. Frequent interaction with friends and relatives can help to maintain that identity. This is made easier when the person is admitted from the local community because friends and relatives are able to drop in more easily.

The environment must include spaces for the resident and their visitors to use within the unit and in its immediate surrounds. These need to be attractive and comfortable to encourage visitors to come and spend time. Stigma remains a problem for people with dementia so the unit should be designed to blend with the existing buildings and not stand out as a 'special' unit. Where possible a 'bridge' should be built between the unit and the community by providing a space that is used by both the community and people with dementia.

Where the unit is a part of a larger site, there should be easy access around the site so people with dementia, their families and friends can interact with other people who live there.

In an early statement of the principles of good design for people with dementia (Fleming & Bowles 1987) it was stated that facilities should be placed close to the community of origin of the person because the identity of a person who has lost their recent memories can be more easily supported by familiar sights and visits from friends and relatives when they are living close to that community. This view has been supported (Chiarelli et al 2005), but despite the increasing attention to the role of the community in supporting people with dementia no empirical investigations of the advantages have been found (Keady et al 2012). The importance of a community to the wellbeing of people with dementia is an emerging field of research. The ongoing contribution that people with dementia make to the community is another important field of study.

RESPOND TO A VISION FOR A WAY OF LIFE

The environment should support people with dementia to lead a life that has meaning and value to them. The choice of this lifestyle, or philosophy of care, will vary between facilities. Some will choose to focus on engagement with the ordinary activities of daily living and have fully functioning kitchens. Others will focus on the ideas of full service and recreation, while still others will emphasise a healthy lifestyle or, perhaps, spiritual reflection. The way of life offered needs to be clearly stated and the building designed both to support it and to make it evident to the residents and staff. The building becomes the embodiment of the philosophy of care, constantly reminding staff of the values and practices that are required while providing them with the tools they need to do their job.

Over the past 25 years there has been extensive interest in providing 'homelike' environments for people with dementia (Verbeek et al 2009). It has almost seemed that the only legitimate approach to providing residential care to people with dementia was by providing them with access to small facilities that emphasise involvement in the ordinary activities of daily living. Recently, however, there has been a move away from this towards larger, more hotel-like environments (Kidd 2012). While this clearly brings challenges to the traditional view of person-centred care it is premature to dismiss it as a mistake. It may well be that the next generation of dementia-specific facility residents will not want to be involved in washing the dishes. They may want an environment that provides them with opportunities to engage in a variety of other activities, such as keeping fit, eating well and enjoying virtual experiences. There is no literature yet to help us design these places but there is substantial support available for those who wish to provide a domestic environment.

In a domestic (homelike) environment the goal of care is to maintain the person's activities of daily living abilities for as long as possible. This requires that they have access to all of the normal household facilities and encouragement to use their abilities (Scott et al 2011). It has been shown that the introduction of a small number of homelike features into an institutional environment resulted in a reduction in pacing, agitation and exit seeking (Cohen-Mansfield & Werner 1998), and improved social interaction and eating behaviour (Melin & Gotestam 1981.)

Access to a homelike environment has been associated with reduction in anxiety and an increase in interest in the surroundings as compared with levels found in residents of traditional nursing homes (Reimer et al 2004). Higher levels of agitation were also found but interpreted as an indication of the greater freedom available to the residents in a homelike environment. Lower levels of aggression have been found in residents of more residential-type units than those who live in more institutional settings (Zeisel et al 2003). Residents in group homes that provide engagement with the ordinary activities of daily living require less help with activities of daily living, have more social engagement, a greater sense of aesthetics and the opportunity to do more than residents in traditional nursing homes (te Boekhorst et al 2009). Support for environmental approaches to encouraging residents to take part in domestic activities have been well described (van Hoof et al 2010).

THE PHILOSOPHY OF CARE

The availability of an evidence base, a set of principles with which to organise it and the means of assessing the quality of physical environments provides a firm foundation for the design of buildings for people with dementia. However, they must be used in relation to a philosophy of care otherwise the building will only be a collection of rooms that people with dementia use. Consider three common types of facilities for people with dementia: one described as homelike; another designed to provide a hotel atmosphere; and the third designed to optimise the delivery of physical care. They can all be designed with reference to the evidence base, the difference between them lies in the differing models, or philosophies, of care. When the philosophy of care is clear—that is, the purpose of the building and the values that underpin that purpose and the evidence is used to help the designer achieve that purpose, the building is likely to be helpful to its users. When the philosophy is not clear and the building is designed without reference to a well-defined purpose or to enable the expression of a clear set of values, the result is likely to be a building that, at best, does not support the staff and residents or, more likely, a building that actually hinders the delivery of care and the enjoyment of life.

It is perfectly possible to build a good homelike environment or a good hotel-style facility or a good care facility for people with dementia by using the evidence that we have. The problem comes when the philosophy is unclear and an unthinking attempt is made to do them all in one building. An even more severe problem occurs when there is an attempt to impose a philosophy on a building that does not really support it. One example of this is to provide satellite kitchens and dining rooms and then operate a centralised hotel-style dining meal service. Another common example of this is trying to insist that a building that has been designed to minimise capital cost and provide basic physical care is a 'homelike' facility.

When the building has been designed to embody a well-formulated philosophy of care it will support the staff in the delivery of the desired care. If it has been designed in the absence of a well-formulated philosophy the chances are that it will frustrate the staff and restrict the residents.

Many organisations have their philosophy of care displayed on a wall in their facilities. Good design requires that the philosophy be practised in every part of the building.

If an organisation lacks a philosophy of care that provides guidance on the design of the buildings there are many ways to develop one. They could start with a global view by referring to the Universal Declaration of Human Rights. This contains many concepts that can be applied directly to the design of a building for people with dementia, for example, dignity, liberty, security of person, privacy, freedom of movement, access to own property, access to participation in the cultural life of the community and the provision of a standard of living adequate for health and wellbeing. A discussion of these values with key stakeholders in the organisation could lead to developing a very strong philosophy of care that would have immediate relevance to the design of the buildings.

Another approach could be to try to look at the world, and the building, through the eyes of the people who will spend their time in the building— people with dementia and staff. A very good start on providing some insight into this is provided by Davis et al (2009) who, through a series of interviews and focus groups, have described life in residential aged care through the lenses of seven experiences: the presentation of self; eating; personal enjoyment; bedroom; family and community connections; end-of-life; and the experience of staff working in the facility. A discussion of these findings could lead to developing a philosophy of care that would inform the design of the building.

The starting point for designing for people with dementia is to clarify what it is that you want to achieve.

THE OBSTACLES TO IMPLEMENTING OUR KNOWLEDGE

While there are examples of good design to be found in Australia and elsewhere (Judd et al 1998) the results of audits of aged care facilities in New South Wales show that many have been designed in a way that does not reflect the application of evidence-based principles (Fleming 2011, Smith et al 2012). This gap between the design of facilities and the evidence base highlights a problem in the translation of dementia design knowledge into practice.

The steps involved in the process of translating knowledge into practice in healthcare have been analysed in several ways. In a very influential paper Pathman et al (1996) provides a useful, four-stage framework for exploring the issues around knowledge translation on a large scale. They suggest that if knowledge is to be translated into practice the potential knowledge users must first become aware of the existence of the evidence, for example, by reading an article or a conference presentation. In the second stage Pathman et al suggest the user must evaluate the new knowledge and come to the conclusion that it is credible and they agree with it. In the third stage the knowledge must be adopted into practice. In the fourth stage, adherence, the new application becomes business as usual, often as the result of the development of regulations to ensure compliance with accepted good practice.

This model of knowledge translation has been used in an investigation of the reasons for the lack of application of the evidence base that we have (Fleming et al 2012). The study involved five facilities in Tasmania and five in New South Wales. In Tasmania a convenience sample of facilities that had been either built or renovated within the last five years was accessed. The New South Wales sample was selected to ensure the facilities had been built within the past two years. The study involved undertaking an audit of each facility using EAT (Fleming 2011, Fleming et al 2003). The data gathered was used to produce a report that highlighted the gaps between the design of the facility and the optimum design as defined by the principles underpinning the EAT. This report was provided to the aged care facility representatives who had been involved in the design process and to the architects. The aged care facility managers and the architects then participated in a semi-structured interview designed to guide the respondent through a discussion of their awareness, acceptance and adoption of the principles of design that underpinned the audit.

Five of the aged care facility managers clearly described an awareness of the principles contained in the report. One claimed to 'have read them in the past' and four responded that they were not aware of the principles of design. All of the managers who were aware of the principles stated that they agreed with them. One of the architects expressed only partial awareness of, and partial agreement with, the principles. The remainder described themselves as being aware of the principles and agreeing with them.

The mean EAT scores of the facilities where the manager was aware of the principles was 73.96, significantly higher (t test, sig. 0.01) than the mean EAT score of 61.82 for those facilities where the manager described themselves as unaware or only partially aware of the principles. This suggests that it is the manager's awareness of the design principles that makes the difference. It appears that the architect's knowledge is overridden by the managers—they write the brief that the architect follows. There is no problem in the agreement phase of Pathman et al's model (1996) because everyone who was aware of the principles agreed with them. The adoption of the principles into practice follows on directly from the agreement.

This finding is of particular importance to registered nurses because the majority of aged care facility managers in Australia are nurses. It highlights the importance of ensuring all nurses who work in aged care facilities have an awareness of the design principles; it is they who can drive the provision of environments that will make life fulfilling for those who live and work in them.

 The managers of aged care facilities, often nurses, are the drivers of the brief and philosophy of care that must inform design. Their knowledge of good design principles can make a significant difference to the quality of the design.

CONCLUSION

While there remains much to be done to tease out the particular contribution of the physical environment to the delivery of high-quality residential care to people with dementia we know enough to design facilities that help us to reduce confusion, depression and agitation while improving social interaction, wayfinding and engagement with life. This knowledge can be structured around 10 principles. The research is increasing in sophistication and is now addressing the complex issues surrounding the interaction between the environment and that most subtle of concepts—quality of life (Garre-Olmo et al 2012, Wetzels et al 2010).

The application of this knowledge is lagging behind. While it is recorded in academic journals it does not appear to be widely known to the people who make the decisions on the designs. These are often nurses.

The availability of easy-to-use tools to help identify the strengths and weaknesses of the environment provides opportunities for managers and staff to take a systematic approach to deciding what can be done to improve their facilities. The challenge that confronts us is to raise awareness of the knowledge that we have so that as and when the opportunity arises to change our environments, we can make sure it is done for the better.

Information about easily accessible resources are provided at the end of this chapter and the following vignettes illustrate how positive changes can be brought about. These vignettes highlight the way the principles of designing for people with dementia can be explored in a new project and when refurbishing a building. They highlight the importance of responding to a philosophy of care, and how there are opportunities to improve the environment even when there is only a small amount of money available to spend.

Vignette

Just maintenance or an opportunity to design for people with dementia?

A residential age care facility had been operating for about 20 years and the building was looking tired and unattractive. It was time to do some maintenance. Rather than just proceed with the obvious things such as painting and installing new carpet and vinyl, the provider began a conversation with an architect who specialised in designing for older people about how they could make the facility more friendly for people with dementia. The first step was a review of the building using an audit tool to see how well the design responded to key design principles. This gave both the architect and the provider a systematic way of reviewing the facility, and highlighted where there was the most potential for improvement. The amount of money they had to spend was limited, and so it was vital to ensure it was spent where it would have the most impact. Discussion also focused on what could be done immediately and what should be identified for the medium and long term, so that the current constraints were recognised but the big picture was not lost.

Everyone agreed it would be good to create rooms with different characters and atmospheres in the facility. This would assist people with wayfinding and give them a variety of experiences to enrich their lives. A range of colours, floor finishes, wall hangings, pictures and light fittings were proposed. Instead of replacing all of the floor vinyl as originally planned, it was decided to spend some of this money on introducing timber panelling in the lounge room and replacing a large window in the dining room with double doors to give people greater access to outside. The furniture in these rooms would also be rearranged to encourage interaction between people and create some private sitting areas. It was decided to contact one of the local service clubs to see if they could create a new patio area outside the dining room and link this to the current garden path. Then residents could walk around outside without coming across dead ends and both the dining room and outdoors would be used more. In so many ways what began as routine maintenance became a chance to improve the environment to meet the needs of people with dementia.

Vignette

Combining key design principles with philosophy of care

An aged care provider wanted to rebuild their facility for people with dementia. They went back to their architects (who had a good understanding of the principles of designing for people with dementia) and set about establishing a multidisciplinary team of managers, care workers, nurses, cleaners and maintenance staff that would brief the architect and work with them during the project. Despite having worked with the client before, the first questions the architect asked were: 'What is your vision for this new facility? How are the older people with dementia to live? What is your philosophy of care?' The architect then sat down and thought about how the key principles of designing for people with dementia could best be interpreted in light of the client's answers.

With much anticipation, the first sketches were presented. Having grappled with key questions during the briefing phase of the project, the client group sat down with the first sketches and 'walked though the building', imagining what each staff member would do, where they would go and how long it would take them to get there. They thought about how residents would move through the building and how they could use each space. Key design principles were discussed and different responses considered. They imagined a typical day for residents such as Joan, Abdullah and Isaac, and how they would live differently in the new facility. Where would they garden? Where would they pray? Where could they listen to music? How could they help to prepare some food? Where would they like to sit? Where would their grandchildren like to be? They prepared initial staffing models and costed them so they understood both how the building would be staffed and what it would cost to provide all the services that would be needed if their plans were to be realised.

This process was repeated by the architect and client a number of times during the project and the design was continually refined. The client's responses to the architect's questions about vision and philosophy of care influenced: the way the building was laid out; the size of the rooms; the resident group size, the types of indoor and outdoor spaces that were provided, the finishes in the facility; the relationship of the building to the site and to the community; and the way a safe and secure environment was created. The way the client and architect approached the design process meant that the building reflected the provider's vision and philosophy of care, and the key principles of designing for people with dementia were integral in the design. The new facility was a great success and the environment was able to fulfill its potential as a key element in the care of people with dementia.

Reflective questions

1. Given that much of the care for people with dementia occurs in buildings that were not specifically designed for them, how would you approach improving these environments?

2. The physical environment should be the embodiment of the philosophy of care. How would you encourage the development of a clear philosophy of care?

3. Which of the principles of design is the easiest to apply to improving the environment in most facilities?

4. How would you go about raising the awareness of the knowledge that we have so that the next generation of facilities are a pleasure to live and work in?

References

Australian Institute of Health and Welfare, 2011. Dementia among aged care residents: first information from the Aged Care Funding Instrument. Aged care statistics series. AIHW, Canberra.

Annerstedt, L., 1993. Development and consequences of group living in Sweden: a new mode of care for the demented elderly. Social Science & Medicine 37, 1529–1538.

Annerstedt, L., 1997. Group-living care: an alternative for the demented elderly. Dementia and Geriatric Cognitive Disorders 8, 136–142.

Atkinson, A., 1995. Managing people with dementia: CADE units … confused and disturbed elderly. Nursing Standard 9, 29–32.

Barnes, S., 2006. Space, choice and control, and quality of life in care settings for older people. Environment and Behavior 38, 589–604.

Bianchetti, A., Benvenuti, P., Ghisla, K.M., et al., 1997. An Italian model of dementia special care unit: results of a pilot study. Alzheimer Disease & Associated Disorders 11, 53–56.

Calkins, M.P., 1988. Design for dementia: planning environments for the elderly and the confused. National Health Publishing, Owings Mills.

Chiarelli, P., Bower, W., Wilson, A., et al., 2005. Estimating the prevalence of urinary and faecal incontinence in Australia: systematic review. Australasian Journal on Ageing 24, 19–27.

Cleary, T.A., Clamon, C., Price, M., et al., 1988. A reduced stimulation unit: effects on patients with Alzheimer's Disease and related disorders. The Gerontologist 28, 511–514.

Cochrane, T.G., 2010. Gardens that care: planning outdoor areas for people with dementia. Alzheimers Australia SA Inc, Glenside.

Cohen-Mansfield, J., Werner, P., 1995. Environmental influences on agitation: an integrative summary of an observational study. American Journal of Alzheimer's Disease and Other Dementias 10, 32–39.

Cohen-Mansfield, J., Werner, P., 1998. The effects of an enhanced environment on nursing home residents who pace. Gerontologist 38, 199–208.

Cohen, U., Weisman, G.D., 1991. Holding on to home: designing environments for people with dementia. Johns Hopkins University Press, Baltimore.

Cox, H., Burns, I., Savage, S., 2004. Multisensory environments for leisure: promoting well-being in nursing home residents with dementia. Journal of Gerontological Nursing 30, 37–45.

Cunningham, C., 2011. Design for people with dementia: audit tool. University of Stirling, Stirling.

Cunningham, C., 2009. Auditing design for dementia. Journal of Dementia Care 17, 31–32.

Davis, S., Byers, S., Nay, R., et al., 2009. Guiding design of dementia friendly environments in residential care settings: considering the living experiences. Dementia (14713012) 8, 185–203.

Day, K., Carreon, D., Stump, C., 2000. The therapeutic design of environments for people with dementia: a review of the empirical research. The Gerontologist 40, 397.

Day, K., Cohen, U., 2000. The role of culture in designing environments for people with dementia: a study of Russian Jewish immigrants. Environment and Behavior 32, 361–399.

Dementia Services Development Centre, 2008. Best practice in design for people with dementia. University of Stirling, Stirling.

Dementia Services Development Centre, 2012a. Dementia Design Audit Tool. University of Stirling, Stirling.

Dementia Services Development Centre, 2012b. Design features to assist patients with dementia in general hospitals and emergency departments. University of Stirling, Stirling.

Dickinson, J.I., Mclain-Kark, J., Marshall-Baker, A., 1995. The effects of visual barriers on exiting behavior in a dementia care unit. Gerontologist 35, 127–130.

Edwards, C.A., Mcdonnell, C., Merle, H., 2012. An evaluation of a therapeutic gardens influence on the quality of life of aged care residents with dementia. Dementia, doi: 10.1177/1471301 211435188.

Elmstahl, S., Annerstedt, L., Ahlund, O., 1997. How should a group living unit for demented elderly be designed to decrease psychiatric symptoms? Alzheimer Disease & Associated Disorders 11, 47–52.

Fleming, R., 2010. The use of environmental assessment tools for the evaluation of Australian residential facilities for people with dementia. Primary Dementia Collaborative Research Centre, UNSW, Sydney.

Fleming, R., 2011. An environmental audit tool suitable for use in homelike facilities for people with dementia. Australasian Journal on Ageing 30, 108–112.

Fleming, R., Bowles, J., 1987. Units for the confused and disturbed elderly: development, design, programmimg and evaluation. Australian Journal on Ageing 6, 25–28.

Fleming, R., Fay, R., Robinson, A., 2012. Evidence-based facilities design in health care: a study of aged care facilities in Australia. Health Services Management Research 25, 121–128.

Fleming, R., Forbes, I., Bennett, K., 2003. Adapting the ward for people with dementia. NSW Department of Health, Sydney.

Fleming, R., Purandare, N., 2010. Long-term care for people with dementia: environmental design guidelines. International Psychogeriatrics 22, 1084–1096.

Garre-Olmo, J., López-Pousa, S., Turon-Estrada, A., et al., 2012. Environmental determinants of quality of life in nursing home residents with severe dementia. Journal of the American Geriatrics Society 60, 1230–1236.

Grant, L.A., Kane, R.A., Stark, A.J., 1995. Beyond labels: nursing home care for Alzheimer's disease in and out of special care units. Journal of the American Geriatrics Society 43, 569–576.

Hagglund, D., Hagglund, D., 2010. A systematic literature review of incontinence care for persons with dementia: the research evidence. Journal of Clinical Nursing 19, 303–312.

Judd, S., Marshall, M., Phippen, P., 1998. Design for dementia: journal of dementia care. Hawker Publications, London.

Keady, J., Campbell, S., Barnes, H., et al., 2012. Neighbourhoods and dementia in the health and social care context: a realist review of the literature and implications for UK policy development. Reviews in Clinical Gerontology 22, 150–163.

Kidd, B., 2012. The wheel turns. Australian Journal of Dementia Care 4.

Kidd, B.J., 1987. Aldersgate Village: an experiment in the design of a client centred nursing home. Architecture in Australia 76.

King's Fund, 2012. Developing supportive design for people with dementia: overarching design principles. The King's Fund, London.

Knapp, M., Prince, M., 2007. Dementia UK. Alzheimer's Society, London.

Lancioni, G.E., Singh, N.N., O'Reilly, M.F., et al., 2010. Technology-aided verbal instructions to help persons with mild or moderate Alzheimer's disease perform daily activities. Research in Developmental Disabilities 31, 1240–1250.

Lawton, M., Fulcomer, M., Kleban, M.H., 1984. Architecture for the mentally impaired elderly. Environment and Behavior 16, 730–757.

Lawton, M., Weisman, G., Sloane, P., et al., 2000. Professional environmental assessment procedure for special care units for elders with dementing illness and its relationship to the Therapeutic Environment Screening Schedule. Alzheimer Disease and Associated Disorders 14, 28–38.

Lekeu F., Wojtasik V., Van der Linden M., et al., 2002. Training early Alzheimer patients to use a mobile phone. Acta Neurologica Belgica 102, 114–121.

Leon, J., Ory, M.G., 1999. Effectiveness of Special Care Unit (SCU) placements in reducing physically aggressive behaviors in recently admitted dementia nursing home residents. American Journal of Alzheimer's Disease and Other Dementias 14, 270–277.

Low, L.F., Draper, B., Brodaty, H., 2004. The relationship between self-destructive behaviour and nursing home environment. Aging & Mental Health 8, 29–33.

Marquardt, G., 2011. Wayfinding for people with dementia: a review of the role of architectural design. HERD: Health Environments Research & Design Journal 4, 75–90.

Marshall, M., 2001. Environment: how it helps to see dementia as a disability. In: Benson, S. (Ed.), Care homes and dementia. The Journal of Dementia Care 6 (1), 15–17.

Melin, L., Gotestam, K.G., 1981. The effects of rearranging ward routines on communication and eating behaviours of psychogeriatric patients. Journal of Applied Behaviour Analysis 14, 47–51.

Moos, R.H., Lemke, S., 1984. Multiphasic Environmental Assessment Procedure (MEAP) manual. Social Ecology Laboratory, Veterans Administration, and Stanford University Medical Center Palo Alto, CA.

Namazi, K.H., Johnson, B.D., 1992. Dressing independently: a closet modification model for Alzheimer's disease patients. American Journal of Alzheimer's Care and Related Disorders and Research 7, 22–28.

Namazi, K.H., Johnson, B.D., 1991a. Environmental effects on incontinence problems in Alzheimer's disease patients. American Journal of Alzheimer's Disease and Other Dementias 6, 16–21.

Namazi, K.H., Johnson, B.D., 1991b. Physical environmental cues to reduce the problems of incontinence in Alzheimer's disease units. American Journal of Alzheimer's Disease and Other Dementias 6, 22–28.

Namazi, K.H., Rosner, T.T., Rechlin, L., 1991. Long-term memory cuing to reduce visuo-spatial disorientation in Alzheimer's disease patients in a special care unit. American Journal of Alzheimer's Disease and Other Dementias 6, 10–15.

Namazi, K.H., Rosner, T.T., Calkins, M.P., 1989. Visual barriers to prevent ambulatory Alzheimer's patients from exiting through an emergency door. The Gerontologist 29, 699–702.

Nay, R., 2003. The dignity of risk. Australian Nursing Journal 9, 33.

Nolan, B.A.D., Mathews, R.M., Harrison, M., 2001. Using external memory aids to increase room finding by older adults with dementia. American Journal of Alzheimer's Disease and Other Dementias 16, 251–254.

Passini, R., Pigot, H., Rainville, C., et al., 2000. Wayfinding in a nursing home for advanced dementia of the Alzheimer's type. Environment and Behavior 32, 684–710.

Passini, R., Rainville, C., Marchand, N., et al., 1998. Wayfinding with dementia: some research findings and a new look at design. Journal of Architectual and Planning Research 15, 133–151.

Pathman, D.E., Konrad, T.R., Freed, G.L., et al., 1996. The awareness-to-adherence model of the steps to clinical guideline compliance. The case of pediatric vaccine recommendations. Medical Care 34, 873–889.

Reimer, M.A., Slaughter, S., Donaldson, C., et al., 2004. Special care facility compared with traditional environments for dementia care: a longitudinal study of quality of life. Journal of the American Geriatrics Society 52, 1085.

Rosewarne, R., Opie, J., Bruce, A., et al., 1997. Care needs of people with dementia and challenging behaviour living in residential facilities. Australian Government Publishing Service, Canberra.

Scott, A., Ryan, A., James, I., et al., 2011. Perceptions and implications of violence from care home residents with dementia: a review and commentary. International Journal of Older People Nursing 6, 110–122.

Sloan, P.D., Mitchell, C.M., Preisser, J.S., et al., 1998. Environmental correlates of resident agitation in Alzheimer's disease special care units. Journal of American Geriatrics Society 46, 862–869.

Sloane, P.D., Mitchell, C.M., Weisman, G., et al., 2002. The Therapeutic Environment Screening Survey for Nursing Homes (TESS-NH): an observational instrument for assessing the physical environment of institutional settings for persons with dementia. Journals of Gerontology Series B-Psychological Sciences & Social Sciences 57, S69–S78.

Smith, R., Fleming, R., Chenoweth, L., et al., 2012. Validation of the Environmental Audit Tool in both purpose-built and non-purpose-built dementia care settings. Australasian Journal on Ageing 31, 159–163.

te Boekhorst, S., Depla, M., De Lange, J., et al., 2009. The effects of group living homes on older people with dementia: a comparison with traditional nursing home care. International Journal of Geriatric Psychiatry epub.

Torrington, J., 2006. What has architecture got to do with dementia care? Explorations of the relationship between quality of life and building design in two EQUAL projects. Quality in Ageing 7, 34.

Van Hoof, J., Kort, H.S.M., Van Waarde, H., et al., 2010. Environmental interventions and the design of homes for older adults with dementia: an overview. American Journal of Alzheimers Disease and Other Dementias 25, 202–232.

Verbeek, H., Van Rossum, E., Zwakhalen, S.M.G., et al., 2009. Small, homelike care environments for older people with dementia: a literature review. International Psychogeriatrics 21, 252–264.

Verbeek, H., Zwakhalen, S.M.G., Van Rossum, E., et al., 2012. Small-scale, homelike facilities in dementia care: a process evaluation into the experiences of family caregivers and nursing staff. International Journal of Nursing Studies 49, 21–29.

Wetzels, R.B., Zuidema, S.U., De Jonghe, J.F.M., et al., 2010. Determinants of quality of life in nursing home residents with dementia. Dementia and Geriatric Cognitive Disorders 29, 189–197.

Wood, W., Harris, S., Snider, M., et al., 2005. Activity situations on an Alzheimer's disease special care unit and resident environmental interaction, time use, and affect. American Journal of Alzheimer's Disease and Other Dementias 20, 105–118.

Woods, B., 1999. The person in dementia care. Generations 23, 35–39.

Zeisel, J., Silverstein, N.M., Hyde, J., et al., 2003. Environmental correlates to behavioral health outcomes in Alzheimer's special care units. The Gerontologist 43, 697.

Zimmerman, S., Sloane, P.D., Eckert, J.K., et al., 2005. How good is assisted living? Findings and implications from an outcomes study. The Journals of Gerontology 60B, S195–S204.

Zuidema, S.U., De Jonghe, J.F.M., Verhey, F.R.J., et al., 2009. Environmental correlates of neuropsychiatric symptoms in nursing home patients with dementia. International Journal of Geriatric Psychiatry 9999, n/a.

Other resources

www.enablingenvironments.com.au

The Alzheimers Australia and University of Wollongong 'Dementia Enabling Environments Project'.

www.health.vic.gov.au/dementia

Davis S., Byers S., Nay R., et al., 2008. Creating dementia-friendly physical and social environments for residential and respite care. Department of Human Services, Melbourne.

Dementia Services Development Centre. Best Practice in Design for People with Dementia—Design Pack

This includes the titles: Designing Gardens for People with Dementia; Designing Interiors for People with Dementia; Designing Lighting for People with Dementia; and Dementia Design Checklist. Available through the DSDC, University of Stirling, http://dementia.stir.ac.uk/design_welcome and www.dementiacentre.com.au.

http://www.health.nsw.gov.au/pubs/2003/adapting_the_ward.html

Fleming R., Forbes I., Bennett K., 2003. Adapting the ward for people with dementia. NSW Department of Health, Sydney.

CHAPTER 22

ASSISTIVE TECHNOLOGY: OPPORTUNITIES AND IMPLICATIONS

Barbara Horner, Jeffrey Soar and Elizabeth Beattie

Editors' comments

Assistive technology is with us and will only get bigger. Health professionals and consumers can use it to their advantage; but to do this it is important to be an integral part of the discussion and not just a recipient. There are ethical issues to be considered and these cannot be left to government and the health industry to work through. Horner, Soar and Beattie outline the advantages, the expected developments and the potential danger signs.

INTRODUCTION

Technology has transformed lives, changed entire industries, eliminated some companies and jobs but created new ones. It has given us products and services, such as in-car navigation devices, telephony over the internet, online social networking and blogging, that have become ubiquitous in little more than the past decade. Information and communications technology (ICT) has affected almost every part of our lives, providing greater convenience, reduced cost, greater safety through automated controls of machinery and improvements in information quality and in our capacity to share information.

There is a plethora of innovative technology available to assist frail older people and people with disabilities. This includes delivery of care and information services into people's homes, tracking devices for people who wander and get lost, robots and smart homes equipped with smart sensor networks and monitors to help keep people safe, socially connected and with immediate access to care services. There is now also the opportunity to take advantage of new transformative technologies such as cloud computing, big data, social networking, green computing and others that are discussed in this chapter. We are witnessing a technological revolution. Innovative technologies are available for use in the home. Terms like 'intelligent home', 'smart home', 'digital home' and 'connected home' are being used to describe the convergence of a range of technologies and their increased use (Essen & Conrick 2007).

This chapter seeks to draw together three major issues—advances in technology in relation to the ageing of the population; advances in the appropriate use of technology in the care of older people; and the need for evaluation of the impact of this technology for user and client within clinical practice.

WHAT IS ASSISTIVE TECHNOLOGY?

Assistive technology (AT) is defined as any product or service designed to enable independence for disabled and older people (FAST 2012). AT devices aim to increase the ability of a person to remain independent, reduce risk and maintain engagement in meaningful activities. They range from simple, low-tech, low-cost products to products designed with a high technological capacity. AT devices may help people deal with the lifestyle changes associated with frailty, illness or disability and therefore increase the ability of the person to maintain independence and be more involved in the activities in their homes, schools and communities (Berry & Ignash 2003).

The aims of AT are to increase the ability of a person to remain independent, reduce risk and maintain engagement in meaningful activities. The term 'assistive technologies' covers a broad range of information and communication technologies. The Assistive Technology Act of 1998 in the United States defines AT devices as any item, piece of equipment or product system, whether acquired commercially, modified or customised, that is used to increase, maintain or improve functional capabilities of individuals with disabilities (United States Congress 1998). ATs include those many devices and implements that have long been used such as wheelchairs, walking frames, hoists, devices for use in the kitchen for helping to prepare food or open jars and cans, and the many innovative products that can be viewed in the independent living centres around Australia and other countries.

The best known intelligence-based ATs are telecare and telehealth. The Telecare Personal Emergency Alarm is the most widely used device and telehealth is beginning to gain greater acceptance, although its use remains low compared with the number of people who might benefit from it. Since the 2012 AT definition above there have been new developments that will be discussed here for their potential to assist the frail aged and people with disabilities. These include applications for smartphones and other handheld devices such as iPads and the equivalent, cloud computing (which has potential to relieve organisations and individuals of some of the burden of acquiring and managing technologies), big data (which offers the potential to detect trends in vast volumes of data), knowledge management, business intelligence, data mining and nano-technologies. Linking the power of these newer innovations might enhance the level of functionality and hence of adoption of telecare and telehealth. In addition most organisations aim to be environmentally sensitive and consequently green computing is discussed in this chapter.

Issues of ageing and frailty that offer opportunities for research include: falls prevention; accidents; medication management and compliance; pain management; incontinence; and cognitive decline. The client environment can be improved in lighting, access, universal design and traffic flow. AT can also assist with financial management, security, social isolation, transport, carer burden and wandering. AT can make work environments more age-friendly and flexible and improve access.

WORK AND FINANCIAL INDEPENDENCE

ATs that can help people remain in the paid workforce despite having a disability are increasingly available. These include voice-to-text computing, specialised computer mice and other pointing technologies. Most independent living centres will have on display many of these technologies as well as disability-friendly workstations, chairs and other accessible office technologies. There is some way to go across industry towards making workplaces age-friendly. This includes physical access and toilets as well as human resources (HR) policies such as allowing greater flexibility that older people might prefer. The technology for teleworking has been with us for more than two decades and is increasingly gaining acceptance.

Apart from a small number of innovators, the aged and community care service sector has been generally slow to embrace the benefits of new technology and information systems, and much of the delivery of services remains labour-intensive. Care in community settings, for example, is often provided by home-visiting care professionals even when the purpose is to check up on an older person or to take vital signs, both of which could be undertaken through technology. There is as yet little adoption by consumers of innovative technology to help them manage their own health, which is a paradox in that accessing health-related information is one of the most popular uses of the internet (Tang & Ng 2006). When telehealth has been provided there is a reported high level of user acceptance and satisfaction, although for ATs there is generally a high level of abandonment (Verza et al 2006).

 Assistive technology aims to increase the ability of a person to remain independent, reduce risk and maintain engagement in activities.

UNDERSTANDING THE ROLE OF ASSISTIVE TECHNOLOGY

Older people often have decreased functional capacity resulting from increased frailty and/or decreasing cognitive ability. One way to offer assistance to an older person through technology is in the form of a range of equipment or devices to *enhance their living environment*, thus extending their ability to operate effectively in the face of decreasing functional capacity and thereby providing an opportunity to maintain their human dignity as they age.

The application of AT should therefore aim to:

- enable those who seek to age in their own home—by maintaining independence, extending capability and productivity, enabling choices
- enable those who live in healthcare facilities and those who care for them— through improvements in communication, access to data and professionals, monitoring and treatment of conditions
- support families to provide the support and care that is needed by an older person and to facilitate their role as part of the care team
- foster innovation that is a response to clinical, social or personal need (as opposed to technology driven).

Intrusive technologies or functions such as the location of technology and monitoring can be of concern, as can be the potential for social isolation, if technologies substitute for human caring. Privacy and confidentiality are critical factors in acceptance of AT. Trust established between a practitioner and an older person will assist individuals to see the benefit of data collection and, with appropriate guidelines, the value of sharing data and experiences with others. Anxiety regarding the perception of 'being watched' by the use of electronic devices is understandable. Surveillance is an uncomfortable concept for most people, particularly someone who is feeling vulnerable or at risk. Careful explanation, clear policies and procedures with rigorous monitoring of adherence to them and regular feedback can all facilitate understanding and acceptance. Engaging the consumer in the selection, establishment and implementation of any AT will encourage acceptance and minimise anxiety.

In future we can expect that technology will transform ageing and aged care, just as it has done for other industries and other aspects of our lives. It will allow greater choice, including remaining safer and more healthy in our own homes, delaying or avoiding a move to institutional care, and choosing to remain socially connected and active.

Philipson and Roberts (2007) identified four key areas where digital technologies can be used to improve the lives of the aged, disabled and chronically ill. These include: self-management of healthcare in home settings with potential savings and other benefits; home automation, which will enhance security, safety and independence at home, and will help maintain quality of life and decrease the demand for carer support hours; communication technologies, which will provide important benefits for people whose mobility is limited, or who live alone; and finally, the various home automation and digital technologies, which can improve quality of life by enhancing independence. Technology has the potential to extend physical independence so that people can stay for longer in their homes. It gives them a more dignified life, and it saves public and private money.

There has also been increasing use of intelligent controls engineered into modern buildings. This includes smoke detectors linked to the building fire sprinkler systems. The elevators are often remotely monitored. Closed circuit television (CCTV) for security is ubiquitous in commercial and public places. The Department of Health in Queensland has begun installing intelligent controls with remote monitoring for some of its hospitals. These control, for example, hot water systems that can monitor use and then reduce energy consumption according to demand. Knowing the periods of peak demand allows scheduling so boilers can prepare in advance. These kinds of controls applied to heating, lighting, air-conditioning and other services can inform patterns of use and reduce energy consumption at quiet times and build up in preparation to periods of peak demand.

The use of technology within the home, however, is not so far advanced. Currently all doors, windows, curtains and light switches need to be operated individually. If we go out and forget to lock the doors there is no embedded intelligence that would recognise the house is vacant and turn off lights and lock doors in the way some modern cars are able. Heating, lighting and air-conditioning systems are dumb, in that they cannot track the movements and numbers of people between rooms and ramp services up or down according to need.

With the widespread concern about the environment there has been the advent of green computing, which encourages the development, use and disposal of technology in a way that is less harmful to the natural environment. Consumers are becoming more sensitised and better educated about these issues (Vine 2008) and older people in particular are concerned not to waste resources, which is, no doubt due to their experiences of difficult economic times. For an organisation, energy efficiency and use of renewable sources can potentially translate into financial savings.

SELECTION OF ASSISTIVE TECHNOLOGIES

While there are many examples of AT in use there is also a high rate of abandonment of existing AT (Reimer-Reiss & Wacker 2000). There is little research into the reasons for abandonment; however, Reimer-Reiss and Wacker (2000) recommend that people be involved in any decisions on AT that they are expected to use. It will be important to learn from experiences in the use of non-intelligent technologies in planning for the evaluation and adoption of intelligent AT. Issues to consider include: the availability of support for the technology; any stigma or embarrassment about its use; availability of people to respond to alerts such as a professional call centre or family carer; whether the potential user has been directly involved in the acquisition; whether it fits conveniently into the living arrangements of the user; and whether our care organisations are ready for the work practice and care model changes that may be necessary for adopting the technology and realising the benefits. Older people's accommodation can be quite small and limit the introduction of, for example, lift chairs.

It will be important to learn from experiences in use of non-intelligent technologies in planning for the evaluation and adoption of intelligent assistive technology.

STEPS FOR SELECTING ASSISTIVE TECHNOLOGIES

When considering the selection and implementation of AT one may be confronted by a plethora of vendor claims and glossy brochures for their products. To facilitate more judicious choices, particularly for care provider organisations, the following steps are suggested.

- Review the research evidence. What have been the experiences of others with this technology?
- Are there arrangements for technical support?
- Who will monitor the signals from the technology? Is there a call centre? If not, what is the capacity of other people to provide 24/7 monitoring?
- Conduct your own pilot research project before wide-scale deployment.
- Develop a business case identifying:
  - details of problems and what the technology is expected to provide
  - identify infrastructure costs—cabling, maintenance support.
- Undertake a cost-benefit analysis.
- Selection processes:
  - Write a detailed specification outlining the problem and the functionality sought.
  - Develop an evaluation matrix to be able to compare alternative products.
  - Invite proposals.
  - Visit places that already have the technology installed to learn from their experiences.
  - Conduct a small-scale pilot of the technology before wide-scale implementation.
- Plan for wide-scale implementation.
  - Do you have expert project management? Has your project manager delivered similar projects previously?
  - Ensure project governance. Develop a steering committee involving key executives.

The following sections will discuss the benefits of AT to both the individual and service provider before addressing possible approaches to evaluation.

UNDERSTANDING AND ACCEPTANCE

FOR THE INDIVIDUAL

AT products can support self-care, enable an individual to accomplish daily living tasks, assist them in communication, work or recreation activities and help them to achieve a level of independence that is necessary for them to remain outside of an institutional care environment.

There is growing evidence to show that supporting self-care leads to a number of positive outcomes:

- improved health and quality of life as the individual feels more 'in control' of their situation

- increased patient satisfaction when the individual feels they can communicate with a health professional and contribute useful information about their health status
- positive impact on the use of services and more appropriate use of services.

AT can be useful for someone who is finding basic household chores difficult or impossible, or who is anxious about their ability to remember events and activities. It is also useful for family members who need to maintain regular contact to 'monitor' heath status, security and safety of the individual who is living alone.

 Assistive technology devices can assist a person who is living at home to better manage their situation and monitor their health status.

Communication is particularly important for someone who has limited mobility, cognitive impairment or who lives a long way from family or friends. AT can provide many different ways for an individual to communicate, to maintain social networks, and to transmit and receive information. Family members and health professionals can monitor health and wellbeing daily and initiate intervention when necessary. AT can manage the risks associated with living alone, as well as monitor lifestyle changes or changes in regular behaviour. Individuals report that they feel better because they can manage their symptoms and respond to changes with, for example, pain management, anxiety and depression.

The following vignettes provide examples of how AT devices can assist a person who is living at home to manage their situation and monitor their health status.

Vignette

Mr A has mild dementia and was starting to forget to turn off the gas when he was cooking. He had a gas detector installed with an automatic shut off valve when gas was detected in the air. This made him feel less anxious about the gas and his memory lapses. His family also felt better because they knew the gas would be detected and turned off if a situation occurred. Eventually the family installed other devices to 'detect' at-risk situations with the water, open doors and lighting.

Vignette

Mrs B had a history of falling. Following an episode in hospital that resulted from a fall, she was provided with a basic bed pressure sensor pad that could detect when she left the bed during the night and automatically turn on the lighting in the bathroom. It then triggered an alarm if she did not return to bed within an agreed time. The program attached to the sensor recorded how many times Mrs B left her bed during the night and this could be checked by the family or visiting carer. At one stage, it was noticed that her visits to the bathroom in the night had increased significantly. Following investigation, it was noted that Mrs B had a urinary tract infection and treatment was commenced.

Carers are usually partners or other family members. Their responsibilities for the dependent person can severely restrict their own activities. They may be unable to leave the dependent person alone if they are prone to wandering, falling or putting themselves at risk in other ways. As a consequence, they can become isolated. Carers often neglect their own nutritional needs and other aspects of their health because they may be too tired to prepare their own meals. They may also be at risk of injury through lifting the dependent person and assisting them in slippery areas like bathrooms.

Caring for someone with cognitive impairment can be particularly stressful. The need to give someone repeated reminders about activities of daily living can be frustrating. The technology that can assist with providing reminders will never become stressed or frustrated. Carers can also use telehealth technology to assist in maintaining their own health as well as that of the person they are supporting.

 The technology that can assist with providing reminders will never become stressed or frustrated.

EXAMPLES OF THE APPLICATION OF ASSISTIVE TECHNOLOGY
TRACKING MOVEMENT

Becoming lost while walking can expose the person to the risk of physical harm, emotional distress and mortality. Understanding why people with dementia walk to excess is only partially understood and as a result developing effective strategies and interventions has been a challenge (Algase et al 2001, 2010, Song & Algase 2008). Some strategies that are implemented with varying degrees of acceptability and success include locking exit doors, installing alarms, surveillance, medication and physical restraint (Dickinson et al 1995, Price et al 2009). However, since it is not possible to predict the initial episode of getting lost in people living with dementia, and individuals lose wayfinding capacity relatively early in the disease course, there is a need for innovations that permit people with dementia to satisfy their need to walk while remaining safe and in contact with carers (McShane et al 1998, Algase et al 2004).

Currently, there is little evidence to support the general use of global positioning system (GPS) tracking for older people in either institutional or domestic settings. Two recent systematic reviews of interventions for wandering behaviour, Robinson et al (2007) and Hermans et al (2007), did not identify any randomised controlled trial of electronic tracking systems for wandering behaviour. The study by Bantry White et al (2010) is the best at this time.

However, a clear example of the effective use of technology can be seen in the application of tracking devices specifically for people with dementia. People with dementia commonly experience walking in excess of that seen in their peers without dementia and while this has benefits there can be a risk of becoming lost, which can result in harm to the person and distress for their families (Aud 2004, Beattie et al 2005, Chiu et al 2004).

There are several technologies available for tracking people including a wearable device with GPS and telecommunications capacity and a web-based tool using Google Maps for identifying location. There are several applications available for mobile phones but this would require the user to remember to take their phone with them when walking. There are also shoes that have a specialised device located at the back of the shoe and in the heel. This would require the user to have only one pair of shoes, remember to wear the GPS shoes for walking and not remove the shoes while away from the home.

One device that is particularly relevant to walking is the satellite-based GPS, which is able to identify a person's location and the time at which they are, or have been, at this location. Not only does this technology have the potential to reduce risk in relation to walking, but it may also increase the ability of a person with dementia to remain independent and engage in meaningful activities. In so doing, it may also help to reduce carer stress related to the risk of the person with dementia becoming lost.

The Alzheimer's Australia Western Australia Safe2Walk Service

Alzheimer's Australia Western Australia (AAWA) provides a tracking service using a device that incorporates GPS technology and a specially designed website for family carers to provide an accurate and reliable location within 10 metres. The device is about the size of a small mobile phone and has one large button which, when pressed, calls and connects with one of three pre-programmed numbers. The button also acts as an SOS—when pressed the location data is sent to the carer's mobile via text message. The GPS allows carers to log on to a secure website to locate the person they care for should they be out later than normal (Grenade 2009).

Engagement of the consumer in the selection, establishment and implementation of any assistive technology will encourage acceptance and minimise anxiety.

TELECARE

Telecare technologies aim to keep people safe. Typically they consist of a hub connected via the home telephone or other telecommunication modality to a call centre. The hub usually has a powerful microphone and speaker, allowing the call centre operator to communicate with the user in their own home. The hub can connect wirelessly to a wearable alarm, flood detector, wearable fall detector, a radio pull-cord in the shower or bathroom, and detectors for gas, flood and falls. A detector is available for the home front door, which, when opened, can trigger an alert and/or an interaction with a call centre operator who can communicate with the resident. This can be useful for people at risk of wandering and the operator can encourage the resident to stay in the home and can call for assistance.

SMART TOILET

Incontinence is a major issue in aged care and a significant factor in decisions regarding admission to aged care homes (Department of Health and Ageing 2003).

There have been several attempts at a smart toilet and a Google search using this term finds more than 500,000 hits reporting primarily on innovations in Japan and Korea. At the Wonju campus of Yonsei University in Korea a toilet has been developed that will undertake pathology tests on wastes. The toilet is also the site for a telehealth consultation where vital signs can be taken. When a person steps up to the toilet their weight is recorded. The toilet is equipped with devices for blood pressure, oximetry and other measures. In countries like Japan and Korea, where almost every home has an electronic bidet-toilet, it is expected that the move to a diagnostic toilet would be a logical step.

 At the Wonju campus of Yonsei University in Korea a toilet has been developed that will undertake pathology tests on wastes and provide information for telehealth consultations.

ROBOTS

Today, robots perform much of the work in manufacturing, including automobile assembly. Work has been underway for many years to build a humanoid robot personal assistant or carer. Honda's Asimo robot may be the most advanced to date and suggests that a robot assistant in homes may not be far off (http://asimo.honda.com/).

There have been other developments of robots as media for telehealth or teleconsultations with clinicians. In 2004 a prototype known as Roy the Robot was built at the Centre for Online Health at the University of Queensland to support Gladstone Hospital, which is about 500 km north of Brisbane. At the time, there was no full-time paediatrician on staff, despite the hospital having a paediatric ward. The robot provided a link with a specialist in Brisbane who could make a virtual ward round.

SMART HOMES

There are smart homes in many countries as research and development laboratories. There is a paradox in that there is a very wide range of technologies available but the adoption is negligible. Chen et al (2007) present an international selection of leading smart home projects, as well as the associated technologies of wearable/implantable monitoring systems and assistive robotics. The extent of work and sophistication of technologies reported on in their paper is impressive; however, it still remains the case that few people are as yet living in a smart home.

ASSISTIVE TECHNOLOGY FOR SERVICE PROVIDERS OR PRACTITIONERS

Effective management of chronic illness and disability among older people requires a close partnership between the individual and all healthcare providers who are involved in their care. The individual who is responsible for their own day-to-day care is best placed to monitor their symptoms and to respond to changes in their condition. They need to be active participants in the treatment and management of their chronic illness.

Compliance with self-management regimens is often not good, which is not surprising if instructions are complex and information confusing. The problem of compliance and the necessity for effective communication between older people and health professionals has led to the need for appropriate, cost-effective information and communication AT.

The management of chronic illness, such as that often experienced by an older person, calls for changes in healthcare delivery and education for health practitioners as part of the 'package' of healthcare. What is needed is AT that will provide rapid access to general health information, reduce duplication of information and services, facilitate portability of records and enhance the quality of the information exchange (Celler et al 2003). Telecommunications and computer-based systems can deliver services, record and transmit data and information, and facilitate communication between an individual and health service or health professional.

It is essential to have clear goals and a clear purpose when health professionals are considering using AT devices that encompass high-level organisational goals as well as clinical need goals (The Royal Society 2006). Examples of high-level goals are:

- provision of a seamless service— to break down barriers between institutions, integrate service delivery and link community and hospital care provision
- ensure interoperability of services, devices, data and external information sources
- provide better communication between health professionals and patients.

Examples of clinical need goals are to:

- assist individuals to better manage their health and their care—provide better information, support self-care, provide more options about treatment
- ensure data available to professionals is accurate, complete, relevant, up to date and readily accessible
- provide a better evidence base for practitioners to make decisions.

Telecommunications and computer-based systems can deliver services, record and transmit data and information, and facilitate communication between an individual and health service or health professional.

Box 22.1 provides an example of such a system that exists in a larger community-based aged care community in Western Australia.

TELEHEALTH

Telehealth refers to the delivery of health services through ICT where the participants are usually physically separated by distance. A telehealth consultation can be automated, with the device prompting a patient with questions, or between a health professional and a patient. In the case of the latter this may be achieved in real-time or using store-and-forward techniques that allow information to be shared asynchronously. Telehealth devices usually involve a hub that most often has a screen, a link to broadband telecommunications and links to peripheral devices such as a blood pressure monitor, oximeter, glucometer, spirometer, thermometer and scales.

Box 22.1

Intelligent building solution

An 'intelligent building' incorporates a range of devices that can record normal behaviour, establish safe limits, monitor and record actual behaviour and provide an alert if that behaviour is outside safe limits, such as length of time in a shower. Such a system can be part of a broader communication system operated through a telephone and monitored in a central server.

For the SwanCare Group, the Intelligent Building Solution supports its commitment to 'create a community environment for seniors which fosters confidence, self-worth and well-being'. Interoperability is the key feature as this system, being able to connect with virtually any application or system because the messaging gateway allows connection to a variety of protocols and interfaces (Schaper & Lapins 2007). This is a highly sophisticated and scalable messaging system that has multiple possible applications. The primary initial use for the system was risk assessment, with the monitoring of smoke, gas, water, electricity use and the detection of 'potential risk' levels of use. When such a level is reached, a message is transmitted via phone. If not responded to, the system alerts a third party. There is also high-speed internet access, voice over internet protocol (VoIP) telephone, security and video services, assistance call and nurse call options. There is also potential for links to external services, health professionals and call centres.

There is as yet a low level of adoption of telehealth services around the world despite its many potential benefits such as giving access to care for people in remote locations, people who might find it difficult to travel to consult a clinician or people who need close and regular monitoring. When telehealth systems have been installed they are often underutilised.

> ### Devices are available that enable vital signs to be captured and stored or else communicated interactively with a carer.

MOBILE DEVICE APPLICATIONS

There is a bewildering array of free or low-cost applications available on mobile devices such as smartphones or tablets.

KNOWLEDGE MANAGEMENT

Knowledge management is software that allows an organisation to manage its knowledge as an asset. This includes knowledge of processes and procedures. Business intelligence helps organisations to continually improve their processes and reduce the risk of loss of knowledge if, for example, there is a turnover of staff. Through business intelligence best practice models can be developed and embedded in organisational processes and procedures that can be continually refined through analysis of data.

CLOUD COMPUTING

Cloud computing refers to the use of ICT resources through the internet and, more particularly, access to software and data storage. The advantages are that an organisation can reduce its need for on-site infrastructure such as servers, software, data storage and even ICT support staff. All that is needed is a link to the internet and an arrangement with a cloud computing provider. Software and data storage costs can be charged on a by-use arrangement such as transaction volume, daily fee or by volume of data downloaded or stored.

This is expected to have great appeal to the aged care sector, which often struggles to find the significant capital costs to acquire and install ICT infrastructure. Attention needs to be paid to the details of contracts, privacy, security, back-up and integrity of data. Cloud services can be located in another country. Aged care organisations need to ensure appropriate arrangements are in place to secure and protect personal healthcare information. What are the back-up and restoration arrangements in the event that the cloud provider goes out of business? Can the software and data be restored? What happens to the data storage devices that contain personal details of your clients and your own confidential financial arrangements?

INTELLIGENT AGENT SOFTWARE

Intelligent agent software can be considered as software robots. The software can be a virtual case manager for older people. It could know details of medication and treatment regimens, activities and patterns of daily living. The intelligent agent will be able to link to a person's health history, be programmed to provide reminders through a range of devices and will be able to learn an individual's patterns of normal living and provide alerts to abnormal events. Through information conveyed from sensors and monitors in the home an intelligent agent can integrate clinical information systems, telehealth and telecare technologies and a response centre, as well as providing links to patients and their families. Agent software can be configurable for each individual and can be used to prompt older people to take their medication and any other everyday things that they would usually need reminding for.

GREEN COMPUTING

The recent advent of 'green' computing reflects the widespread interest in environmental issues. This includes energy conservation, promoting the use of renewable sources, recycling and reducing the negative impact of the disposal of technology products. There is now greater interest in disposing of electronic waste in a more responsible way; this includes the toxic components of ICT, including batteries. The term covers the manufacture of technologies so as to reduce adverse impacts on the environment.

In aged care many providers are interested in this concept as part of being a good corporate citizen. Practical activities might include reducing avoidable travel through the substitution of videoconferencing and telehealth. ICT products often have a short life of around three years so provision needs to be made for the responsible disposal and potential recycling of devices and materials. ICT has the potential to reduce the use of paper through making information more readily available on electronic devices. Many organisations have finally made the long-awaited move to being paperless through reducing the availability of printers.

CALL CENTRES AND MONITORING

An essential component of AT and smart homes is the arrangements for responding to an event or signal. There is often a presumption that the person receiving the messages will be a family member or general practitioner. If messages and alerts are directed to a family member, then protocols need to be developed; for example, what will happen if a carer's mobile phone battery is flat or they are somewhere that they cannot hear the call? For GPs to receive telehealth information and monitor signals there would need to be arrangements for funding and accountability and insurers would need to agree to reimburse these services. Those changes are not likely to happen in the near future.

There are companies that already provide the alert button that is widely used by frail older people and people with disabilities. Some of these are moving more into telecare and telehealth services. It is critical that these services operate according to standards and protocols. Consideration needs to be given towards what signals can be responded to by the software and what requires a human operator, especially given that many older people may not be comfortable with automatic voice response systems. In addition, some health authorities operate telephone triage and may also wish to extend into the home and AT monitoring market.

STANDARDS

Recognition of the need for international standards to guide the development of AT has led to establishing the Continua Health Alliance (www.continuaalliance.org). This aims to develop and promote the adoption of standards to ensure that technologies are interoperable—that is, they can connect and exchange information and that the information has the same meaning to the sender and receiver. This will be critical for safety as well as for managing costs, ease of training and reducing the potential for consumers to be locked into the products of a particular supplier.

Further work in standards is required to ensure the quality of call centre services, security and privacy, and also for protocols for operation; for example, at what point is it reasonable for a remote operator to activate web cameras and potentially invade a person's privacy?

SOME POSSIBLE APPLICATIONS OF ASSISTIVE TECHNOLOGY

This section outlines some examples and how they can be used as a strategy to educate practitioners and draw their attention to how some of the 'less complex' devices might be utilised in practice to address common areas of concern. Not all options will work for everyone, but options are worth investigating for individuals and individual situations.

TRACKING PEOPLE AND OBJECTS

Hand-held devices and mobile phones can be utilised to track a person with a tendency to wander. Wandering behaviour often creates anxiety for the partner or carer who finds themselves in conflict over a security and behaviour management issue. An individual wearing this type of device can leave home alone but not be 'lost' as their movement can be monitored. They can be spoken to and can call a preset number if they become confused or concerned, providing they are able to remember how to do this.

 Hand-held devices and mobile phones can be utilised to keep in contact with, and track if required, a person with a tendency to wander.

There is a device that will monitor the front door and provide an alert to a carer as well as an audible message to the dependent person if they attempt to leave their home alone. That way the person can be encouraged to return to the house and the carer can be alerted.

SENSOR TECHNOLOGIES, PERSONAL HEALTHCARE DEVICES

Devices that are based on low-cost computer technology and bought over the counter or on the internet are available. These currently include pedometers (monitor an exercise regimen), scales, thermometers, heart-rate monitors, blood pressure monitors, body fat analysers and blood sugar monitors. Information can be collected, stored and transmitted to another person. Other technologies that would enable a person to live independently in their home for longer include passive infrared detectors, door entry systems, bed and chair sensors, and emergency monitoring systems.

MOBILITY AND FALLS MONITORING

Home monitoring devices such as sensor pads have been around for some time. They have been fitted in homes in places where a person is more likely to fall such as by the bed, at the foot of a chair and in the bathroom. Similar devices can be worn on the body and networked to monitor physiological state, or sewn into clothing.

Vignette

Mr O lives alone in a retirement unit. He was diagnosed with Parkinson's disease some time ago and, although managing very well on his own with Meals on Wheels and home help, his family is becoming increasingly worried about him because he seems to be more unsteady on his feet and reports that he is falling over quite a lot, particularly when he gets out of his chair or out of bed to go to the toilet at night. In discussion with his visiting nurse, Mr O agrees to have sensors fitted to several places in his home; adjacent to his chair in the dining room where he has his meals, in the lounge room where he watches the TV, and in the bedroom. He also agrees to an 'alert system' connected to a central service. The sensors give the family peace of mind and he feels 'better protected' without losing his independence.

BEHAVIOUR PATTERNS AND MONITORING

As mentioned, 'smart homes' are being piloted in a number of countries. Simple surveillance technology can observe and record routine behaviour within an individual's home, for example, when they get up, when they are in the kitchen, their sleep patterns and when they leave the home. Routine activity and behaviour patterns can be analysed and interpreted with the intention that mechanisms can be put into place to recognise potential risk and 'alert' the individual or a third party when a situation requires intervention.

Vignette

Mrs C lives alone with help from her family and a Home and Community Care Package. She has some deficit in her left arm and hand from a stroke about three years ago and mild cognitive impairment but not a diagnosis of dementia. She manages well and is very proud of her independence. She is sociable and has many friends; she 'loves a chat'. Her family were getting concerned that Mrs C was not coping quite as well as she had been, and in particular, forgetting things and getting side-tracked. With the assistance of a private company, they enrolled her in a program that develops patterns of her usual behaviour and identified potential risk areas and events, like when she was cooking and had the stove on. The program installed a 'voice-over' action that was alerted by certain events and time patterns. The value was demonstrated with one particular event. Mrs C was cooking at the stove, getting her dinner ready. The door bell rang—it was Mrs D from another unit. They struck up a conversation about activities planned for the next day. Mrs C completely forgot she was cooking. Suddenly, an alarm sounded and a loud, programmed voice said, 'Please go to the kitchen immediately; there is a problem at the stove'. This was repeated several times. Mrs C responded to the alert, left Mrs D and returned to the kitchen, turned off the gas burner, and chastised herself for forgetting what she was doing. As soon as the 'risk' was eliminated, the voice alert ceased.

BARRIERS TO USING ASSISTIVE TECHNOLOGY

From an industry perspective, low market awareness and visibility, lack of standards and uncertainty can limit take-up of AT. Older people may have limited knowledge of possible products and their application. Consumer education and awareness is not common. There is limited literature on product reviews or comparison of products to inform consumers. There is also limited literature on comparative user requirements such as economic factors, gender issues, income levels or environmental factors. A lack of a systematic approach to market developments leads to high costs for research and market validation (Commission of the European Communities 2007). Innovative small-scale implementation due to fragmented approaches to risk-sharing and a lack of forward-looking activity limit good practice.

From the perspective of the consumer, there are other concerns. Older people, when faced with new technologies, can find themselves in a difficult, vulnerable position. This may be due to their personal situation—income, location, health, disability. The complexity of the technology may be overwhelming, the equipment not available or difficult to access. Products are sometimes not adapted to meet specific needs of older people, directions are in small print or not in print at all. This can increase an existing sense of frustration and vulnerability and close down any desire to 'try something new'. Instead of being empowering, taking control of a challenging situation and managing a health condition, AT can be 'the last straw' for an older person and just too much to take on.

Barriers and challenges can be considered under several categories.

ATTITUDES TO TECHNOLOGY

Physical disabilities that restrict accessibility to the user interface limit the ability to handle the device, just as cognitive barriers can limit the understanding of procedures and navigation.

ETHICAL CONCERNS

Intrusive technologies or functions, such as the location and monitoring, can be of concern, as is the potential for social isolation if technologies substitute for human caring.

Given that global developments in technology are fast-paced, ongoing and unlikely to be reversed, issues about the ethical use of available ATs in the healthcare sector is a pressing issue. This is particularly the case for those who are frail and vulnerable and reliant on others for care. The core ethical principles of autonomy, beneficence, non-maleficence and justice have been used by some authors to raise important ethical questions inherent in technology use in healthcare and in research with older people (Borges 2008, Feil-Seifer & Matarić 2011, ICT & Ageing 2009, Magnusson & Hanson 2003, Pollack 2005). However, significant questions still remain about how to build ethical sound protections into new and evolving technologies and how these will shape the acceptability of technologies. Several core principles emerge from this literature.

- Technological options must not become a substitute for the meaningful human interaction that underpins quality healthcare. Rather, technology needs to be considered as an adjunct to existing acceptable and evidence-based practices, one option among a number of others in most situations.
- Technology that engenders discomfort or fear in older adult users is unacceptable.
- Where a technology has been shown to improve the health and wellbeing via robust research, every effort needs to be made to ensure equality of access to that technology.
- Where technology is selected for use, the objectives, scope, timing, function and review of the technology use needs to be stipulated by guidelines and policies directed by decision makers.
- Potentially negative aspects of technology use need to be recognised such as: autonomy, privacy, confidentiality and security issues; loneliness and isolation; dependence on technology; and the conferring of social stigma.
- The option must be retained to discontinue the use of products and services if they prove to be unsuccessful for the user.

CONFIDENTIALITY AND PRIVACY

Transmission of personal data to other providers or professionals can be seen to be an invasion of privacy. Essen's (2008) study in Sweden, seeks to offer an account of how older people experience electronic care surveillance in relation to their privacy. The study was based on in-depth interviews with older people who participated in a telemonitoring project and who had experience of being continuously actively monitored in their own homes. The findings suggest that older people can perceive electronic care surveillance as freeing and as protecting their privacy in the sense that it enables them to continue living in their own home rather than moving to a nursing home. One individual, however, experienced a privacy violation and the surveillance service was interrupted at her request. This illustrates the importance of built-in possibilities for individuals to exit such services. In general, the study highlights that e-surveillance can be not only constraining but also enabling. The study therefore supports a notion of the dual nature of surveillance.

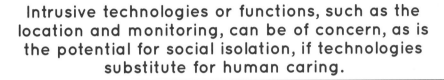

Intrusive technologies or functions, such as the location and monitoring, can be of concern, as is the potential for social isolation, if technologies substitute for human caring.

EVALUATION OF ASSISTIVE TECHNOLOGY

It is essential that health professionals give thought to the evaluation of these technologies to ensure that appropriate devices are selected for clients and intended outcomes are achieved. Such evaluation may be achieved by examining both the technologies themselves and their impact upon individuals. Lindenberger et al (2008) suggest three main principles for evaluating AT. Importantly, they suggest examining how such technologies make provision for person specificity rather than taking an off-the-shelf approach whereby the technology is matched with a problem not a person. Second, they highlight the need to consider the impact in resource allocation, an area examined by Mann et al (1999) who suggested that the use of AT slows the rate of functional decline while also reducing both institutional and in-home personnel costs. Last, Lindenberger et al (2008) also stress the importance of interim and regular evaluation. This commonsense advice simply means that clinicians are advised to evaluate early and often and seek to discover any problems at an early stage when remediation should be easier and more cost-effective.

Evaluation of these technologies and their impact upon individuals is essential to ensure appropriate devices are selected for clients and intended outcomes are achieved.

When considering how well an assistive device or technology meets the criterion of person-specificity and impacts upon resource allocation, one evaluation approach that can prove useful is multi-attribute evaluation theory (MAUT), which was specifically developed to evaluate complex scenarios. It also allows the evaluation task to be broken down into manageable segments and provides a score to indicate users' overall degree of satisfaction with both the evaluation object and its constituent attributes, which in this case would be an example of AT. MAUT has been in use for many decades, but more recently it has been used as an evaluation tool for such diverse aged care issues as satisfaction with home care (Samuelsson 2000), diagnostic decision support in aged care (Koch 2004) and selection of atypical antipsychotics (Bettinger et al 2007).

Lee et al (2003) recognised that many healthcare decisions are problematic because of their complexity and in turn their important consequences on both the quality of life of individuals and on the allocation of limited resources. They also observe that traditional healthcare decision modelling is often inadequate to properly assess these decisions and suggest that approaches such as MAUT may provide a more useful alternative. Readers wishing to further explore the types of problems best suited to evaluation using MAUT should consult Olson (1995) for a detailed analysis of the approach. Additionally, the AT devices that provide physiological measures for the individual may lend themselves to such evaluation. Examples of issues that could be ranked for importance and scored for performance could include:

- cost
- durability
- ease of use
- impact on client independence
- impact on treatment compliance
- meets intended purpose
- portability.

From the above discussions it is evident that using ATs seeks to empower individuals by maintaining their sense of independence, autonomy, self-determination, self-respect and self-reliance by providing support for tasks vital for daily living.

Many readily available tools that focus on an individual's functional ability can assist health professionals in assessing either the need for, or the impact of, ATs on clients. Such tools also serve several other useful purposes such as profiling clients' progress over time, considering pre- and post-implementation scores, reflecting on outcomes of rehabilitation planning, impact upon carer burden and allowing national and international benchmarking using these commonly used reliable and validated tools.

CONCLUSION

Searches using the *Cumulative Index to Nursing and Allied Health Literature* (CINAHL) and online search engines will yield a wide variety of other assessment tools that will assist clinicians in their choice of interventions including ATs. These tools cover myriad issues such as cognitive function, level of social support, pain perception, quality of life, satisfaction with care support and self-esteem. Useful discussion of the interaction of these variables and their impact on client assessment is provided by both Arnadottir & Mercer (1999) and Savard et al (2006).

The tools may also be downloaded from a variety of internet sites but it should be noted that the copyright status of instruments does change over time.

Some instruments that were previously in the public domain and free to use have subsequently been commercialised and require a licence fee for use. Readers should check the conditions of use of individual instruments prior to their use for clinical practice or research purposes. A useful repository of tools is provided by Lichtenberg (1999) who highlighted a range of reliable and valid assessment for assessing functional status, psychosocial health, comorbidity and behavioural issues, along with case examples to illustrate their use. An additional challenge for evaluation is the speed of development of AT, which in turn is likely to require clinicians to find alternative and appropriate means of evaluation that focus on the impact on the end user, as opposed to simply accepting the claims of developers and vendors who are likely to have a quite different agenda for adopting their products.

FUTURE DIRECTIONS

This chapter has provided an overview of the actual and potential application of AT and evaluation strategies that are available in the care of older people. There are still many questions that need to be explored to ensure that we:

- adopt appropriate research strategies to accompany AT innovation, design and implementation
- work towards common language and ontology to provide a basis for standards, performance indicators, evidence-based practice and for benchmarking
- devise and apply tools for impact assessment to provide a fuller and fairer picture of true costs and benefits
- inform policy at government and service sector levels.

There is also need for multidisciplinary research to bring technology development in line with socioeconomic realities of health systems and user expectations and to share successes and challenges.

Reflective questions

1. How can busy age care providers keep up with the latest in assistive technology?

2. Is there a planning process happening in your workplace to consider the use of this technology?

3. Consider how much technology is impacting on your life in the community at present. Street surveillance, shopping centre surveillance, bank transactions, airport ticketing, computer linkages between government departments, such as Centrelink and Immigration, and eBay purchasing. Most older people have adjusted to card banking and Medicare cards; many are using computers. What are the main difficulties in the use of assistive technology?

4. Are there ethical issues in the use of assistive technology?

References

Algase, D., Beattie, E., Therrien, B., 2001. Impact of cognitive impairment on wandering behavior. Western Journal of Nursing Research 23 (3), 283–295.

Algase, D., Beattie, E., Antonakos, C., et al., 2010. Wandering and the physical environment. American Journal Of Alzheimer's Disease And Other Dementias 25 (4), 340–346.

Algase, D.L., Son, G.R., Beattie, E., et al., 2004. The interrelatedness of wandering and wayfinding in a community sample of persons with dementia. Dementia and Geriatric Cognitive Disorders 17 (3), 231–239.

Arnadottir, S., Mercer, V.S., 1999. Functional assessment in geriatric physical therapy. Issues on Aging 22 (2), 3–12.

Aud, M., 2004. Dangerous wandering: delopement of people with dementia from long-term care facilities. American Journal of Alzheimer's Disease & Other Dementias 19 (6), 361–368.

Bantry White, E., Montgomery, P., McShane, R., 2010. Electronic tracking for people with dementia who get lost outside the home: a study of the experience of familial carers. British Journal of Occupational Therapy 73 (4), 152–159.

Beattie, E., Song, J., LaGore, S., 2005. A comparison of wandering behavior in nursing homes and assisted living facilities. Research & Theory for Nursing Practice 19 (2), 181–196.

Berry, B., Ignash, S., 2003. Assistive technology: providing independence for individuals with disabilities. Rehabilitation Nursing 28 (1), 6–14.

Bettinger, T.L., Schuler, G., Jones, D.R., et al., 2007. Schizophrenia: multi-attribute utility theory approach to selection of atypical antipsychotics. The Annals of Pharmacotherapy 41 (2), 201–207.

Borges, I., 2008. Older people and information and communication technologies: an ethical approach. The European Older People's Platform, Brussels. Online. Available: http://www.age-platform.org/EN/IMG/pdf_AGE__Ethics_and_ICT_Final-2.pdf, 1 May 2013.

Celler, B.G., Lovell, N.H., Basilakis, J., 2003. Using technology to improve the management of chronic disease. The Medical Journal of Australia 179 (1), 242–246.

Chen, M.H., Hsieh, C.L., Mao, H.F., et al., 2007. Differences between patient and proxy reports in the assessment of disability after stroke. Clinical Rehabilitation 21, 351–356.

Chui, Y., Algase, D., Whall, A., et al., 2004. Getting lost: directed attention and executive functions in early Alzheimer's disease patients. Dementia & Geriatric Cognitive Disorders 17 (3), 174–180.

Commission of the European Communities, 2007. Ageing well in the information society: an I2010 initiative. COM Brussels 14 Jun 2007.

Department of Health and Ageing, 2003. Incidence of incontinence as a factor in admission to aged care homes. National Continence Management Strategy. Department of Health and Ageing, Canberra. Online. Available: http://www.health.gov.au/internet/main/publishing.nsf/Content/0B09434227835C36CA256F190010BC30/$File/execrpt.pdf, 30 Sep 2012.

Dickinson, J., McLain-Kark, J., Marshall-Baker, A., 1995. The effects of visual barriers on exiting behavior in a dementia care unit. The Gerontologist 35 (1), 127–130.

Essen, A., 2008. The two facets of electronic care surveillance: an exploration of the views of older people who live with monitoring devices. Social Science and Medicine 67 (1), 128–136.

Essen, A., Conrick, M., 2007. Visions and realities: developing 'smart' homes for seniors in Sweden. Journal of Health Informatics 2 (1), 2.

FAST, 2012. Definition of assistive technology from King's Fund consultation 2001. Online. Available: http://www.fastuk.org/home.php, 29 Sep 2012.

Feil-Seifer, D.J., Matari&#x0017;, M.J., 2011. Ethical principles for socially assistive robotics. IEEE Robotics & Automation Magazine, Special issue on Roboethics, Veruggio. J. Solis and M. Van der loos 18 (1), 24–31.

Grenade, L., 2009. Evaluation of the use of gps to promote safe walking among people with dementia (safe2walk)—pilot study evaluation report. Curtin Health Innovation Research Institute, Perth.

Hermans, D.G., Htay, U. Hla., McShane, R., 2007. Non-pharmacological interventions for wandering of people with dementia in the domestic setting. Cochrane Database of Systematic Reviews 2007, Issue 1. Art. No.: CD005994. DOI: 10.1002/14651858. CD005994.pub2.

ICT & Ageing, 2009. Compilation report on ethical issues in EU ICT & ageing: users, markets and technologies. Online. Available: www.ict-ageing.eu, 29 Sep 2012.

Koch, B., 2004. Contemporary care planning issues. In: Nay, R., Garratt, S. (Eds.), Nursing older people: issues and innovations. Elsevier, Sydney.

Lee, R.C., Donaldson, C., Cook, L.S., 2003. The need for evolution in healthcare decision modeling. Medical Care 41 (9), 1024–1033.

Lichtenberg, P.A., 1999. Handbook of assessment in clinical gerontology. John Wiley, New York.

Lindenberger, U., Lövdén, M., Schellenbach, M., et al., 2008. Psychological principles of successful aging technologies: a critical review. Gerontology 54 (1), 59–68.

Magnusson, L., Hanson, E.J., 2003. Ethical issues arising from a research, technology and development project to support frail older people and their family carers at home. Health and Social Care in the Community (5), 431–439, Blackwell, Oxford.

Mann, W.C., Ottenbacher, K.J., Fraas, L., et al., 1999. Effectiveness of assistive technology and environmental interventions in maintaining independence and reducing home care costs for the frail elderly: a randomized controlled trial. Archives of Family Medicine 8, 210–217.

McShane, R., Gedling, K., Keene, J., et al., 1998. Getting lost in dementia: a longitudinal study of a behavioral symptom. International Psychogeriatrics 10 (3), 253–260.

Olson, D.L., 1995. Decision aids for selection problems. Springer, Berlin.

Philipson, G., Roberts, J., 2007. Caring for the future: the impact of technology on aged and assisted living (Invited Paper). Journal of Health Informatics 2 (1), edn1.

Pollack, M., 2005. Intelligent technology for an aging population. The use of AI to assist elders with cognitive impairment. AI Magazine 26 (2), 9–24.

Reimer-Reiss, M.L., Wacker, R.R., 2000. Factors associated with assistive technology discontinuance among individuals with disabilities. The Journal of Rehabilitation 66 (3), 44–50. CA-DDS 7.01.

Robinson, L., Hutchings, D., Dickinson, H.O., et al., 2007. Effectiveness and acceptability of non-pharmacological interventions to reduce wandering in dementia: a systematic review. International Journal of Geriatric Psychiatry 22, 9–22.

Samuelsson, G., 2000. The quality of home care services in Sweden: consumer expectations and changing satisfaction. In: Warnes, A.M., Warren, L., Nolan, M., (Eds.), Care services for later life: transformations and critiques. Jessica Kingsley Publishers, London.

Savard, J., Leduc, N., Lebel, P., et al., 2006. Caregiver satisfaction with support services—influence of different types of services. Journal of Aging and Health 18, 3–27.

Schaper, L., Lappins, M., 2007. Implementation of an intelligent building solution within an Australia residential aged care facility. Paper presented at the 2nd International Conference on Technology and Ageing. 16–19 June 2007. Toronto, Canada.

Song, J.A., Algase, D., 2008. Premorbid characteristics and wandering behavior in persons with dementia. Archives of Psychiatric Nursing 22 (6), 318–327.

Tang, H., Ng, J., 2006. Googling for a diagnosis—use of Google as a diagnostic aid: internet based study. BMJ 333, 1143.

The Royal Society, 2006. Digital healthcare: the impact of information and communication technologies on health and healthcare. The Clyvedon Press, Cardiff, UK pp. 7–60.

United States Congress, 1998. Assistive technology act. Online. Available: http://www.section508.gov/docs/AssistiveTechnologyActOf1998Full.pdf, 31 Jul 2012.

Verza, R., Lopes Carvalho, M.L., Battaglia, M.A., et al., 2006. An interdisciplinary approach to evaluating the need for assistive technology reduces equipment abandonment. Multiple Sclerosis 12 (1), 88–93.

Vine, E., 2008. Breaking down the silos: the integration of energy efficiency, renewable energy, demand response and climate change. Energy Efficiency 1 (1), 49–63.

CHAPTER 23

INNOVATIVE RESPONSES TO A CHANGING HEALTHCARE ENVIRONMENT

Rhonda Nay, Benny Katz and Michael Murray

Editors' comments

Recent government reports acknowledge the need for innovative approaches to the practice and education of health practitioners; these issues are addressed in this chapter along with the need for changes in how health professionals work. The issue of access for older people and health professionals who live in rural areas is raised and different approaches to meeting their needs are described in the vignettes. These models will be closely watched for application to other sites.

INTRODUCTION

This chapter acknowledges the sweeping changes in healthcare demand, the projected workforce shortages and the need for innovative responses. It argues for new care delivery models, flexibility and innovation in educational preparation of health professionals, and presents examples of creative responses to perceived shortages in specialist expertise and growing demand from an ageing population.

CHANGES IN DEMAND

There have been, and continue to be, enormous changes in the healthcare environment and healthcare demands. There are several factors that contribute to increased demands beyond those driven by the ageing of the population. Consumers have a higher expectation of service, of effective health outcomes, and are expecting increased participation and engagement in their own care and the care of their families. Fast declining, except perhaps among the old–old, are the days of meekly responding 'yes, doctor' or 'yes, nurse'. Expectations, fuelled in part by general societal changes, are underpinned by more accessible information (often web–based), formation of disease–focused associations and a steady flow of information in newsprint. Consequent upon the information explosion and broad availability of health information we have a much more informed public; we know knowledge is power, and so a better informed consumer results in higher expectations. Although there is little evidence to substantiate increasing success in aged care related litigation, the *fear* of litigation and loss of reputation has driven a concomitant aversion to risk and attention to risk management.

There have been, and continue to be, enormous changes in the healthcare environment, workforce and healthcare demands.

As noted elsewhere in this book, health professionals and organisations are required to base clinical practice on the best available evidence and to embed clinical governance, consumer participation in healthcare decisions and continuous quality improvements (Fetherstonhaugh et al 2010, Muir Gray 2001, Swage 2003). The ageing of the population, predominantly through the reduction in infant, child and to a lesser extent young adult mortality, health promotion and public healthcare measures have seen the major burden of disease now coming from chronic disease and disability. Nearly half of those aged 65–74 years have five or more long–term physical health conditions and we know from Chapter 2 that the number in this age group is rapidly increasing. Life expectancy in Australia now is around 79 for men and 84 for women. Among older people the greatest cause of disability and the biggest killer is dementia (Australian Institute of Health and Welfare (AIHW) 2012a). And yet our health professionals receive little to no specific dementia education.

People over 65 years of age represent 13% of the Australian population yet occupy more than 47% of public hospital beds (Australian Bureau of Statistics (ABS) 2011, Gray et al 2004). The ageing of the population will continue to increase the demand for health services at a time when health providers are under increasing funding pressures. Community demand and healthcare costs led to an emphasis away from care in acute hospitals towards more self and supported care in the community. Older people are likely to have comorbid conditions, many of which will reduce functional ability, but with appropriate services independence may be preserved.

This major shift in type and place of service delivery requires a major rethink in how services are delivered, who should deliver them, and what skills are required (Stone & Benson 2012). Numerous reviews and innovative programs have been funded to address workforce issues, reduce admission to hospital, shorten the length of stay and prevent readmission (e.g. see www.health.gov.au and www.aihw.gov.au). While creative solutions should accommodate the present, more visionary planning focused on the future is needed. It will take at least 10 years to bring about any major change as educational institutions will also need to incorporate industry expectations into curriculum.

> **This major shift in type and place of service delivery requires a major rethink in how services are delivered, who should deliver them, and what skills are required.**

Information and assistive technologies have changed the way we do business generally, caused workforce reengineering, and aided in the independence of many individuals who previously depended on high levels of support (see Ch 22). New technologies constantly arrive on the market and, although expectations often exceed reality, they will inevitably enable even more choice and independence for future generations.

CHANGES IN SUPPLY

The literature leaves no doubt that workforce shortages are a current reality internationally and will worsen as the baby boomers retire (Commonwealth of Australia 2012, Frank & Weiss 2012, Productivity Commission 2005, 2011, World Health Organization (WHO) 2006). Medicine, nursing and most areas of allied health are reporting demand exceeding supply, especially in rural areas. While demand is increasing because of the bulge in the population of older people and expected increase in the old-old, the relatively smaller populations of generations X and Y equals demand outstripping supply. Additionally the feminisation of the medical workforce has been associated with more part-time workforce participation and some literature suggests that generations X and Y are more interested in lifestyle balance than previous generations—again reducing effective full-time (EFT) working health professionals. The trend to more flexible working arrangements may have benefits for both employer and employee, although it is associated with a reduction in EFT employed health professionals. This fact needs to be taken into consideration when planning training places to cater for future workforce needs.

> **The literature leaves no doubt that workforce shortages are a current reality internationally and will worsen as the baby boomers retire.**

New models of service delivery, new education models and incentives are required to ensure that these pressures do not drive down the quality of care of older people.

> **The increasing average age of the health workforce also suggests a looming crisis as the baby boomers retire.**

INNOVATION IN THE CARE OF OLDER PEOPLE

Innovation in the care of older people is not a new concept. In the 1930s Dr Marjorie Warren, a medical officer at the West Middlesex Infirmary, was given the responsibility for the care of 714 chronically ill patients at the nearby Poor Law Infirmary. She created the first geriatric medical unit in the United Kingdom (UK), instituting medical treatment, rehabilitation and discharge planning for a previously neglected population. She was able to increase the turnover three times the previous rate and reduce the need for chronic beds to 240 (Barton & Mulley 2003).

In 1979 Rubenstein et al established an inpatient unit to provide diagnosis, rehabilitation and discharge planning for older hospital inpatients at high risk of nursing home discharge. Patients treated in this unit had a one-year mortality rate of 23.8% compared with 48.3% for those who had received usual care, in addition to lower rates of nursing home discharge (26.9% versus 26.7%) (Rubenstein et al 1984). A meta-analysis of 28 randomised controlled trials involving 9871 participants confirmed the reduction in institutional admission and mortality at six months of patients who had undergone comprehensive geriatric assessment (Stuck et al 1993). Other innovative approaches have included specialist inpatient units for older people including orthogeriatric units and acute care units. Community Aged Care Assessment Teams (ACATs) now cover the whole of Australia, providing assessment of the accommodation and care needs of older people and those with disabilities in their own homes. Specialist outpatient services have been developed including memory clinics, continence clinics, falls and balance clinics, pain clinics and wound clinics.

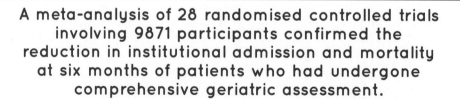

A meta-analysis of 28 randomised controlled trials involving 9871 participants confirmed the reduction in institutional admission and mortality at six months of patients who had undergone comprehensive geriatric assessment.

The development of innovative care models for older hospital patients has largely occurred in larger metropolitan hospitals with established geriatric services, and to a lesser extent in major regional centres. Access to these services has been difficult or impossible for people living in more remote areas. It is simply not feasible to replicate a metropolitan model of geriatric care in all locations, particularly with a shortage of specialist geriatricians, nurses and allied health staff with expertise in aged care.

About one-third of Australians aged older than 65 years live in rural areas, including outer regional (86%), remote (10%) and very remote (4%) sites (Davis & Bartlett 2008). People aged over 65 years in Australia make up 12.3% of people in major cities, 14.1% in inner regional areas, 12.8% in outer regional areas, 9.7% in remote areas and 7.7% in very remote sites (Larson 2006). Older adults from rural areas are typified by self-reliance, stoicism, hardiness and a preference for informal networks and accordingly have less frequent use of, and delays in using, health services. Increased geographical distances to access services and decreased use of health services combine to exacerbate risk for disease already increased by excess weight, smoking, drinking and occupational and environmental dangers inherent in rural areas (Davis & Bartlett 2008).

People living in rural regions frequently endure a lack of health services and insufficient community and economic resources compared with their urban counterparts and the criteria for service provision derived from urban settings fail to meet the needs of rural older people (see Ch 4). Providers of aged care health services in rural areas need to have awareness of the structure and operation of rural aged care and the special needs of older people in rural areas, such as transport (Davis & Bartlett 2008). For example, older women in rural areas are less likely to consult general practitioners (GPs), specialists and allied health professionals despite similar quality of life and disabilities compared with urban older women. This is associated with higher rates of hospitalisation and greater use of community and respite services (Byles et al 2006).

There is now established evidence that comprehensive geriatric medical assessment, backed up by specialised geriatric services, can provide better management and outcomes for frail older people (Dainty 2007). The resources to provide such services are scarce in smaller or more rural communities where practitioners need to garner a wide range of interdisciplinary skills, particularly when the service system is fragmented into different sectors, agencies and institutions, none of which can provide the specialised focus that this segment of the population needs (Crilly et al 1999).

Since 1999 many (e.g. Nay & Closs 1999, Nay & Pearson 2001, Pearson et al 2002, Haesler et al 2007, Hodgkinson et al 2011) have argued for more flexible staffing models and education programs for nurses. They have called for health professionals to put client need ahead of protection of professional boundaries. The Australian Government and state governments have established numerous committees to advise on workforce developments in health and funded various trials including extended scope of practice, substitution and new expanded roles (Department of Human Services 2007, Nay 2003, National Health Workforce Taskforce 2009, Productivity Commission 2011). These changes have not of course progressed in a linear or untroubled manner. Some advocates of nursing, medicine and allied health have fought loudly and vigorously to maintain traditional professional boundaries and argued simply for government to provide more money, more university places and better conditions (Van Der Weyden 2007). In our view this is marching into the future backwards! More of the same is not a solution when all around you is changing. Having a doctor diagnose and prescribe does not guarantee public safety; having enrolled nurses administer medications does not mean the end of registered nurses (RNs) in aged care—although to read the media and quotes from unions you could believe this to be the case.

> **The Australian Government and state governments have established numerous committees to advise on workforce developments in health, and have funded various trials including extended scope of practice, substitution and new expanded roles.**

Getting it right into the future surely requires planning to start with an emphasis on public health measures, health education and other preventative measures. Planning should reflect healthcare need, not health professional need. We contend principles and evidence, rather than vested interests, provide a firmer basis from which to make decisions on care delivery.

> **Planning should reflect healthcare need, not health professional need.**

Following this approach, starting with client need and the published evidence, numerous interested stakeholders, most notably VAHEC,[1] developed a set of principles to guide staffing and skills mix for residential aged care facilities (RACFs) in Australia.[2] These principles were revised in 2010.

Exactly how the principles are implemented would be dependent upon such factors as:
- resident mix and care needs
- facility size, location and design
- skill availability
- the philosophy of the organisation.

The principles specific to direct care (Department of Human Services, unpublished) included the following.
- Staffing decisions will take account of:
  - resident dependency, needs and accreditation standards
  - staff experience and competencies and the need to support staff development
  - preferences of staff as far as possible to ensure reasonable workload, a work/life balance and occupational health and safety (OH&S) standards are met
  - financial resources
  - the context and model of care
  - the need to provide clinical leadership and evidence-based practice
  - the capacity to share resources across services
  - assessment of demand—acuity, peaks and troughs and flexibility to ensure adequate coverage of high demand times (e.g. sundowning)
  - availability of different skills.

....

[1]VAHEC was one of the industry representative organisations in Victoria.
[2]Residential aged care in Australia includes what is generally known as nursing home (high) and hostel (low) levels of care; some RACFs are associated with acute and other services and others are stand-alone services.

- All residents will have access to an RN for assessment and monitoring and, where the complexity/acuity of care requires it, care delivery. This requirement is to be determined by an RN or GP assessment.
- All high-care residents will be assessed by an RN on admission, on a regular basis, and whenever there is a significant change in condition.
- All high-care (nursing home) facilities will have 24-hour RN coverage preferably onsite. Where it can be demonstrated that such onsite coverage, is impossible because of unavailability of RNs, an enrolled nurse (EN) with medication endorsement and appropriate educational preparation, experience and competency will be onsite with ready access to an RN.
- All RACFs will have access to psychiatric expertise concomitant with resident needs.
- All RACFs will have a director of nursing (DON) responsible for nursing care; however, the DON may be shared across services and not necessarily be based on site.
- Regardless of the model used, nursing will have direct input into budget and other policy and practice decisions impacting on resident outcomes.
- RACF care teams may include ENs and personal care attendants (PCAs)/assistants in nursing (AINs) with care responsibilities delegated according to their educational preparation and competence.
- All RACFs will include activity/therapy hours sufficient to ensure resident lifestyle needs are met and accreditation standards achieved.
- In the absence of more sophisticated data, team size and mix could be decided upon evaluation of care mix based on the preceding 12 months' data; high care would be expected to have RNs or ENs as team leaders and a higher proportion of qualified staff overall than low care.
- Staff will be educationally prepared and competent to undertake the various responsibilities.
- Specific educational preparation will be provided in the staffing methodology, delegation and leadership.

As can be seen, these principles encourage staffing models that are determined first and foremost by client need and staff competency rather than professional territorial claims. Who does what and when is determined by educational preparation and competence rather than tasks allotted according to professional title. In the future gerontic nurse practitioners could typically join a GP/geriatrician/allied health team and provide services to older people across the continuum of care. This will reduce waiting times, avoid hospitalisation and improve outcomes for older people. Or perhaps more creatively we will see transdisciplinary education and health professionals such as the nurse social work practitioner being prepared in the US (Schneiderman et al 2008).

Who does what and when is determined by educational preparation and competence rather than tasks allotted according to professional title.

The following vignette provides an example of how flexibility and innovation can address a gap in geriatric services.

Vignette

Wangaratta Base Hospital is a 222-bed hospital servicing north-eastern Victoria. Specialist services for older people include a 31-bed geriatric evaluation and rehabilitation unit, an aged psychiatry service, a community rehabilitation centre, and continence, falls and memory clinics. This service had advertised for several years for a geriatrician without success. They approached Nay to discuss other options for meeting client needs. A model using local nurse practitioners, medical staff and a Melbourne-based geriatrician was considered an exciting option. Murray and Katz were then recruited to provide the Melbourne-based geriatric services.

The two senior medical staff on the geriatric evaluation and rehabilitation ward, GPs by training, enrolled in a Master of Gerontology course by distance education. The hospital also appointed two gerontic nurse practitioner candidates enrolled at Deakin University.

The development of the nurse practitioner model of gerontic care is an innovative approach to deal with local issues in a regional heath service and the broader issue of health needs of an ageing population. The aim was to ensure that the care of older patients, particularly those with multiple and complex problems, is not jeopardised by increasing specialisation within the hospital system and the shortage of geriatric medical specialists or related expertise. Progressively the nurse practitioners became competent to assess, order investigations and prescribe medications for defined conditions within a specified group of patients. This was not restricted to the aged care and rehabilitation unit, but available to all older people initially within the hospital and over time to the emergency department, community and residential aged care, with a further two nurse practitioner candidates being appointed in early 2009. The nurse practitioners will become the leaders of the multidisciplinary team caring for older patients.

In collaboration with the Department of Geriatric Medicine at St Vincent's Hospital, Melbourne, consultant geriatricians attended Wangaratta Base Hospital for one day every two weeks over a five-year period. Their role was to mentor and support the hospital doctors and nurse practitioner candidates, and to enhance the models of aged care being delivered in Northeast Health Wangaratta through education and implementation of practice guidelines. The geriatricians also undertook consultations on patients throughout Northeast Health Wangaratta in addition to multidisciplinary teaching ward rounds during these visits. These consultations not only focused on the clinical care of patients with complex care needs but are used as examples to develop best practice disciplinary and transdisciplinary care upon which education is based. In 2008 the model was expanded through teleconferencing between the nurse practitioner candidates and consultant geriatricians on alternate weeks to the visits. By 2012 three nurse practitioner candidates had graduated, and taken up positions not only within Wangaratta Hospital but in other regional hospitals in north-eastern Victoria. At this stage Wangaratta Hospital was able to employ its own medical specialist, enabling the visiting geriatricians to withdraw. The innovative model of care had been established, and will be ongoing.

Enhancing the skills and knowledge of the staff working in aged care at Wangaratta Base Hospital has involved a multifaceted approach. Mentoring complements the academic approach of the university courses and addresses some of the problems associated with distance education, creating a collegiate environment and providing early feedback on progress. The mentors ensure that the theoretical knowledge is applied practically in the clinical setting, and areas that need additional attention are identified.

The role being developed at Wangaratta Base Hospital for nurse practitioners in aged care is not simply to make up for a shortage of medical practitioners in aged care. The role focuses on the detection and management of common problems in older people that often remain under-recognised in a hospital system that is becoming increasingly more specialised. It is competency based, building on the existing holistic skills of nursing; assessing older patients at risk and implementing early interventions may reduce the severity or even prevent these common geriatric problems.

Older people are often considered in terms of their frailty, complexity of their medical problems and resultant disability. These describe the population as a whole but are more difficult to quantify in an individual patient. An easier approach to individual patients is based on identifying common geriatric syndromes, specifically immobility, instability (falls), incontinence and impaired intellect/memory (delirium/dementia), described by Sir Bernard Isaacs as the 'giants of geriatric medicine' (Isaacs 1965). Isaacs asserted that, if you look closely enough, all common problems with older people relate back to one of these giants. Best practice guidelines for these syndromes are widely available (e.g. see www.health.vic.gov.au/acute-agedcare). Through a focus on detecting the geriatric giants, early multidisciplinary intervention can be introduced to optimise the outcome of the hospital admission.

DELIRIUM

Delirium affects about 30% of older patients at some time during their hospitalisation, and as many as 73.5% of postoperative patients and those in intensive care units (Dyer et al 1995, Francis 1992). Delirium is predictive of longer hospital admissions and worse outcomes including nursing home discharge and death. Guidelines for screening, identification, prevention and management of delirium are widely available (e.g. see the Australian and New Zealand Society for Geriatric Medicine 2012, Department of Human Services 2006). Multicomponent approaches have been shown to increase the detection of delirium and reduce the total number of days with delirium and the total number of episodes of delirium (Inouye et al 1999). Though they are not the only health specialty that could develop necessary competencies to holistically manage complex older patients, nurse practitioners are ideally suited to identifying and implementing management guidelines to deal with Isaac's 'geriatric giant' given that in reality they are likely to be the best equipped of the health specialties to adopt an expanded scope of practice.

The nurse practitioner role can be positioned to play a pivotal role in the multidisciplinary approach to aged care. Working in close collaboration with the treating doctor the nurse practitioner is able to assess, order investigations and treat a range of medical conditions. Problems are identified early, whereas in the traditional model they may have gone unrecognised or not detected until later. In close collaboration with nursing and allied health staff, functional maintenance programs are introduced, aimed at preventing functional decline associated with illness, hospitalisation and bedrest (Clinical Epidemiology and Health Service Evaluation Unit 2007).

Our experience is that nurse practitioners are able to cross traditional boundaries, adding capacity to a range of health disciplines, often more effectively than the hospital medical officers who are frequently on their own steep learning curve as they move through multiple hospital rotations. Nurse practitioners liaise closely with community service providers to ensure optimum care continues following discharge.

The nurse practitioner role can be positioned to play a pivotal role in the multidisciplinary approach to aged care.

The care of older people is not solely confined to specialists in aged care. Indeed, even in institutions with full-time geriatricians, only a small proportion of older people are managed by specialist geriatricians. With the population ageing it is becoming increasingly important that all health practitioners gain expertise in the care of older patients. Opportunities for training are limited.

Vignette

The Victorian Geriatric Medicine Training Program[3] was established to address the training needs of specialist geriatricians as well as other doctors, nurses and allied health staff treating older people. It has established an internet-based program to address the educational needs of doctors in the first few years after graduation. The initial tutorials cover topics such as dementia, delirium, incontinence, mobility and falls, drug therapy, pain, end-of-life care, legal aspects, healthy ageing and comprehensive geriatric assessment. Each module contains core educational material, case studies and interactive learning components. Although written with junior doctors in mind, nurses and allied health staff also find them valuable. They are available online at <www.anzsgm.org/vgmtp>. Innovative and accessible dementia education has also been supported for all disciplines through the Australian Government-funded Dementia Training Study Centres.

While we have outlined examples of innovations with which we have had personal involvement, there are of course many others that have been evaluated and can be accessed through the various government websites; examples include physiotherapists in emergency departments, pharmacists in disease management units, orthoptists in diabetes clinics and general practice nurses. And yet, the potential for creative models is unrealised. Why, for example, do we not have GPs able to claim for email consultations? Many people

....
[3]The Victorian Geriatric Medicine Training Program was established by the Australian and New Zealand Society for Geriatric Medicine and funded by the Victorian Government Department of Human Services.

self-manage chronic conditions and require limited support. The time, cost, and often discomfort wasted traveling to the surgery and sitting in the waiting room for what may be an answer to one question could be reduced to a one-minute email resulting in better outcomes for the consumer and the busy GP.

CONCLUSION

Ageing, changes in healthcare demands, emerging technology and evolving workforce issues require innovative planning and responses if we are to provide 'world class care'. Importantly, new models need to add value to health outcomes and to be sustainable. Health services must look beyond short-term funded trials and, subject to evaluation, incorporate innovative roles and models into service plans. The risk otherwise is a project mentality that is ad hoc, term-defined, reactive to funding opportunities, outside usual business and fails to realise long-term benefits.

We have tried in this chapter to suggest that the changes do not represent a crisis but rather opportunities for new ways of thinking about care delivery models. At the heart of our argument is a belief that best practice is an issue of competency not craft and if we keep older people 'front and centre' we will continue to successfully develop innovative responses to a changing healthcare environment.

Reflective questions

1. Consider the emergence of new roles for practitioners and discuss this with your colleagues.

2. Given the changes in the health workforce how can other workers be used to fill gaps and support the professional practitioner?

3. How should healthcare delivery be evaluated and by whom?

4. Mentorship programs work well for new practitioners. How could you use such an approach for keeping yourself and staff skilled and competent?

5. Maintaining client-driven care is the future challenge for all healthcare providers. Is your organisation considering this challenge?

References

Australian and New Zealand Society for Geriatric Medicine, 2012. Position statement 13: delirium in older people. Online. Available: http://www.anzsgm.org/documents/PS13DeliriumstatementRevision2012.pdf, 1 May 2013.

Australian Institute of Health and Welfare, 2012b. Dementia in Australia. Cat. no. AGE 70. AIHW, Canberra.

Department of Human Services, 2007. Better skills, best care—stage 1 final report. Online. Available: http://www.health.vic.gov.au/workforce/downloads/bsbc_report_stage01_2007.pdf, 17 Oct 2012.

Department of Human Services, 2004. (unpublished report) Innovative workforce responses to a changing aged care environment. Department of Human Services, Victoria.

Australian Bureau of Statistics, 2011. Population by age and sex, regions of Australia. Online. Available: http://www.abs.gov.au/Ausstats/abs@.nsf/mf/3235.0 17 Oct 2012.

Australian Institute of Health and Welfare, 2012a. Australia's health 2012. Australia's health series no.13. Cat. no. AUS 156. Online. Available: http://www.aihw.gov.au/WorkArea/DownloadAsset.aspx?id=10737422169, 14 Oct 2012.

Barton, A., Mulley, G., 2003. History of the development of geriatric medicine in the UK. Postgrad Med Journal 79, 229–234.

Byles, J., Powers, J., Chojenta, C., et al., 2006. Older women in Australia: ageing in urban, rural and remote environments. Australasian Journal On Ageing 25, 151–157.

Clinical Epidemiology and Health Service Evaluation Unit, 2007. Best practice approaches to minimise functional decline in the older person across the acute, sub-acute and residential aged care settings: update 2007. Melbourne Health. Online. Available: http://docs.health.vic.gov.au/docs/doc/0A1A42D295F67742CA257852000ECC48/$FILE/functional-decline-update.pdf, 1 May 2013.

Commonwealth of Australia, 2012. Living longer, living better. Australian Government, Canberra, pp. 38.

Crilly, R., Harris, D., Stolee, P., et al., 1999. A framework for development of geriatric services in rural areas. Gerontology And Geriatric Education 20, 59–72.

Dainty, P., 2007. Comprehensive geriatric assessment. British Journal of Hospital Medicine 68 (8), M133–M135.

Davis, S., Bartlett, H., 2008. Healthy ageing in rural Australia: issues and challenges. Australian Journal On Ageing 27, 56–60.

Department of Human Services, 2006. Clinical practice guidelines for management of delirium in older people. Victorian Government, Melbourne.

Dyer, C., Ashton, C.M., Teasdale, T.A., 1995. Postoperative delirium. A review of 80 primary data collection studies. Archives of Internal Medicine 155 (5), 461–465.

Fetherstonhaugh, D., Nay, R., Winbolt, M., 2010. Evidence-based health care. In: Liamputtong, P., (Ed.), Research methods in health: a practical guide for the health professions. Oxford University Press, Melbourne, pp. 269–285.

Francis, I., 1992. Delirium in older patients. Journal Of American Geriatric Society 8, 829–838.

Frank, J., Weiss, J., 2012. Public health workforce: preparing for an aging society. In: Prohaska, T., Anderson, L., Binstock, R., (Eds.), Public health for an aging society. The John Hopkins University Press, Baltimore, pp. 275–298.

Gray, L., Yeo, M.A., Duckett, S.J., 2004. Trends in the use of hospital beds by older people in Australia: 1993–2002. MJA 181 (9), 478–481.

Haesler, E.J., Nay, R., O'Donnell, M., et al., 2007. Effectiveness of staffing models in residential/subacute/extended aged care settings (Protocol). Cochrane Database of Systematic Reviews, Issue 3.

Hodgkinson, B., Haesler, E., Nay, R., et al., 2011. Effectiveness of staffing models in residential, subacute, extended aged care settings on patient and staff outcomes.

Cochrane Database of Systematic Reviews, Issue 6. Art. No.: CD006563. DOI: 10.1002/14651858.CD006563.pub2.

Inouye, S.K., Bogardus Jr., S.T., Charpentier, P.A., et al., 1999. A multicomponent intervention to prevent delirium in hospitalized older patients. New England Journal Of Medicine 340 (9), 669–676.

Isaacs, B., 1965. An introduction to geriatrics. Balliere, Tindall And Cassell, London.

Larson, A., 2006. Rural health's demographic destiny. Rural And Remote Health 6, 551–559.

Muir Gray, J., (Ed.), 2001. Evidence-based healthcare. Churchill Livingstone, London.

National Health Workforce Taskforce, 2009. Health workforce in Australia and factors for current shortages. KPMG April 2009.

Nay, R., (Chair) 2003. Aged care enrolled nurse working party report to the minister for ageing. CoA.

Nay, R., Closs, B., 1999. Staff and quality in non-acute facilities, In: Nay, R., Garratt, S., (Eds.), Nursing older people: issues and innovations. MacLennan & Petty, Sydney.

Nay, R., Pearson, A., 2001. Educating nurses to protect the past or to advance health care? A polemic. Australian Journal of Advanced Nursing 18 (4), 37–41.

Pearson, A., Nay, R., Koch, S., et al., 2002. Recruitment and retention of nurses in residential aged care—final report. Commonwealth Department of Health & Aged Care, Canberra.

Productivity Commission, 2005. Australia's health workforce, research report, Canberra, Australian Government Productivity Commission: 397. Online. Available: http://www.pc.gov.au/__data/assets/pdf_file/0003/9480/healthworkforce.pdf, 1 May 2013.

Productivity Commission, 2011. Caring for older Australians, draft inquiry report. Australian Government, Canberra, pp. 507.

Rubenstein, L.Z., Josephson, K.R., Weiland, D., et al., 1984. Effectiveness of a geriatric evaluation unit. New England Journal of Medicine 311, 1664–1670.

Schneiderman, J.U., Waugaman, W.R., Flynn, M., 2008. Nurse social work practitioner: a new professional for health care settings. Health And Social Work 33 (2), 149–154.

Stone, R.I., Benson, W.F., 2012. Financing and organizing health and long-term care services for older populations. In: Prohaska T.R., Anderson L.A., Binstock R.H., (Eds.), Public health for an aging society. Johns Hopkins University Press, Baltimore. pp. 53–73.

Stuck, A., Sui, A.l., Weiland, G.D., et al., 1993. Comprehensive geriatric assessment: a meta-analysis of controlled trials. The Lancet 342, 1032–1036.

Swage, T., (Ed.), 2003. Clinical governance in health care practice. Butterworth Heinemann, Edinburgh.

Van Der Weyden, M., 2007. Challenges and change in medical training: the Australian curriculum framework for junior doctors. Medical Journal of Australia 186 (7), 332–333.

World Health Organization, 2006. International action needed to increase health workforce. WHO, Geneva. Online. Available: http://www.who.int/mediacentre/news/releases/2007/pr05/en/print.html, 12 Oct 2012.

CHAPTER 24

MY JOURNEY OF HEARTBREAK: MY PARENTS AND ALZHEIMER'S DISEASE

Jennifer Carr

Editors' comments

Evidence-based practice is essential to better practice; the client experience and choice are central to evidence-based practice. This chapter is critical for hearing the voices of people living with dementia. Health professionals are frequently criticised for imparting their expertise while forgetting the real experts are the people living with dementia—or any other condition.

This chapter relates the experience of one family faced with both parents developing dementia. The story is presented in a chronological time frame and illustrates the complex maze of interacting forces involved in providing care. Personal feelings of helplessness, frustration, anger and despair are shadowed by love and caring.

This story also highlights the importance of early diagnosis and initiation of support for all concerned. Current information about the illness trajectory, regular medical checks and family discussion are necessary to understand the issues families face. Without a clear pathway for assistance the family is left with increasing anxiety and indecision. The realisation that dementia is a terminal illness and that each person has a different pathway, but palliation will ultimately be necessary, needs to be made clear from the beginning. Unfortunately this is not often the case and families are left floundering. End-of-life issues such as power of attorney, guardianship and admission to care facilities are left until a crisis ensues, often with family disagreements.

There are many issues raised in this story that illustrate the lack of knowledge of healthcare providers. A lack of proper referral and follow-up impacts on how the family copes and ultimately influences the life of the person living with dementia.

INTRODUCTION

In 1987 my husband, Ian, and I made the decision to relocate to Taree, the town of our births where Mum and Dad had always lived. We had enjoyed the opportunities of city life for 10 years. When our first child arrived, a daughter, we were happy to contemplate the more relaxed country lifestyle.

My father had recently undergone surgery for malignant melanoma: this fact provided the immediate impetus for the move. He was approaching the age of 60—Ian could help manage his pharmacy business while Dad could, we assumed, ease himself into retirement at his own pace. Mum was a cancer survivor who had fought through many operations, the legacy of which was an ileostomy. The daily routine required to live with the results of this operation was a burden that Mum faced with strength and bravery.

Two sons soon completed our family, and we enjoyed living in a close-knit, friendly community. Although we didn't 'live in each other's pockets', we saw Mum and Dad regularly. The kids enjoyed having their grandparents nearby. Over the years, Mum and I made a routine of 'our Friday': hairdresser first, shopping, a coffee shop lunch, more shopping, pick the kids up from school, then home. It became sacred and treasured 'us' time.

MY FATHER TED'S STORY

Dad turned 72 in the year 2000. He had worked as a pharmacist all his life, played a major role in community organisations and served as secretary and elder in his church. We started noticing Dad was easily distracted, starting jobs at the pharmacy and leaving them, never to finish. He found it difficult, and sometimes impossible, to learn new computer or workplace procedures. He began to spend more time in his back office, paying bills and doing church correspondence.

Ian and I soon purchased the business outright. Dad hadn't planned for 'retirement', nor did Mum want Dad under her feet as she kept to her rigid daily housekeeping routines. Dad still had a need to attend 'work' every day, so a nearby first-storey office was furnished for him where he could attend to his church business. Once no longer a part of his beloved pharmacy business, Dad sank into a deep depression, feeling he was no longer 'useful'. His doctor put him on antidepressants and anti-anxiety medications, and Dad slowly returned to a semblance of his old self.

Dad loved to play lawn bowls and often won playing pairs' competitions. When knee pain forced him to stop playing, he had a total knee replacement in the local private hospital. It was here we noticed more of Dad's memory issues. He didn't retain instructions, and therefore forgot to buzz the nurses for pain relief. Against orders, he tried to walk himself to the ensuite toilet. At the time, I put this down to depression and the pain of the operation. Dad's recovery wasn't totally successful, and he never returned to bowls or his upstairs office.

OCTOBER 2005

Mum and Dad celebrated their 50th wedding anniversary at a party for family and friends. Our gift to them was a weekend away in the Hunter Valley. Mum was an avid gardener, so I booked a hotel close to the Hunter Gardens: a two and a half hour drive from home that they had taken on several occasions. I checked that Dad's mobile phone was on and charged, gave them a simple

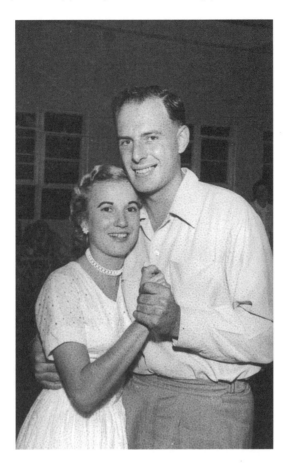

Figure 24.1

Mum and Dad's engagement

printed map with written instructions and phone numbers, and farewelled them, with a request to phone me when they arrived. I estimated this should be around 4 pm.

When I had heard nothing by 6 pm, I rang Dad's mobile phone: no answer. The hotel then rang me, asking if Mum and Dad were still coming. Assuring them they were, I asked the hotel to keep me informed, telling myself I would ring the police if I hadn't heard by 8 pm. When the phone rang at 7.30 pm it was Dad. They had been lost for over two hours. I asked why he hadn't rung me or the hotel for directions. He replied that they were fine and he had forgotten about the mobile. Obviously, so had Mum! Thankfully, the return trip resulted in no further dramas.

Dad was constantly losing things at home, mislaying keys and notes, driving himself and Mum to distraction. He forgot how to use his camera and his laptop computer, so our son Tim wrote out simplified instructions and placed

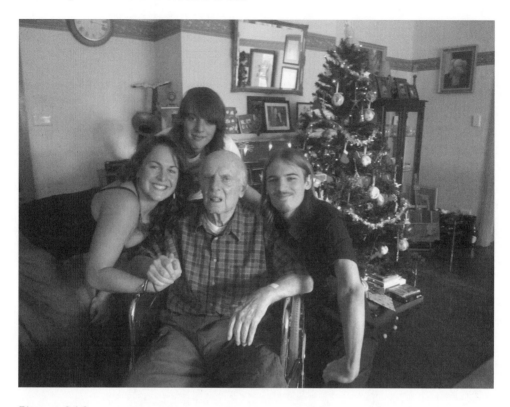

Figure 24.2

Christmas with children

coloured stickers on buttons and keys that Dad needed to use. Tim spent many hours patiently helping Dad, who would ring up at all hours when his devices 'stopped working'. It was usually necessary for Tim to go around and help in person, as telephone instructions were impossible to communicate.

EARLY 2007

Dad's memory was worrying him and us, and his general practitioner (GP) referred him to a specialist physician, not because he thought Dad had dementia but because he thought Dad needed his medications reviewed. This doctor was very understanding and reassuring with Dad, discussed his memory problems, gave him his first mini-mental test and overviewed his medications. Dad had monthly visits. He started Aricept therapy, which seemed to keep him on a plateau for some time. We were told Dad had 'memory issues'; dementia wasn't mentioned. I looked up Aricept and found it was for Alzheimer's disease. I then checked the Alzheimer's Australia website and found out as much as possible about the disease.

OCTOBER 2007

Ian and I spent a week in New Zealand visiting our daughter. While we were away, Dad told Mum he felt unwell and complained of bad headaches. (I had never in my life heard Dad complain of a headache.) On the anniversary of my maternal grandmother's death, Mum and I would always visit her grave and place some flowers. In my absence, Mum asked Dad to drive her. Dad still had the headache but drove to the cemetery nonetheless. As he drove home, Dad told Mum he couldn't see but they continued slowly on, praying that God would get them home safely, Mum directing Dad as he drove. After this, Dad slept all afternoon.

That night, a Friday, he drove downtown to pick up a takeaway meal. As he exited his car, his legs gave way and he fell onto the neighbouring vehicle. Luckily, some friends witnessed the incident and drove Dad home. When Dad's best friend, Alan, called in the following Sunday afternoon, Dad's headache was still present and he was obviously confused. Alan escorted Dad to an emergency department at once but because he was unaware of the recent episodes couldn't relate a full history. After a few hours, Dad was discharged and told to contact his own doctor the next day. By the time a CT scan was arranged, at least a week had elapsed since his sudden headache, and results weren't conclusive. I believe Dad had had a transient ischaemic attack (TIA), possibly his first.

MAY 2008

Our daughter's contemporary dance troupe was to perform in Noumea, New Caledonia, so Ian and I took Mum and Dad and the two boys for a tropical break. We noticed Dad having trouble using his ATM and credit cards, forgetting passwords and even failing to recognise which were which. Back home Dad became quieter, preoccupied and was misplacing things constantly. He took me aside one day and told me: 'I know they're hiding things from me, but I'm not going to let the buggers beat me'. He said he couldn't see them but he knew they were there, hiding his keys, pens and notes. As 2008 progressed, Dad's hallucinations increased but changed to be auditory: the voices sang his favourite songs and hymns to him, and this made him happy.

I convinced Dad to stop driving at night and organised friends to taxi him to Rotary meetings and other gatherings. Both Mum and Dad were upset with me 'putting my foot down' about this issue, which increased to outright anger when I suggested Dad stop driving altogether. Mum could see only that her independence was being taken away—she was in denial about Dad's illness. As Dad continued to drive around town, we did receive reports about the erratic nature of his driving, which we forwarded (anonymously) to the authorities, trusting that the system would at least lead to a re-evaluation of his driving skills. This didn't occur!

JANUARY 2009

Ian, the boys and I were in the middle of planning a European adventure for the Easter school break. We had approached aged care to assess Dad for a 'care package' during our four-week absence. One evening after dinner Mum collapsed in her bedroom. Dad rang me in a panic, unsure of what to do. When I arrived, Mum was on the floor, very hot and semiconscious. The ambulance took her to emergency and I followed with Dad, knowing he would be very anxious waiting alone at home. Mum was discharged from hospital the next day after being rehydrated. We were given no firm diagnosis. She spent the next couple of days in bed as I looked after them both. There were no referrals to specialist assessment or care.

MARCH 2009

Ian had taken Dad to buy himself a new, easier-to-use camera and a TV that displayed subtitles, both of which were becoming increasingly necessary. I joined them at the optician's where Dad collected his new glasses, and he and I headed for the supermarket a short distance up the street. Dad seemed very quiet and started having trouble walking. By the time we got to the supermarket he was shuffling and, when I asked if he was OK, he couldn't answer me. I guided him to a bench and sat him down. After a few minutes I suggested we go home, but he was unable to get up from the bench. With Ian's help, I got him into the car. At home, I strapped Dad's electronic blood pressure machine on him. The reading was very low, so I drove him straight to the doctor's, where they confirmed the blood pressure reading and gave an electrocardiogram. Again, there was no firm diagnosis except a probable TIA.

APRIL 2009

While Ian and I were in Europe with the boys, Dad handed in his driver's licence. To renew it, he needed to take a full driving test, and he recognised the impossibility of this challenge. I was pleased that he was able to make that decision for himself, though it was not a happy one. While we were away the home nursing arranged through aged care were to visit every second day. After two visits, Mum cancelled the service, explaining to me later: 'We didn't need them, and besides I don't like strangers in my house'. In hindsight, it is clear that Mum was having problems of her own, of which I had little suspicion.

JUNE 2009

Early one morning I received an urgent and panicked phone call from Mum. The scene she described, had it not been so immediately serious, could have been a vaudevillian piece of physical comedy. Dad had fallen asleep on the lounge. Mum went over to wake him and tell him to go to bed. Eventually rousing, Dad found he couldn't move his legs, so Mum (150 cm tall) attempted to support Dad (185 cm and quite stocky) as they headed towards the bedroom end of the house. It took many attempts, much effort and about an hour for the pair to stumble up the hallway into the bedroom. Once on the bed, Dad slipped to the floor, immobile. Acknowledging defeat, Mum fetched some quilts and joined Dad and Chocky, the dog, on the floor for the night.

After this (presumed) TIA, Dad's voice hallucinations became more agitated, keeping him awake at night and telling him frightening things. He started pacing at night, keeping Mum up with questions and concerns, often about money. One night, Dad was very agitated and confided to Mum that the voices were telling him to jump in the swimming pool and stay there and not get out. It was after dinner and a wintry winter's night. Mum quickly locked all the doors and called us. Ian and I seemed able to calm Dad down where Mum could not.

As time passed, there were many similar crises. It was very tiring for Mum; she and Dad were arguing a lot. Her attitude to Dad and his illness was becoming quite hostile. Soon Dad was having trouble keeping track of his medication. We changed to a Webster pack dosette system, which worked well for a while. Before long, though, Mum was finding missed tablets on the kitchen floor, and we found that Dad was pushing the wrong day's tablets out, missing some and doubling up on others. I was very upset to see my amazing Dad, a pharmacist for 56 years, unable to cope with his own medications.

When I asked Mum to take charge of his medications, she became very angry, saying that she wasn't going to do any more for him. Again, in hindsight, I should have recognised the warning signs of Mum's struggle to cope. Rather, I was upset with Mum for not wanting to care for Dad the way he had always cared for her.

A FRIDAY INCIDENT

It was on one of my Fridays shopping with Mum. As usual, the first stop was her hairdresser appointment. Mum was ready and waiting when I drove by to pick her up, but I didn't see Dad because he had slept late and was still showering. Once at the hairdresser's, I received a mobile phone call from Ian. Dad had been ringing him at his work, in a panic as to where we were. When I rang him, he explained that his first thought (presumably triggered by a recent news report) was that we had been kidnapped by terrorists. I reassured Dad, but we never left him alone after this incident. One of Dad's friends would spend Fridays with him, taking him on drives where they would enjoy a coffee or ice-cream.

In October 2009 Dad's lifelong best friend Harry passed away after a long battle with Parkinson's disease. By this time, Dad's long experience of public speaking had deserted him, and his words at the funeral were quietly spoken, nervous and a bit confused. Harry's death was a huge blow to Dad and he became sadder, quieter and more withdrawn. In December, the specialist geriatrician told us that Dad's MRI showed the results of many small bleeds over a period of years and a brain image consistent with Alzheimer's.

CARERS' MEETINGS

Mum and I started attending monthly Alzheimer's Australia carers' meetings at a nearby church hall. I gained much help and support from these meetings and enjoyed them.

Mum, on the other hand, found the meetings difficult and used them as a release for her negativity. She would become annoyed if other carers' problems were more trivial than her own. She would tell the group how hard her life was, that she didn't see her retirement being like this. Her life was ruined; being sole carer was just too hard.

The group was well aware that Mum had a great deal of family support. When she claimed the title of 'sole carer', it made Mum sound ungrateful for everything my brother Peter and I were doing. At this point I was managing all finances, paying bills, making appointments, shopping and much more. Peter visited every evening, helped in the garden and had dinner with Mum and Dad every night. Again, I missed clues that Mum wasn't coping well and was in denial about her own problems as much as Dad's.

APRIL 2010: A BEACH HOLIDAY

Our long-time family friend Bruce offered to drive Mum and Dad the 550 km to the Gold Coast for a fortnight's stay at their favourite beachside holiday resort. Bruce was able to stay for the first week and would then return after the second week to drive them home. Driving North, Dad became very anxious and wanted to turn back. Mum wouldn't hear of it. I phoned every night to talk to Mum and Dad but also get a report from Bruce. He was able to tell me that things were not good. Mum and Dad argued often; Mum was sometimes abusive, calling Dad 'stupid' and 'an idiot'. When I spoke to Mum she complained about Dad. When I spoke to Dad, he told me he was always in trouble and that Mum didn't like him.

PRIVATE HOSPITAL

Once home, Dad's hallucinations seemed to be taking over. He couldn't sleep; the voices were loud and distracting. He couldn't sit still to eat his dinner. When Mum insisted he sit down, Dad became angry because he was only doing what 'they', the voices, were telling him. The geriatrician had Dad admitted to the mental health wing of the local private hospital. We didn't foresee that as Dad left his home of 55 years to go to hospital, he would never return.

The psychiatric team at the hospital were wonderfully caring. Dad didn't understand why he was there. I told him it was to treat his depression and that they were going to review his medications. Unfortunately, weeks of adjusting doses and changing to new drugs seemed to do little for Dad's depression or the hallucinations. I was asked to approve a course of electroconvulsive therapy (ECT). Though sceptical, I was assured that good results were possible and that if the depression eased other problems may be more manageable. Dad responded poorly to the ECT, and the course was stopped prematurely.

Dad spent seven weeks in the mental health ward. His hallucinations were increasingly insistent and even more terrifying. At a meeting with the mental health team, we were told they didn't think a return home would be possible. The team were aware of the hostile atmosphere between Mum and Dad, having witnessed a few incidents themselves.

Dad was present with the family when his psychiatrist and his team outlined their treatment plan. He would move to a nursing home, conveniently just across the road from the hospital, for respite care. We explained that Mum wasn't well enough to care for him at home. Whether he believed this entirely,

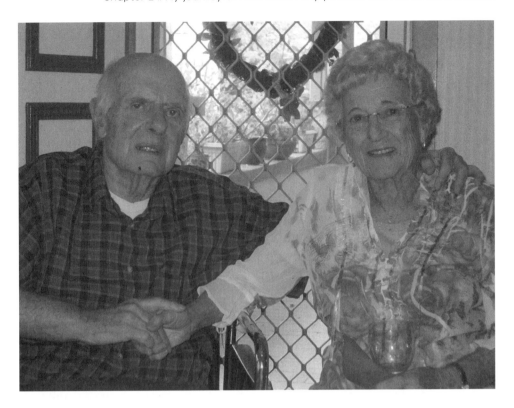

Figure 24.3

Mum and Dad at Christmas

I'm not sure, but Dad seemed to understand his situation: he had the presence of mind to utter a disappointed 'Aw, shit'.

The nursing home was a modern, pleasant place with large outdoor decks and a barbecue area. Dad's friend Harry had lived there and he knew a number of the residents. Dad grew more withdrawn but was happy to have us visit every day and didn't want us to go home. When my brother visited, he would bring Dad's dog, Chocky, which made it a special time for both of them.

SEPTEMBER 2010

Dad's respite time at the home was almost over. I met with the administrator to organise a permanent placement for Dad. Dad's respite time had been in low care, so I was somewhat shocked to be told that Dad was now considered high care. I was informed there had been 'incidents'; Dad had been walking into other residents' rooms at night in a state of undress. I had myself witnessed him running up and down the hallways because the voices told him if he didn't run a kilometre there would be 'consequences'. They said, 'Run, Teddy boy, or else!'.

That same night, Dad was found on his floor, unresponsive. After a few days in hospital, he returned to the home, this time to his permanent room in the dementia-specific wing. Dad's room was down a long corridor, the furthest room from the nurse's station. Though it was quiet, I feel that it reduced Dad's opportunities to interact with other residents and staff. Dad was often a difficult patient. One day, four nurses were required to shower him. I hated the thought of Dad being so disturbed and terrified.

He had obviously taken a big step down after the last TIA. He could no longer care for himself. He had to be reminded to come to meals. He was overwhelmed with hallucinations, which were now sensory as well as auditory. He refused food and was afraid that drinks would 'mix with his blood' and kill him. He believed he couldn't breathe unless he was lying down with his feet raised up against the wall. He claimed his chest was full of woodchips and his legs were filling up with froth.

One male nurse especially took Dad's case to heart and was very proactive and encouraging with Dad. He would call in the hospital's mental health team when things were rough and kept me well informed about Dad's wellbeing, even phoning me to keep me updated. Generally, we felt that the care provided was of a good standard, though it appeared to me that some personnel needed better dementia-specific training. While Mondays to Fridays seemed quite adequately staffed, Saturdays and Sundays seemed to have a skeleton 'locum' staff, less experienced and not familiar to the residents.

Eventually, I made sure I timed a daily visit to help Dad with his lunch. By evening, Dad had little appetite for dinner: 'sundowning' was by now an issue.

It wasn't long before Dad could no longer have his meals in the communal dining room. He was refusing food or spitting it out, and refusing to drink. Dad lost a lot of weight; I had to keep buying smaller, elastic-waisted trousers.

At this stage of my life my two sons were still at home, Ian was working a six-day week and Mum was making many demands on me. I felt this was taking a toll on my own health. By December, Dad had had a couple more trips to emergency for rehydration. He was now frail and needed a wheelchair.

We brought Dad to our house for Christmas dinner. He was anxious on the drive from the nursing home. Despite much coaxing, he refused all offers of food and drink. He was agitated and concerned for his breathing. However, he spent two hours at our home and some lovely family photos were taken. When it was clear that Dad could cope no more, my brother Peter and daughter Lauren drove him back to the home. Lauren returned in tears. Dad had refused to let go of her arm; Peter had to prise open Dad's still-strong grip on her. It was very upsetting for all.

I felt Mum's behaviour throughout this time was strange. Having made a few friends of other carers in the dementia wing, she was happier talking to them than attending to Dad. She wouldn't sit close to him in his room, or hold his hand. She kissed him briefly, only as we were leaving. She became cranky with Dad 'fussing about' with his food, which in turn upset him. It became more practical for me to visit twice: the first time to help Dad, the second time to bring Mum. Dad always wanted me to help him. He would say, 'Jenny, help me, help me', which broke my heart because he could no longer tell me what help he needed.

It was 'policy' for the nursing home to ring the primary carer if a resident had a fall. I began getting calls at all hours about this issue. However, Dad

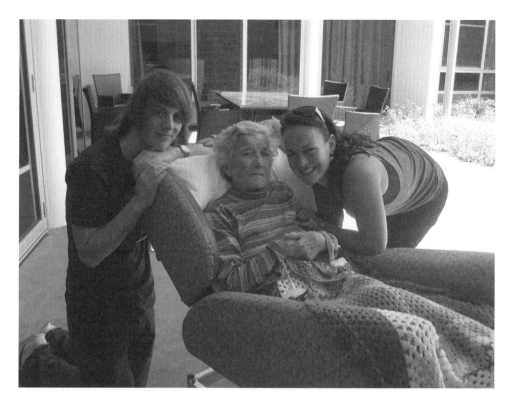

Figure 24.4

Mum with her grandchildren

wasn't falling: he was getting himself down on the ground and crawling, as he had become afraid of falling out of bed and therefore felt safer close to the ground. As Dad's condition deteriorated, he spent most of his time on his bed, not wishing to come out of his room at all. Dad never forgot who we were, or our names, though he did little talking by now. He slept a lot both day and night, and refused food and drink. The only help he accepted was when I gently cleaned his mouth with a lemon swab.

We could see his time was very close. I signed the 'living will' instructing 'Do not resuscitate', one of the most difficult things I have had to do on my own. Dad passed away on 4 March 2011. I had been with him all day. I held his hand as he took his last breath. Mum and Peter, Ian, the boys and my cousins had been in and out all day. A minister friend called and prayed over him. His two most special friends also prayed and sang him hymns before he passed.

Farewell, Dad. You were my hero and inspiration, a devoted husband and father, an adoring grandfather, loving brother, brother-in-law, uncle and loyal friend. You were a successful businessman, pharmacist, community worker, dedicated Christian servant, church secretary and elder.

I miss you so much, but could never wish you back to suffer as you did during those last nine months.

MY MOTHER RUTH'S STORY

During Dad's last few months, had I not been directing most of my energies to his care, I might have been quicker to notice a decline in Mum. There were isolated incidents: she wasn't ready when I picked her up for appointments, or she had been ready for hours, having mistaken the time. She seemed to get lost in the supermarket aisles, once even telling me 'Coles is all back-to-front'.

Soon after Dad's funeral, Mum underwent a dental operation that required a general anaesthetic. Given the option, I booked her in to stay overnight because I was concerned how the anaesthetic might affect her. When I called by to pick her up from home, she was still fussing with her suitcase. Checking, I found she had packed several sets of clothes but forgotten her toiletries and ileostomy gear.

The operation to remove a tooth went well. However, on my arrival the head nurse, G, called me aside. I was shocked when he asked me whether we had had Mum assessed for dementia. Mum had been very upset, confused and angry with the staff overnight. It was clear that the anaesthetic had affected her badly. G suggested we have Mum assessed sooner rather than later. I went to Mum's room fearing the worst and asked her if she was ready to go. She replied angrily: 'No! I feel sick. No one has even come near me today: no doctor, no food and no medication'. In reality, she had enjoyed a big breakfast, and the doctor had seen her that morning. G said he had often observed a huge effect with anaesthetics, even on patients with the mildest dementias.

Having postponed my own knee replacement operation for the duration of Dad's illness, I arranged to have this operation in a Sydney hospital during May 2011. In my absence, Ian and Peter were looking in on Mum regularly, but it was clear she was more anxious than usual without me close by. I didn't realise the extent to which I had become her 'security blanket', usually only a phone call and three-minute drive away.

A week after my operation I was still in Sydney recuperating. It was 8.30 am when Ian received a call from Sandra, Mum's cleaning lady, who couldn't get Mum to answer the door and let her in. Ian soon arrived with spare keys and found Mum in bed, her voice almost inaudible, saying she couldn't move. Ian and Sandra managed to get Mum into her lounge chair, where she was given a cup of tea and seemed to recover well. When Sandra left, Peter arrived to make Mum some lunch, stayed a couple of hours and left.

When Ian and Peter turned up that evening at about 6 pm, Mum hadn't moved from her chair, so they offered to call her doctor. She said she would wait and see. Ian had been home only a few minutes when Peter rang, alarmed, saying he thought Mum was having a stroke. He had been talking to her when she suddenly lost consciousness. The ambulance soon arrived. By that time, Mum had come around and she was duly admitted to hospital on 14 May 2011.

It was obvious Mum was battling multiple problems, the most immediate of which was that her ileostomy, known as a Koch pouch, had collapsed. In this operation, no longer performed, a living pouch is formed at the end of the gut to provide storage for waste. The waste is removed by inserting a tube into the stoma (opening) and a stoma pad reapplied. Most Koch patients had their operations 'converted' to other types over the years.

It was unfortunate that no local surgeon was familiar with Mum's operation. Furthermore, Mum hadn't seen a gastrointestinal specialist since the retirement of her previous one. Through my best friend, a medical professional in Sydney, we located a surgeon who had even trained with Dr Koch, inventor of the operation. The local surgeon liaised by phone and gave Mum a temporary operation that allowed her pouch to be emptied and pressure relieved. Her condition was still serious, so I discharged myself from my own knee rehab and was driven home by my sister-in-law in the company of Ian's mum.

Though her conversation was mostly lucid, Mum reported the oddest delusions, which we put down to her illness and her pain medication. It was arranged for Mum to be sent to Liverpool Hospital by air ambulance. She was there from 31 May until 30 June, when she was transferred to Taree's Mayo Hospital. We couldn't accompany her, so we waved her goodbye in Liverpool. She was smiling and chirpy and enjoying a joke with the driver as she was loaded in. We followed, as immediately as we could, by car. When we arrived at the hospital six long hours later, it was a different Mum who greeted us. She was furious with us: 'How could you leave me here in this *prison*?' We managed to explain things sufficiently, and she calmed down.

We retired to our hotel, dined and I went to bed exhausted and in pain. The next day at the hospital Mum was miserable, said everyone hated her and wanted to go home. However, she brightened up on meeting her specialist, who explained how he planned to fix Mum's operation. She would be put on a liquid diet for a week or two in preparation. Ian and I decided to stay nearby for the length of Mum's hospitalisation. This turned out to be very necessary, as I was receiving phone calls from frantic nurses most mornings requesting that we come quickly. Mum was upset and crying and wouldn't settle until we arrived at about 10 am. Apart from an excursion for lunch, we usually stayed until 7 pm.

Hospitals are simply not equipped to deal with dementia patients. Although Mum hadn't been 'officially' diagnosed, I was constantly asked by doctors and nurses about her dementia. As for me, it was a blow that was just too hard to face so soon after Dad's passing. Finally, two weeks after Mum's admission to Liverpool, Ian and I were waiting in our hotel room for the results of Mum's 'reconstruction' surgery when the specialist rang through. The news was shattering. The envisaged operation wasn't possible due to multiple internal adhesions. The specialist, too, was bitterly disappointed. The only course had been to place a permanent catheter, which would drain into an external ostomy bag.

I rang my brother and Mum's two sisters with the devastating news. We had had such high hopes but now I wondered if Mum would ever be able to live a normal life in her own home. After the operation, Mum was allocated a bed in a shared room with three other patients. She was very anxious and confused, saying she was useless to everyone now. She seemed to understand the implications of the bad news from the specialist. However, this wasn't the feisty, demanding woman who had spent half her life tossing aside adversity. I had never known Mum to be depressed, but she was now quite miserable.

The stoma nurse visited Mum every day to train her into her new routine. The nurse told me Mum was surprised by the bag every time she was taken into the bathroom. 'Does your mother have dementia?'. After four weeks in Liverpool, Mum was discharged to the care of the local private hospital. Closer to home, I thought Mum's outlook and physical condition would improve. She had missed Peter very much and she had many friends who could visit. Mum was convinced she could cope at home. We doubted this, and were relieved that she wouldn't be discharged until she could use her new ostomy bag properly.

Despite daily counselling from the stoma nurse, Mum could never remember that she had a new type of bag. On many occasions, she took herself to the bathroom, pulled off the new bag and attempted her old procedure. Once, she tore out the new, sewn-in catheter, which meant replacement under anaesthetic, followed inevitably by days of confusion. In a final attempt to prevent Mum self-damaging, signs were placed in her room urging her not to empty her bag, and ring for the nurse. We soon realised Mum couldn't remember the call button or how to use it.

During one visit around the third week of this hospital stay, I noticed that Mum's whole body was shaking; she was confused and having trouble talking. When I got home, the hospital phoned to say Mum had had a grand mal seizure, her electrolytes were 'a mess' and she had been placed on a drip. She was sleeping peacefully. The next morning, the story was quite different. Mum had revived to such an extent that she had climbed out of a railed bed and fallen. She seemed to have suffered only a bump or two, but was taken for an x-ray as a precaution.

I had been in touch with Mum's two sisters about her decline, and this was to be the weekend of their visit. Mum was so excited to see them; she was alert and in the best mood I had seen her for months. There was much laughter, many stories of the old days and many hugs. The goodbyes were very emotional and as soon as the visitors had gone, Mum was back in her sad mood.

At that point, the head nurse reported to me that the x-ray had revealed that Mum had fractured her pelvis in the fall. There was no treatment: it would have to heal itself. They had organised for Mum to be transferred to a nursing home the following day. Two weeks before, I had been advised to find Mum a nursing home. I explained that I had hoped Mum could live at home, perhaps with assistance from home nursing. Reluctantly, I agreed that this option was now impossible. The family decided it would be better to place Mum in a different facility from the one that had cared for Dad. We had chosen a newly built, light and airy place surrounded by a large garden.

Mum's move into the home by ambulance was a little traumatic, resulting in pain from her fracture, so she went to bed while I filled out the necessary admission forms with the staff. When we visited the next morning, Mum was comfortably seated in a recliner chair in the vast common room and in good spirits. She introduced us to everyone: 'I've had a lovely trip,' and, pointing to a male nurse, 'That one flew the plane, those others helped me with my luggage'. How amazing it was that we had found her there!

Mum continued to be happy there. The staff was exceptionally devoted to the residents and would always pleasantly greet residents and visitors. In Mum's memory, past and present seemed to fuse. All her loved ones were there with her; her grandma, mother, aunts and my dad joined us in the present day. The daily visiting routine included a leisurely stroll once or twice around the garden,

Mum being pushed in her recliner. Mum could never remember that she had fractured her pelvis and constantly tried to get up from her chair. When we had to leave, she couldn't understand why she couldn't come home with us.

Mum's catheter fell out every two weeks or so. Her GP was able to repair it at the home a couple of times, but the skin around the stoma site was losing condition so the next repair was done by the surgeon in hospital. Again, the general anaesthetic seemed to take a toll and Mum went another step down. I could see Mum moving through the dementia stages week by week.

Mum's emotional lability was extreme. She would cry with joy when she saw us, be instantly cantankerous if we stopped her rising from her chair, and angry when we explained that she couldn't go home with a broken bone. In the late afternoons she became very agitated so Mum spent most evenings in her recliner near the nurses' station, even being wheeled alongside as they did their rounds. She often spent much of the night awake, and her management proved a real challenge for the staff and her doctors.

I arrived one day to find Mum nursing a baby doll. Unaware that this was considered a therapy for dementia patients, I found this sight upsetting and confronting. I was told that the doll had been given to Mum the previous night as a last resort to calm her down. I granted my permission to continue the doll therapy. In Mum's mind, Blue Boy was her real baby and she guarded him jealously. At this time, Mum's speech deteriorated quite suddenly. All she could do was constantly repeat short phrases: 'come on, come on, come on'. If any of us asked Mum a question, she would repeat her phrase as if it were appropriate to the conversation.

Trying to escape the confines of her chair, Mum had a few falls while at the home. After one fall, I had to accompany Mum to her doctor's surgery in a wheelchair taxi so a big gash to her forehead could be stitched. At the doctor's, and despite the presence of Blue Boy, Mum was very agitated, thrashing around and yelling. I had to physically restrain her myself, one of the most distressing things I have been asked to do.

The next day, Mum hovered between sleep and agitation, and the nurses decided to send Mum to hospital as a precaution, thinking that the fall might have led to a serious bleed. I went directly to the emergency department where I found four staff trying to hold Mum down. Though she had been sedated in preparation for x-rays and scans, Mum was still resisting enough that she had to be held down for them by a burly security guard. I was shaking with distress at this point, and had a headache. Mum was being kept in, so the doctor suggested I go home and get some rest. Mum spent a couple of days in hospital, mostly asleep. A family member had to be there at mealtimes because the catering staff simply delivered the trays. There was no staff available to sit and feed patients in Mum's condition.

On day three, we met the doctor as he did his rounds. The x-rays and scans had found no new problems, but we were finally given confirmation that Mum's brain had signs of atrophy typical of Alzheimer's. She was to be discharged back to the nursing home. To multiply Mum's indignities, her hospital visit had resulted in a crush injury to her left thumb. When swabbed and tested, it turned out to be golden staph. To stop Mum interfering with the dressing, her hand was bound up tightly in a sock taped securely onto her wrist. Though we attended to help feed Mum as many meals as we could and help her drink, she was losing a lot of weight. She slept most of the day and tended to stay awake at night.

On 17 September 2011 our youngest son turned 18. Though Mum was asleep when Ian, Lauren, Jeremy and I arrived, we woke her gently to share a celebratory cake and take some photos. We positioned her recliner outside overlooking the garden. She was very happy to see us and, as we started to sing *Happy Birthday*, she joined in with enthusiasm. It was a wonderful moment. It had been weeks since Mum had spoken more than single words.

In early October Ian and I spoke at some length with the home's consultant geriatric psychiatrist. As we had presumed and feared, she told us that Mum was 'a very sick woman' and that her body had already started the process of 'shutting down'. We were told to prepare ourselves for 'the call'. That event came sooner than we imagined. Early on 9 October, the home called us in. Mum's vital signs were very low. Ian and I arrived to find Mum wrapped in blankets, shaking and jerking, waving her arms around. We heard her shout 'Margaret' (her sister's name) loudly, but that was the last thing she spoke.

The nurse asked if I wished to send her to hospital. I preferred that she stay. It was the attitude of the staff that Mum was in her home, and they wanted to look after her there. Once again, I signed the 'do not resuscitate' paperwork. Peter arrived, and though he was aware of Mum's fast decline, he was quite shocked and disbelieving when I told him of what was happening. The GP arrived to organise a morphine pump, and Mum was settled into bed. I was told she had perhaps 24–48 hours.

We started making phone calls to relatives and friends from the room. Peter, presumably finding it hard to cope, left after an hour or so. Ian fetched our boys to farewell their grandma. The home's kitchen provided a tray of beautiful sandwiches, cakes and drinks for us. The nurses took exceptional care of Mum, brushing her hair, putting cream on her lips, treating her with love and respect. One of my dearest friends, Kim, arrived, and stayed while Ian took the boys home. Other friends came and went, by then, I was numb.

As Kim left to make us some dinner, Ian arrived. A mobile phone call took him out of the room. I looked over at Mum. She looked peaceful; I felt peaceful. I could see her lips were turning purple. She had gone, and I kissed her.

Vignette

Hallucinations are a false perception having no relation to reality and not accounted for by any exterior stimulus. They may be visual, olfactory, auditory, tactile or gustatory (Taber's Cyclopedic Medical Dictionary 2001). The person experiencing a hallucination is unable to distinguish between the real and imaginary. Hallucinations may be brought on by feelings of isolation, loneliness, abandonment or alienation (Ebersole et al 2007). The origins of hallucinations are often difficult to separate but specific areas of brain activity are the basis for the types of hallucinations.

Mrs Brown was admitted to a nursing home because of her deteriorating mental health state. She presented with signs of dementia—wandering, calling out and poor cognitive ability. She also had a diagnosis of age-related macular degeneration (AMD). The staff had to constantly remind her where she was and to try to help her exclude the hallucinations she exhibited. One repeating hallucination was that her bedroom was her childhood room and had wallpaper of daisies and fairies on all walls. She would ask the staff whether they liked the paper and told them her father had put it up for her when she was five or six. Staff agreed they all liked the wallpaper and tried to prompt Mrs Brown to tell them other stories about her childhood. She wasn't agitated about this hallucination but as her dementia progressed and her blindness became worse the visual disturbances became more frightening. These visual hallucinations occurred regularly until she changed to a terminal state of dementia.

Diagnosing hallucinations due to dementia or because of visual disturbances are not usually attempted. In people who are not experiencing dementia they can understand that what they are seeing is not real; however, with the added burden of dementia with no insight this is not possible. With AMD the possibility of Charles Bonnet syndrome (CBS) being the cause of the visual hallucinations because of loss of sight is not considered because there is no medical cure.

The things people see with CBS fall into two categories:

- simple repeating pattern
- complex hallucinations of people, landscapes or objects (RNIB 2011). The only treatment is to recognise the symptoms as a disease and not a mental health problem. Unfortunately, combined with dementia, the use of drugs to influence behaviour often exacerbates visual hallucinations.

The intervention of staff to move the person to another environment, changing the level of lighting, ensuring the person is not left alone and listening to try to defuse the concern can help. Hallucinations are usually frightening occurrences and require genuine understanding from care staff that the reality of the person has changed. Requesting eye checks for suspected AMD should be regularly conducted by an ophthalmologist.

Reflective questions

1. Diagnosing dementia is often difficult. What are the two most important assessment tasks to consider in forming a diagnosis?
2. What could be done to improve family support following diagnosis?
3. Differentiate between hallucinations, delirium and depression.
4. Consider what could be done to improve care in the acute hospital environment for people who have a dementia.
5. Examine your state's legal position on end-of-life directions, such as enduring power of attorney, guardianship, living wills and advance care planning.

References

Ebersole, P., Hess, P., Touhey, T., et al., 2007. Toward healthy aging: human needs and nursing response. Mosby, St Louis.

RNIB, 2011. Charles Bonnet syndrome. Online. Available: http://www.rnib.org.uk/eyehealth/eyeconditions/conditionsac/pages/charles_bonnet.aspx, 23 Jan 2013.

Taber's cyclopedic medical dictionary, nineteenth ed. 2001. F A Davis & Co, Philadelphia.

Further reading

Alzheimer's Australia information publications at www.alzheimers.org.au.

Bryden, C., 1998. (Revised edition 2012) Who will I be when I die: dementia from an insider's perspective. Jessica Kingsley Publishers, London.

Bryden, C., 2005. Dancing with dementia. Jessica Kingsley Publishers, London. Further information can be obtained from www.christinebryden.com.

Davidson, A., 2006. A Curious kind of widow: loving a man with advanced Alzheimer's. Fithian Press, McKinleyville, CA.

Fazio, S., 2008. The enduring self in Alzheimer's disease: getting to the heart of individualised care. Health Professions Press, Baltimore.

Hudson, R., (Ed.), 2003. Dementia nursing: a guide to practice. Ausmed Publications, Melbourne.

Kitwood, T., 1998. Dementia reconsidered: the person comes first. Open University Press, Buckingham.

Long, C., 2009. Palliative care for advanced dementia—approaches that work. Journal of Gerontological Nursing 35 (11), 19–24.

Pieters-Hawke, S., Flynn, H., 2003. Hazel's journey: a personal experience of Alzheimer's. Macmillan, Sydney.

CHAPTER 25

VISIONARY LEADERSHIP FOR A 'GREYING' HEALTHCARE SYSTEM

John Daly, Debra Jackson and Rhonda Nay

Editors' comments

For any of the ideas discussed in this book to be translated into everyday policy and practice there is a requirement for great leadership. Doing things differently is always difficult and there are always the barriers and groups of resistance. In order to support the change the philosophy, culture, system and processes all need to be aligned with each other and staff have to see the change as a good thing. Great leadership will understand people as whole, human beings—not things to be restructured! Great leadership will sell the change so staff and all stakeholders see it as logical, engaging and meaningful.

INTRODUCTION

Our healthcare system, consumers and providers, are ageing. People over the age of 65 years use the most bed days, consume the most community care, and are the majority of residents in long-term care. Health professionals are increasingly over the age of 45 years. To ensure resources are used appropriately and consumers receive quality care requires visionary leadership. This is not a time for doom and gloom, but it is necessary that government, health professionals, industry providers, researchers, and educators 'do things differently'. More money for more of the same is not the answer. Too often management prevails and leadership is forgotten as individuals in leadership positions who lack leadership qualities and skills bounce from managing one crisis to the next. This book is about improving care for older people; for the ideas and innovations to flourish, leadership is essential. So what do we know about leadership in healthcare?

WHAT DO WE KNOW ABOUT LEADERSHIP IN THE HEALTHCARE CONTEXT?

Despite widespread acknowledgment of the importance of effective and responsive leadership in the healthcare context (Daly et al 2010, Jackson 2008a, Schwartz & Tumblin 2002), the scholarly discourses around leadership in healthcare are still relatively scant. In 2004 Dowton (2004) considered articles indexed over more than 30 years in five Australian journals (*The Medical Journal of Australia, Australian & New Zealand Journal of Surgery, Australian & New Zealand Journal of Psychiatry, Australian Family Physician*, and the *Journal of Internal Medicine* and its predecessor) and could barely find 50 articles dealing with leadership. Furthermore, very few of these 50 articles, editorials or letters provided substantial information or commentary on the makings of leadership. One regionally relevant and accessible electronic archive of medical interest, the electronic *Medical Journal of Australia*, does not index 'leadership', and in more than 3800 entries has but three items with 'leadership', 'lead' or 'leader' in the title (Dowton 2004 p 2).

Vance and Larson (2002) undertook a review of leadership research in healthcare and business for the period 1970–1999. From a review of 6628 articles they concluded that, to date, the literature on leadership in the discourses around health and business has been primarily 'descriptive'. Writing more than a decade later on transformational leadership, Hutchinson and Jackson (2013) also note that the literature is largely uncritical and generally devoid of gendered and cultural considerations. Although work in the social sciences indicates that leadership styles can have a major influence on performance and outcomes, minimal transfer of this work to the health system is evident. Limited research on leadership and healthcare outcomes exists, such as changes in patient care or improvements in organisational outputs (Hutchinson & Jackson 2013). In this era of evidence-based practice, such research, though difficult to conduct, is 'urgently needed' (Vance & Larson 2002 p 165).

On the other hand, Hamlin notes that:

> ... *much research has been done over the past thirty years or so concerning the study of managerial and leadership behaviour. However, the majority of studies have almost exclusively been focused on the 'absolute' or relative 'frequency' of observed behaviours, or on the amount of time devoted to particular activities, and not on the 'quality' or 'mastery' of specific behaviours associated with either effective or ineffective management and leadership.*

(Hamlin 2002 p 248)

Nursing—as opposed to healthcare generally—has a more established literature on leadership that has likely been brought about by the pressures faced by the discipline over the past two decades. In the Australian context these pressures have been caused (at least in part) by the transfer of education from hospitals to the education sector. This transfer resulted in a loss of a layer of senior nurse leaders from the health sector, as many educators and tutor sisters moved from health into education (Mannix et al 2006). Furthermore, the transfer created a need to ensure that leadership models to support the entry of new graduates were in place. Internationally, nursing has been grappling with acute and chronic shortages of nurses, particularly in specialty areas. These pressures have resulted in exploration of various leadership models that might assist in retaining staff and developing a sustainable workforce (e.g. see Jackson 2008a, Thyer 2003). The nursing literature identifies various models and styles of leadership, ranging from the very bureaucratic and autocratic styles of leadership, through to the charismatic and relationship-based approaches. The latter approaches have found particularly fertile ground in nursing (Jackson 2008b) and we have seen the emergence of models that embrace concepts such as mentoring and a focus on creating and enhancing collegial relationships and personal growth (Grossman 2007). However, though there is considerable literature on leadership in nursing, it has been dominated, rather uncritically, by transformational leadership, and there has only been very limited examination of the 'darker' sides of leadership (Hutchinson & Jackson 2013).

HOW DOES THE CURRENT AND FUTURE HEALTHCARE CONTEXT AFFECT LEADERSHIP?

Leaders in healthcare are challenged to lead constituents within the context of an ever-changing, highly politicised and volatile environment (Jackson & Daly 2011). The health system in Australia has undergone enormous change in the past two decades. It is clear that this change will continue as governments strive to meet current and projected challenges while working to create new systems of care that are cost-effective, based on evidence, equitable, accessible, responsive and of good quality. Health disparities exist in Australia, and Indigenous and other marginalised people in particular have needs that must be addressed so that their health outcomes match those of the mainstream population. The needs of the population for healthcare are predicted to increase due to a number of factors, for example, population growth, ageing and the growing incidence and burden of chronic disease. Growth in the prevalence of chronic disease is likely to be influenced by alcohol and drug abuse, poverty, socioeconomic disadvantage, unhealthy lifestyle and diet, and possibly climate change (Australian Government 2008).

Leaders in healthcare are challenged to lead constituents within the context of an ever-changing, highly politicised and volatile environment.

In 2006 people aged older than 65 years constituted 13% of the Australian population, and this is predicted to increase to 24% by 2036 (Australian Government 2008). The burgeoning costs of acute care and management of chronic diseases (many of which are a consequence of lifestyle) are currently under scrutiny. Without changes in health involving the community, these costs may become unaffordable. A re-conceptualisation of health and healthcare may see more expenditure on disease prevention and health promotion, which has been held at low levels in the past. It is clear from the recent Australia 2020 Summit that healthcare reform is on the agenda.

Change in the Australian health system in the past two decades has presented significant challenges for health professional groups and required them to adapt to: new health service policy environments; professional role changes; new models of care; diminishing resources for health with concomitant increases in demand for health services; workforce supply and demand issues; the rise of consumerism; rising levels of litigation in healthcare; and greater levels of uncertainty. This is a global phenomenon across developed countries. Leatt and Porter note that:

> In the last decade, healthcare throughout the world has experienced broad strategic management strategies, such as re-structuring, regionalisation, downsizing of personnel, reduced bed capacity, and decreased funding. At the same time consumers are expecting higher quality services, more information about treatment options, as well as more accountability for performance. At the service delivery level, health professionals are burnt out, feel undervalued and under-rewarded, have lost trust in their employers and governments, and appear dissatisfied. Health service workers appear more resistant to change and less open to creativity and to innovation.

(Leatt & Porter 2003 p 22)

Conflict has also been a feature of the healthcare landscape in Australia in the past decade, often between senior clinician leaders in healthcare and health bureaucrats, because of differing perceptions regarding the most appropriate distribution of resources for healthcare, health service priorities and sometimes resentment at what may be seen as unnecessary interference by government in roles and accountabilities of health professionals. Philosophical incongruence (rhetoric versus reality) can also impact on harmonious development and delivery of healthcare. Many health professionals are, for example, educated in a person-centred approach, a principle embedded in the rhetoric of many healthcare systems, which then demand tight economic efficiency in resourcing to a level where it becomes impossible to operationalise the aspiration of 'person-centredness' in actual practice (Jackson & Raftos 1997, Lumby & Duffield 1994). The driver can become a systems focus on leanness and getting tasks completed quickly. The notion of multidisciplinary teams is also a part of the rhetoric, yet team dysfunction often undermines efforts to assure quality care. Indeed the notion of team in healthcare remains contested, and not all health professionals subscribe to the notion of multidisciplinary healthcare as appropriate to all contexts (Saltman et al 2007). This is problematic and adverse events in healthcare can be attributed to a number of factors, including poor collaboration and communication in healthcare teams (Manojlovich et al 2008).

Philosophical incongruence between person-centred approaches and high levels of tight economic accountability can impact on harmonious development and delivery of healthcare.

Manojlovich et al observe that:

> Research from other disciplines interested in finding solutions has been recently focused on two key areas: conceptualizing the hospital as a high-reliability organisation and developing a safety component in the overall organisational culture. In both cases, teamwork and collaboration are stressed … and nursing collaboration is becoming more prevalent in safety culture studies.

(Manojlovich et al 2008 p S12)

Recent expert deliberations about how the health system of the future will need to be structured foreshadow a system that is much more focused on prevention and primary care—one that is 'person centric' rather than 'hospital and physician centric' (Talsma et al 2008 p S19). In Australia the National Health and Hospitals Reform Commission will address a number of key themes in its work in efforts to re-shape healthcare systems. It will provide advice on the framework for the next Australian Health Care Agreements (AHCAs), including robust performance benchmarks in areas such as (but not restricted to): elective surgery, aged and transition care, and quality of healthcare; reducing inefficiencies generated by cost-shifting, blame-shifting and buck-passing; better integrating and coordinating care across all aspects of the health sector, particularly between primary care and hospital services around key measurable outputs for health; bringing a greater focus on prevention to the health system; better integrating acute services and aged care services and improving the transition between hospital and aged care; improving frontline care to better promote healthy lifestyles and prevent and intervene early in chronic illness; improving the provision of health services in rural areas; improving Indigenous health outcomes; and providing a well-qualified and sustainable health workforce into the future (Council of Australian Governments 2007 p 5).

The scale and breadth of these issues, which may be embraced in any health system reform agenda, appear daunting. Workforce in health will continue be one of the major issues into the future. This is a global challenge that will need to be met to enable adequate delivery of healthcare (World Health Organization 2006). Numerous national and international strategies have been developed in attempting to address workforce shortages; however, if ambitious reforms to healthcare and its delivery are to be realised, then role changes and the nature of health work broadly will need to be re-shaped. The model for the health workforce and health professions (including how they are educated) as it currently exists is unlikely to be able to deliver what will be needed in healthcare delivery in the future.

If ambitious reforms to healthcare and its delivery are to be realised, then role changes and the nature of health work broadly will need to be re-shaped.

The health environment is also challenged by chronic and acute staff shortages and an ageing workforce (Jackson 2008c, Watson 2005).

This challenges leaders to work to create optimal environments that are supportive and contribute to healthy and positive workplaces. Indeed, the need for good leadership in current healthcare systems has been acknowledged across a range of health professional groups (Daly et al 2010, Davidson et al 2006, Dowton 2004, Firth-Cozens & Mowbray 2001, Jackson 2008a, Leatt & Porter 2003). In addition, the dearth of leaders in clinical practice in health systems and the need for growth in leadership capacity have also been clearly articulated as fairly urgent priorities in healthcare (Garling 2008).

Leadership capacity is seen as an important part of the solution to inefficient, suboptimal management, poor coordination of services in healthcare, improved patient/client care, and the realisation of improved health outcomes (Firth-Cozens & Mowbray 2001, Wong & Cummings 2007). Effective leadership is essential in order to support both the development of a skilled and ethical workforce and support optimal clinical outcomes. Failures by leaders to respond appropriately to clinical and workplace concerns have been linked to negative working and clinical environments (Jackson et al 2012). However, it has been argued that existing governance models in healthcare are anachronistic and not appropriate to contemporary management challenges and needs (Schwartz & Tumblin 2002). In considering doctors as leaders, Gregor (2006) observes that medical practitioners are required to shift from traditional models of care to those that foster integrated care delivery, development of collaborative partnerships and relationships and facilitate patient self-management. Effective leadership is needed to smooth the progress of these cultural changes. Dowton argues that:

> Leadership is ultimately a social function within an organisation or group. Any consideration of leadership which begins with aphorisms about influence, control, motivation, inspiration, leading by example and so forth, avoids the need to consider the nature of organisations of the modern world. Regrettably, the role of leaders in modern professional and service organisations often continues to focus on a hierarchical view of leadership as a part of the mechanical view of organizations (i.e., thinking of an organisation as a machine in which all parts can be understood in detail). In such a view, power, control and outcomes arise through the division of labour and differentiation of functions—the command and control model. Significant parts of healthcare systems in Australia remain locked in this paradigm.

Source: S Bruce Dowton. Leadership in medicine: where are the leaders?. Med J Aust 2004;181(11):652–654. © Copyright 2004 The Medical Journal of Australia—reproduced with permission

Healthcare is an extremely complex and highly political area. Effective leadership will be crucial in achieving any improvements in the health system and in healthcare in the future. This has implications for health professional education and the sustainability of health systems and the future of discrete health disciplines. Capacity building for leadership roles in healthcare needs to be firmly on the agenda. There is evidence to support the view that the current model of health system and healthcare can actually constrain efforts to provide effective leadership in many settings (Jackson et al 2012). Power, influence, control and tradition are factors in this, and achieving sustainable change at system, organisational or unit level requires some examination of these issues.

Medical practitioners are required to shift from traditional models of care to those that foster integrated care delivery, development of collaborative partnerships and relationships, and facilitate patient self-management.

WHO CAN BE A LEADER?

The capacity to provide effective leadership should not be seen as linked to positional power only; all members of a team can exercise timely and effective leadership (Daly et al 2010, Jackson 2008a, Kouzes & Posner 2002). Leaders without positional power exert influence through persuasive means (Jackson 2008a), and so would likely have highly developed interpersonal skills. Indeed, in understanding that leaders can emerge from any level of an organisation, there is recognition that leadership is associated more with activities, personal qualities and characteristics than position and status (Jackson 2008a).

All members of a team can exercise timely and effective leadership.

In arguing the merits of leadership as an 'activity', Ronald Heifetz—a psychiatrist and leadership academic at Harvard University—notes:

This allows for leadership from multiple positions in a social structure. A president and a clerk can both lead. It allows for use of a variety of abilities depending on the demands of the culture and the situation. Personal abilities are resources for leadership applied differently in different contexts. As we know, at times they are not applied at all. Many people never exercise leadership, even though they have the personal qualities we might commonly associate with it. By unhinging leadership from personality traits, we permit observations of the many ways in which people exercise plenty of leadership everyday without 'being leaders'.

(Heifetz 1994 p 20)

Within the complex field of healthcare, leadership capacity is perhaps best guided by agreed levels of legitimacy (Heifetz 1994), competency and scope of practice within clinical care teams. In recent times, frameworks that guide clinical decisions across levels of health workers in some fields could assist in this regard. Individuals need, however, to be taught to exercise good leadership. As Dowton (2004 p 2) notes, '[c]linical mastery or eminence in discipline-specific research does not necessarily translate into an ability to lead'.

BEING AND GROWING LEADERS

Leadership is a complex activity and an in-depth discussion of all theories of leadership is beyond the scope of this chapter. Kouzes and Posner (2002) define leadership, in part, as 'an identifiable set of skills and practices that are available to all of us, not just a few charismatic men and women' (p 20). Leadership can be conceptualised in many ways, for example, as an activity (Heifetz 1994) or a relationship (Kouzes & Posner 2002).

Leaders are said to have a range of qualities that they bring to bear in leading. Leaders are said to have 'initiative, self-control, commitment, talent, honesty, credibility and courage' (Kelley 1988 p 146), emotional intelligence and vision (Jackson 2008a). They are able to demonstrate credibility (Kouzes & Posner 2002) and exercise 'power and authority and influence' (Heifetz 1994 p 20). Effective leaders can facilitate the development of high-performing teams, which is reflected in organisational performance and work environments that are conducive to good performance and high levels of job satisfaction for many employees. They are able to inspire commitment to organisational goals, and motivate and enthuse staff. Good leaders are also concerned with development and maintenance of work environments that promote psychological and physical safety where staff retention is optimised. Sutton (2007) argues that civility in the workplace has a bearing on organisational performance and so there is an imperative on leaders to actively promote workplace civility and appropriately manage incivility.

Though leadership qualities held by individuals will often become apparent, even in very hierarchical and bureaucratic environments, there are certain leadership styles that will facilitate and nurture the leadership potential of constituents, while other leadership approaches can have the opposite effect (Jackson 2008a). There is quite a body of evidence that leadership style can greatly influence culture and outcomes in the health environment (Jackson et al 2012). It is important that individuals therefore reflect on the sort of leadership they want to show (Cummings 2012). Good leaders facilitate the development of leadership potential in others in the organisation. This can be achieved through providing opportunities to lead and in ensuring mentoring or other supportive frameworks are in place to support individuals to develop leadership skills.

There are certain leadership styles that will facilitate and nurture the leadership potential of constituents.

Kelley makes the point that:

> We are convinced that corporations succeed or fail, compete or crumble, on the basis of how well they are led. So we study great leaders of the past and present and spend vast quantities of time and money looking for leaders to hire and trying to cultivate leadership in the employees we already have ... Leaders matter greatly. But in searching so zealously for better leaders we tend to lose sight of the people these leaders will lead. Without his armies, after all, Napoleon was just a man with grandiose ambitions. Organisations stand or fall partly on the basis of how well their followers follow.

(Kelley 1988 p 142)

He suggests that:

> ... *effective followers share a number of essential qualities:*
> * *they manage themselves well;*
> * *they are committed to the organization and to a purpose, principle, or person outside themselves;*
> * *they build their competence and focus their efforts for maximum impact;*
> * *they are courageous, honest, and credible.*

(Kelley 1988 p 144)

Some of the great leaders include John F Kennedy, Martin Luther King, Emily Pankhurst, Nelsen Mandella, Mahatma Ghandi and Aung San Sui Kyi. Although they fought for different things, in different ways they shared the capacity to get others to see their vision and follow their dreams. All suffered extraordinarily for their dreams. Leaders in our healthcare system are not asked to die or be imprisoned for their beliefs, but it does take courage to lead in any context. Ours is a society that by and large does not like change—leadership inevitably brings change. By definition leaders face resistance, hostility, criticism and constant opposition. Sharing the vision and the leadership across all levels of an organisation (from the gardener to the board chair) increases buy-in and, as Taoist philosopher Lao Tzu (600 BC—531 BC) is reported to have said, a leader 'is best when people barely know he exists. When his work is done, they will say: we did it ourselves' (Thinkexist.com 2013). The following vignette demonstrates how visionary leadership in the care of older people might look.

Vignette

Covey (2005 p 21) argues that 'human beings are not things needing to be motivated and controlled; they are four dimensional—body, mind, heart and spirit' and leadership is about working to unleash their full potential. How apt is such a view in the context of this chapter?

Let yourself imagine or recall a case where the leadership was lacking:

The mood of the place is low. Staff grumble; there is never any laughter in the corridors. Everyone is worried about their job. Managers are pushed to find more and more savings—cuts in budgets are unpredictable except that they keep happening. There is no rationale or plan given for why the cuts occur where they do. The CEO has changed three times in the past four years. No one seems to know where the place is headed. On the rare occasion when the boss is seen she does not greet staff, patients or families and looks entirely miserable. Indeed, staff are quite sure she does not even know who they are or what they do. There is no enthusiasm or creativity. Why take a risk in this environment? Keep your head low and hope it does not get chopped.

There is a registrar who hates working with older people, especially those with dementia. Her response to any call for assistance is to order more antipsychotics. Never are any issues investigated as 'they are going to die anyway and they are blocking beds more deserving and interesting cases should have'. The other staff discuss the appalling care

but decide whistleblowers would not be tolerated—might hit the
newspapers and damage the service's reputation. The last person to
raise a concern was made redundant very smartly!

Of course when it is coming up to accreditation we get paint
slapped around and appear to have the required equipment, staff and
other resources—wish it happened every week.

We have to take students from the university—they just take up
tearoom space and want to observe everything; get in the road more
likely. The person who is supposed to supervise them can never be
found and they only stay a few hours and bugger off. None of them
really know what they can and can't do. I just send them to do
showers.

We used to have a nice place where staff, families and patients
gathered (smokers) and it was amazing how much you learned about
them—seemed to relax. Now we have to walk for miles and stand on the
road in the rain. Apparently it is a 'health promotion' thing. I don't feel
very healthy standing out here freezing to death. As for the poor
buggers from palliative care—guess they can save on morphine 'cos
they will die of pneumonia. Anyway I can retire soon.

Now turn that around and imagine great leadership:

The mood of the place is alive. Staff are busy but happy; there is
laughter in the corridors. Everyone is excited about their job. Managers
are pushed to find more and more savings but this has all been
discussed with us and we understand. Together we identified areas when
we could make savings without loss of jobs while still maintaining good
care. We have had the same management team for years and they are
fantastic. They are forever coming around, know us by name and what
we do. Jean always comes around and visits the patients and we have to
tell her all about them—in front of them—and then they tell us if we
missed anything. It helps rapport and makes us more person centred I
reckon. There is so much enthusiasm and creativity. We are encouraged
to take risks—so long as no one suffers—and if there is a stuff up no one
gets the blame; we just look for another solution.

As soon as staff got suspicious about polypharmacy it was reported
to our manager. Audits were done and when it was evidenced that
indeed this was polypharmacy at its worst and older people were not
receiving appropriate evidence-based care the doctor was reported and
given a choice of undertaking specialist dementia training with a
geriatrician or face disciplinary action. The whistleblowers received an
award for saving lives and having the ethics and courage to come
forward.

Accreditation is never a worry here 'cos we go well beyond
compliance; we're all so proud to show and speak out about our better
practices.

We love to take students from the university—they keep us on our toes
and reflecting on our practices. We have worked with the university to
develop the curriculum and clinical expectations. We also worked on the
assessment. So everyone knows what is expected and we are on the
same page. It is such a shame we can't have students all year round—
it's just great fun.

With the new regulations around smoking the hospital had to move
us from where we gathered for tea and lunch breaks. We understood
that as health professionals we should give up—but we negotiated a plan
with management and they have provided a nice space protected from
the elements provided we all attend the Quit program. Even the families
and patients come along. Some have given up.

Reflective questions

1. Where would you want to work?

2. What are the elements of leadership that you can identify from these vignettes?

3. At what level of the organisation are they apparent?

CONCLUSION

Though it is seldom easy, leadership can be challenging and rewarding. Effective leadership in today's volatile health context requires courage, vision and the ability to create care environments in which organisational objectives can be achieved, while simultaneously ensuring positive and supportive working settings for staff. In care of older people, there is real scope for leaders to make a difference and contribute to creating high-quality, flexible and responsive living and care settings, as well as stimulating, rewarding and exciting working environments.

Reflective questions

1. Change of direction in any system of care delivery takes courage and commitment. How can boards and chief executive officers influence a visionary approach to person-centric care delivery?

2. A complex system not only has to provide care for clients but also has to value its staff. How can an organisation become person-centric for all concerned in the system?

3. Daring to be different is often tried but not sustained. Consider the factors that can impede a new vision from being followed.

4. New ways of doing work are needed in aged care services. The workforce is ageing itself and younger workers are not being attracted to the field. Various incentives are currently being offered to attract health professionals to work in aged care. Consider the advantages as well as the disadvantages of aged care work. Sell your job to a new prospective employee.

References

Australian Government, 2008 Australia 2020 Summit long-term health strategy. Unpublished, Canberra.

Council of Australian Governments, 2007. National health and hospitals reform commission terms of reference, communique. Online. Available: http://www.coag.gov.au/coag_meeting_outcomes/2007-12-20/cooag20071220.pdf, 18 Aug 2008.

Covey, S., 2005. The 8th habit. Free Press, New York.

Cummings, G., 2012. Your leadership style—how are you working to achieve a preferred future? Journal of Clinical Nursing 21, 3325–3327.

Daly, J., Speedy, S., Jackson, D. (Eds.), 2010. Nursing leadership. Churchill Livingstone, Sydney.

Davidson, P.M., Elliott, D., Daly, J., 2006. Clinical leadership in contemporary clinical practice: implications for nursing in Australia. Journal of Nursing Management 14, 180–187.

Dowton, S.B., 2004. Leadership in medicine: where are the leaders? The Medical Journal of Australia 181, 652–654.

Firth-Cozens, J., Mowbray, D., 2001. Leadership and quality of care. Quality in Healthcare 10, ii3–ii7.

Garling, P., 2008. Final report of the Special Commission of Inquiry into Acute Care Services in NSW Public Hospitals. NSW Government, Sydney.

Gregor, A., 2006. Doctors as leaders in the NHS. Clinician in Management 14, 163–166.

Grossman, S., 2007. Mentoring in nursing: A dynamic and collaborative process. Springer, New York.

Hamlin, R.G., 2002. A study and comparative analysis of managerial and leadership effectiveness in the National Health Service: An empirical factor analytic study within an NHS Trust hospital. Health Services Management 15 (4), 245–263.

Heifetz, R.A., 1994. Leadership without easy answers. Belknap Press, Cambridge.

Hutchinson, M., Jackson, D., 2013. Transformational leadership in nursing: towards a more critical interpretation. Nursing Inquiry 20 (1), 11–22.

Jackson, D., 2008a. Servant leadership: a framework for developing sustainable research capacity in nursing. Collegian 15 (1), 27–33.

Jackson, D., 2008b. Random acts of guidance: personal reflections on professional generosity. Journal of Clinical Nursing 17 (20), 2669–2670.

Jackson, D., 2008c. Retiring from nursing: can we avoid the retirement brain drain? Journal of Clinical Nursing 17 (22), 2949–2950.

Jackson, D., Daly, J., 2011. All things to all people: adversity and resilience in leadership. Nurse Leader 9 (3), 21–22, 30.

Jackson, D., Hutchinson, M., Peters, K., et al., 2012. Understanding avoidant leadership in healthcare: findings from a secondary analysis of two qualitative studies. Journal of Nursing Management DOI: 10:1111/j.1365-2834.2012.01395.

Jackson, D., Raftos, M., 1997. In uncharted waters: confronting the culture of silence in a residential care institution. International Journal of Nursing Practice 3 (1), 34–39.

Kelley, R.E., 1988. In praise of followers. Harvard Business Review November-December, 142–148.

Kouzes, J.M., Posner, B.Z., 2002. The leadership challenge, third ed. Jossey Bass, San Francisco.

Leatt, P., Porter, J., 2003. Where are the healthcare leaders? The need for investment in leadership development. Health Care Papers 4 (1), 14–31.

Lumby, J., Duffield, C., 1994. Caring nurses: The dilemmas of balancing costs and quality. Australian Health Review 17 (2), 72–83.

Mannix, J., Faga, P., Beale, B., et al., 2006. Towards sustainable models for clinical education in nursing: an on-going conversation. Nurse Education in Practice 6 (1), 3–11.

Manojlovich, M., Barnsteiner, J., Burns Bolton, L., et al., 2008. Nursing practice and work environment issues in the 21st Century: a leadership challenge. Nursing Research 57 (1S), S11–S14.

Saltman, D.C., O'Dea, N.A., Farmer, J., et al., 2007. Groups or teams in health care: finding the best fit. Journal of Evaluation in Clinical Practice 13 (1), 55–60.

Schwartz, R., Tumblin, T., 2002. The power of servant leadership to transform health care organisations for the 21st century. Archives of Surgery 137, 1419–1427.

Sutton, R., 2007. The no asshole rule: building a civilised workplace and surviving one that isn't. Sphere, London.

Talsma, A., Grady, P., Feetham, S., et al., 2008. The perfect storm: patient safety and nursing shortages within the context of health policy and evidence-based practice. Nursing Research 57 (1S), S15–S21.

Thinkexist.com, 2013. Lao Tzu quotes. Online. Available: http://thinkexist.com/quotation/a_leader_is_best_when_people_barely_know_he/214091.html, 1 May 2013.

Thyer G., 2003. Dare to be different: transformational leadership may hold the key to reducing the nursing shortage. Journal of Nursing Management 11 (2), 73–79.

Vance, C., Larson, E., 2002. Leadership in business and health care. Journal of Nursing Scholarship 34 (2), 165–171.

Watson, R., 2005. The global shortage of registered nurses. Journal of Clinical Nursing 14 (4), 409.

Wong, C.A., Cummings, G.G., 2007. The relationship between nursing leadership and patient outcomes: a systematic review. Journal of Nursing Management 15, 508–521.

World Health Organization, 2006. The world health report 2006: Working together for health. Online. Available: www.who.int/hrh/whr06/en, 18 Aug 2008.

INDEX

Page numbers followed by 'f' indicate figures, 't' indicate tables, and 'b' indicate boxes.